T0263236

Therapeutics

Editor

YVONNE R.A. VAN ZEELAND

VETERINARY CLINICS OF NORTH AMERICA: EXOTIC ANIMAL PRACTICE

www.vetexotic.theclinics.com

Consulting Editor
JÖRG MAYER

May 2018 • Volume 21 • Number 2

ELSEVIER

1600 John F. Kennedy Boulevard • Suite 1800 • Philadelphia, Pennsylvania, 19103-2899
http://www.vetexotic.theclinics.com

VETERINARY CLINICS OF NORTH AMERICA: EXOTIC ANIMAL PRACTICE Volume 21, Number 2
May 2018 ISSN 1094-9194, ISBN-13: 978-0-323-58380-0

Editor: Colleen Dietzler
Developmental Editor: Meredith Madeira

Veterinary Clinics of North America: Exotic Animal Practice (ISSN 1094-9194) is published in January, May, and September by Elsevier, Inc., 360 Park Avenue South, New York, NY 10010-1710. Subscription prices are $276.00 per year for US individuals, $492.00 per year for US institutions, $100.00 per year for US students and residents, $324.00 per year for Canadian individuals, $593.00 per year for Canadian institutions, $347.00 per year for international individuals, $593.00 per year for international institutions and $165.00 per year for Canadian and foreign students/residents. To receive student/resident rate, orders must be accompanied by name of affiliated institution, date of term, and the *signature* of program/residency coordinator on institution letterhead. Orders will be billed at individual rate until proof of status is received. Foreign air speed delivery is included in all *Clinics* subscription prices. All prices are subject to change without notice. **POSTMASTER:** Send address changes to *Veterinary Clinics of North America: Exotic Animal Practice*, Elsevier Health Sciences Division, Subscription Customer Service, 3251 Riverport Lane, Maryland Heights, MO 63043. **Customer Service: Telephone: 1-800-654-2452** (U.S. and Canada); **1-314-447-8871** (outside U.S. and Canada). **Fax: 1-314-447-8029. E-mail: journalscustomerservice-usa@elsevier.com (for print support); journalsonlinesupport-usa@elsevier.com (for online support).**

Reprints. For copies of 100 or more of articles in this publication, please contact the Commercial Reprints Department, Elsevier Inc., 360 Park Avenue South, New York, New York 10010-1710. Tel.: 212-633-3874; Fax: 212-633-3820; E-mail: reprints@elsevier.com.

Veterinary Clinics of North America: Exotic Animal Practice is covered in *MEDLINE/PubMed (Index Medicus).*

Contributors

CONSULTING EDITOR

JÖRG MAYER, Dr med vet, Msc
Diplomate, American Board of Veterinary Practitioners (Exotic Companion Mammals); Diplomate, European College of Zoological Medicine (Small Mammals); Diplomate, American College of Zoological Medicine; Associate Professor of Zoological Medicine, Department of Small Animal Medicine and Surgery, University of Georgia College of Veterinary Medicine, Athens, Georgia, USA

EDITOR

YVONNE R.A. VAN ZEELAND, DVM, MVR, PhD, CPBC
Diplomate, European College of Zoological Medicine (Avian, Small Mammal); Division of Zoological Medicine, Department of Clinical Sciences of Companion Animals, Faculty of Veterinary Medicine, Utrecht University, Utrecht, The Netherlands

AUTHORS

GUNTHER ANTONISSEN, DVM, MSc, PhD
Postdoctoral Researcher, Departments of Pharmacology, Toxicology and Biochemistry, and Pathology, Bacteriology and Avian Diseases, Faculty of Veterinary Medicine, Ghent University, Merelbeke, Belgium

ELS M. BROENS, PhD, DVM
Veterinary Microbiologist, Head of Veterinary Microbiology Diagnostics Center, Department of Infectious Diseases and Immunology, Clinical Infectiology, Faculty of Veterinary Medicine, Utrecht University, Utrecht, The Netherlands

SUE CHEN, DVM
Diplomate, American Board of Veterinary Practitioners (Avian); Gulf Coast Avian and Exotics, Gulf Coast Veterinary Specialists, Houston, Texas

THOMAS COUTANT, Dr med vet, IPSAV (Zoological Medicine)
Zoological Medicine Service, Department of Clinical Sciences, CHUV (Centre Hospitalier Universitaire Vétérinaire), Faculté de Médecine Vétérinaire, Université de Montréal, Saint-Hyacinthe, Québec, Canada

GIGI DAVIDSON, BS Pharm
Diplomate, International College of Veterinary Pharmacists; Director of Clinical Pharmacy Services, North Carolina State University College of Veterinary Medicine, Raleigh, North Carolina, USA

KATIE W. DELK, DVM
Diplomate of the American College of Zoological Medicine; Senior Veterinarian, Veterinary Services, The North Carolina Zoo, Asheboro, North Carolina, USA

SARA DIAS, DVM, MSc
Resident ECZM (Small Mammal), Exotic Animals Department, Hospital Clínic Veterinari, Universitat Autònoma de Barcelona, Barcelona, Spain

CLAIRE D. ERLACHER-REID, DVM
Diplomate of the American College of Zoological Medicine; Sr. Staff Veterinarian, SeaWorld Orlando, Orlando, Florida, USA

BRENNA COLLEEN FITZGERALD, DVM
Diplomate, American Board of Veterinary Practitioners (Avian Practice); Associate Veterinarian, Medical Center for Birds, Oakley, California, USA

JENNIFER GRAHAM, DVM
Diplomate, American Board of Veterinary Practitioners (Avian/Exotic Companion Mammal), Diplomate, American College of Zoological Medicine, Department of Clinical Sciences, Cummings School of Veterinary Medicine at Tufts University, North Grafton, Massachusetts, USA

J. JILL HEATLEY, DVM, MS
Diplomate, American Board of Veterinary Practitioners (Avian, Reptilian, Amphibian); Diplomate, American College of Zoological Medicine; Associate Professor, Veterinary Small Animal Clinical Sciences, Schubot Exotic Bird Health Center, College of Veterinary Medicine & Biomedical Sciences, Texas A&M University, College Station, Texas, USA

MELODY HENNIGH, RVT, KPA CTP
Medical Center for Birds, Oakley, California, USA

ISABELLE LANGLOIS, DMV
Diplomate, American Board of Veterinary Practitioners (Avian); Zoological Medicine Service, Department of Clinical Sciences, CHUV (Centre Hospitalier Universitaire Vétérinaire), Faculté de Médecine Vétérinaire, Université de Montréal, Saint-Hyacinthe, Québec, Canada

AN MARTEL, DVM, MSc, PhD
Diplomate, European College of Zoological Medicine (Wildlife Population Health); Professor, Department of Pathology, Bacteriology and Avian Diseases, Faculty of Veterinary Medicine, Ghent University, Merelbeke, Belgium

JAUME MARTORELL, DVM, PhD
Diplomate, European College of Zoological Medicine (Small Mammal); Professor of Departament de Medicina I Cirurgia Animlas, Facultat de Veterinaria, Universitat Autònoma de Barcelona, Head of Exotic Animals Department, Hospital Clinic Veterinari, Barcelona, Spain

JESSICA A. MARZIANI, DVM, CVA, CVC, CCRT
CARE Veterinary Services PLLC, Houston, Texas, USA

CHRISTINE M. MOLTER, DVM
Diplomate of the American College of Zoological Medicine; Staff Veterinarian, Veterinary Clinic, Houston Zoo, Inc, Houston, Texas, USA

BERNICE MUNTZ
Dierentrainer, Leidschendam, The Netherlands

SETH C. OSTER, DVM
Assitant Clinical Professor, Department of Clinical Science, Auburn University, Auburn, Alabama

SUSAN PAYNE, PhD
Associate Professor, Veterinary Pathobiology, Schubot Exotic Bird Health Center,
College of Veterinary Medicine & Biomedical Sciences, Texas A&M University,
College Station, Texas, USA

OLIVIA A. PETRITZ, DVM
Diplomate, American College of Zoological Medicine; Assistant Professor of Avian and
Exotic Animal Medicine, Department of Clinical Sciences, North Carolina State University
College of Veterinary Medicine, Raleigh, North Carolina, USA

LAUREN V. POWERS, DVM
Diplomate, American Board of Veterinary Practitioners (Avian Practice); Diplomate,
American Board of Veterinary Practitioners (Exotic Companion Mammal Practice);
Service Head, Avian and Exotic Pet Service, Carolina Veterinary Specialists, Huntersville,
North Carolina Adjunct Assistant Professor, North Carolina State University College of
Veterinary Medicine, Raleigh, North Carolina, USA

NICO J. SCHOEMAKER, DVM, PhD
Diplomate, European College of Zoological Medicine (Small Mammal & Avian); Diplomate,
American Board of Veterinary Practitioners-Avian; Associate Professor, Division of
Zoological Medicine, Utrecht University, Utrecht, Netherlands

BRIAN L. SPEER, DVM
Diplomate, American Board of Veterinary Practitioners (Avian Practice); Diplomate,
European College of Zoological Medicine (Avian); Medical Center for Birds, Oakley,
California, USA

IAN TIZARD, BVMS, PhD, DSc
Diplomate, American College of Veterinary Microbiologists; Distinguished Professor,
Veterinary Pathobiology, Schubot Exotic Bird Health Center, College of Veterinary
Medicine & Biomedical Sciences, Texas A&M University, College Station, Texas

INGEBORG M. VAN GEIJLSWIJK, PhD, PharmD
Hospital Pharmacist, Director of Pharmacy, IRAS Veterinary Pharmacology and
Therapeutics Group, Pharmacy Department, Faculty of Veterinary Medicine, Utrecht
University, Utrecht, The Netherlands

YVONNE R.A. VAN ZEELAND, DVM, MVR, PhD, CPBC
Diplomate, European College of Zoological Medicine (Avian, Small Mammal); Division of
Zoological Medicine, Department of Clinical Sciences of Companion Animals, Faculty of
Veterinary Medicine, Utrecht University, Utrecht, The Netherlands

**CLAIRE VERGNEAU-GROSSET, Dr med vet, IPSAV (Zoological Medicine),
CES (Avian Pathol)**
Diplomate, American College of Zoological Medicine; Zoological Medicine Service,
Department of Clinical Sciences, CHUV (Centre Hospitalier Universitaire Vétérinaire),
Faculté de Médecine Vétérinaire, Université de Montréal, Saint-Hyacinthe, Québec,
Canada

MARIKE VISSER, DVM
Graduate Student, Department of Anatomy, Physiology and Pharmacology, Auburn
University, Auburn, Alabama

ASHLEY ZEHNDER, DVM, PhD
Diplomate, American Board of Veterinary Practitioners (Avian), Department of Biomedical
Data Science, Stanford, California, USA

Contents

> Pharmacokinetic (PK) and pharmacodynamic (PD) publications provide scientific evidence for incorporation in evidence-based veterinary medicine, aiding the clinician in selecting doses and dosing intervals. PK and PD studies have reported wide variations within exotic species, owing to physiologic differences in absorption, distribution, metabolism, and excretion. PK studies offer species-specific data to help tailor doses and dosing routes to individual patients, minimize toxicity, and provide a cornerstone for PD studies to determine drug efficacy. This article reviews the application of PK parameters and the challenges in determining the PD activity of drugs, with a particular emphasis on exotic species.

> Lack of species-specific pharmacokinetic and pharmacodynamic data is a challenge for pharmaceutical and dose selection. If available, dose extrapolation can be accomplished via basic equations. If unavailable, several methods have been described. Linear scaling uses an established milligrams-per-kilogram dose based on weight. This method does not allow for differences in species drug metabolism, sometimes resulting in toxicity. Allometric scaling correlates body weight and metabolic rate but fails for drugs with significant hepatic metabolism and cannot be extrapolated to avians or reptiles. Evidence-based veterinary medicine for dose design based on species similarity is discussed, considering physiologic differences between classes.

> Extralabel drug use is the use of a Food and Drug Administration (FDA)-approved drug in a manner different from what is stipulated on the approved label. Compounding is the process of preparing a medication in a manner not indicated on the label to create a formulation specifically tailored to the needs of an individual patient. Extralabel drug use and compounding are vital aspects of safe and effective drug delivery to patients in exotic animal practice. There are few FDA-approved drugs for exotic animal species, and many approved drugs for other species are not available in suitable formulations for use in exotic animals.

preshipment examinations, quarantine, and a rigorous necropsy protocol are vital tools to maintain a healthy collection.

Claire D. Erlacher-Reid

Aquatic species live most of or all their lives in water; therefore, the health of the environment is intimately connected to their health and medical care. Understanding and maintaining appropriate husbandry and nutrition for the housed aquarium species are essential to sustain health. Most diseases of fish are secondary opportunistic infections; prevention and early diagnosis are recommended. Treatments involve environmental and/or nutritional management first, followed by targeted pharmacologic treatment to control a specific pathogen. Pharmacokinetic research evaluating the effects and safety of medications in fish are greatly needed in the peer-reviewed literature.

Olivia A. Petritz and Sue Chen

The selection and dosing of medications for exotic pets are often challenging because most drugs are used in an extralabel manner without pharmacokinetic and pharmacodynamic studies. Doses are often extrapolated from common domestic animals, and safety data are often lacking in exotic species. Just as the bioavailability and therapeutic levels are different for each species, what may be a safe and commonly used medication in one species can be deadly in another. Various drugs with documented contraindications in certain exotic pet species are outlined in this article, and the pathophysiology, clinical signs, and treatment options are described when applicable.

Els M. Broens and Ingeborg M. van Geijlswijk

Reduction of antimicrobial use can result in reduction of resistance in commensal bacteria. In exotic animals, information on use of antimicrobials and resistance in commensals and pathogens is scarce. However, use of antimicrobials listed as critically important for human medicine seems high in exotic animals. Ideally, the selection of a therapy should be based on an accurate diagnosis and antimicrobial susceptibility testing. When prescribing antimicrobials based on empiricism, knowledge of the most common pathogens causing specific infections and the antimicrobial spectrum of antimicrobial agents is indispensable. Implementing antimicrobial stewardship promotes the prudent use of antimicrobials in exotic animals.

Gunther Antonissen and An Martel

The use of antifungals in birds is characterized by interspecies and interindividual variability in the pharmacokinetics, affecting drug safety and efficacy. Oral antifungal drug absorption is a complex process affected by drug formulation characteristics, gastrointestinal anatomy, and physiology. New antifungal drug delivery systems can enhance drug stability, reduce off-target side effects, prolong residence time in the blood, and improve efficacy. Topical administration of antifungals through nebulization shows promising results. However, therapeutic output is highly influenced by drug formulation and type of nebulizer, indicating that these factors should be taken into account when selecting this medication route.

Ashley Zehnder, Jennifer Graham, and Gunther Antonissen

> Treatment options for animals with cancer are rapidly expanding, including in exotic animal medicine. Limited information is available about treatment effects in exotic pet species beyond individual case reports. Most cancer treatment protocols in exotic animals are extrapolated from those described in humans, dogs, and cats. This article provides an update on cancer treatment in exotic animal species. The Exotic Species Cancer Research Alliance accumulates clinical cases in a central location with standardized clinical information, with resources to help clinicians find and enter their cases for the collective good of exotic clinicians and their patients.

Jessica A. Marziani

> The nontraditional therapies of traditional Chinese Veterinary Medicine and chiropractic care are adjunct treatments that can be used in conjunction with more conventional therapies to treat a variety of medical conditions. Nontraditional therapies do not need to be alternatives to Western medicine but, instead, can be used simultaneously. Exotic animal practitioners should have a basic understanding of nontraditional therapies for both client education and patient referral because they can enhance the quality of life, longevity, and positive outcomes for various cases across multiple taxa.

VETERINARY CLINICS OF NORTH AMERICA: EXOTIC ANIMAL PRACTICE

THE CLINICS ARE NOW AVAILABLE ONLINE!
Access your subscription at:
www.theclinics.com

Preface

Therapeutics

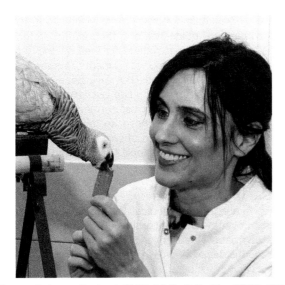

Yvonne R.A. van Zeeland, DVM, MVR, PhD, Dip. ECZM, CPBC
Editor

Seventeen years ago, Stephen Fronefield served as guest editor of the *Veterinary Clinics of North America: Exotic Animal Practice* issue on Therapeutics. Since then, medical treatment options for exotic animal species have increased tremendously, not in the least part because of the availability of more advanced diagnostic techniques, which facilitate correct disease diagnosis, but also because new types of drugs have become available. Nevertheless, we are still facing similar challenges as we did two decades ago, as the number of controlled studies evaluating the safety and efficacy of pharmaceutical agents in exotics remains scarce, and little to no drugs have been approved for use in exotic, wildlife, and zoo species. Moreover, from information that is available, we learn that extrapolating dosages from other species is not as simple and easy as one may have hoped as there are great anatomic and physiologic differences between the species we are treating. Even within the same order, dosing regimen can differ tremendously, as exemplified by the difference in pharmacokinetic parameters of meloxicam in Grey parrots (*Psittacus erithacus*) versus Hispaniolan Amazon parrots (*Amazona ventralis*), which respectively require 0.5 mg/kg every 24 hours and 1.5 mg/kg every 12 hours orally

Vet Clin Exot Anim 21 (2018) xiii–xv
https://doi.org/10.1016/j.cvex.2018.02.001
1094-9194/18/© 2018 Elsevier Inc. All rights reserved.

to achieve similar plasma levels. While consulting exotic animal formularies, it is therefore especially important to thoroughly investigate how these dosages were established and critically evaluate whether and which dose applies best to the individual patient.

Compounding of drugs, which is often necessary for accurate and easy drug delivery, may further complicate the establishment of effective treatment protocols as this process can greatly affect the bioavailability of drugs. As a result, we need to continue to critically evaluate our treatment guidelines and therapeutic protocols and carefully monitor responses of the individual patient as well as the group that may be treated alongside. During the evaluation, we furthermore need to be aware of the potential harm we can do to the animal, not only because of the potential adverse effects that can result from the drug itself but also because of the potential stress and anxiety that medicating an animal can induce. Similarly, we need to be aware that our treatments can also have an impact on human health and the environment. The rapid rise and spread of antibiotic resistance in particular is one of the biggest threats to global health, food security, and development today, which urges us to use these drugs in a sensible and responsible manner.

This issue of the *Veterinary Clinics of North America: Exotic Animal Practice* addresses these and other topics related to the medical treatment of exotics. In contrast to other issues, which often cover the different groups of animals in separate articles, this issue comprises sixteen papers that cover both basic considerations and guidelines with regard to therapeutic decision making (ie, from pharmacokinetics to low-stress medication techniques and administration routes for both individual patients and groups) as well as updates and current insights on some of the more common therapies in exotic animal medicine, including antimicrobial, cardiovascular, and contraceptive drugs, and oncologic therapy. As exotic pet owners are increasingly turning to nontraditional therapies, a separate article is allocated to this topic to aid the general practitioner in getting a better understanding of what these therapies comprise.

Given the growing number of drugs that are being used in exotic animals, this issue does not attempt to provide a complete overview of the drugs and dosages that are used in exotics. For this purpose, the reader is referred to the *Exotic Animal Formulary* by J. Carpenter of which the fifth edition has been released in the fall of 2017. For any veterinarian dealing with exotics, this is an absolute must have to look up a drug dose in any of the commonly seen exotic species. With the information provided in this issue, however, it is hoped that practitioners, researchers, and students will obtain guidelines on how to make the correct decisions while designing a therapeutic plan.

A special thanks goes out to all the authors who contributed to this issue and who have devoted a significant portion of their time and energy on presenting the most up-to-date information in a clear and comprehensible manner. Similarly, I would like to thank Elsevier for providing me the opportunity to serve as a guest editor of this issue and Meredith Madeira and the rest of the editorial team for their support and guidance during the preparation of this issue. It has been a great learning experience and a real pleasure to work with these people, and I truly appreciate the valuable contributions that everyone has made to this issue. And last, I hope that the combined wisdom of your peers may help guide you during the process of decision making and that you value the information they have provided. Enjoy!

Yvonne R.A. van Zeeland, DVM, MVR, PhD, Dip. ECZM, CPBC
Division of Zoological Medicine
Department of Clinical Sciences of Companion Animals
Faculty of Veterinary Medicine
Utrecht University
Yalelaan 108
Utrecht 3584 CM, The Netherlands

E-mail address:
Y.R.A.vanZeeland@uu.nl

Translating Pharmacokinetic and Pharmacodynamic Data into Practice

Marike Visser, DVM*

KEYWORDS

- Pharmacokinetic • Pharmacodynamic • Study design • Drug movement

KEY POINTS

- Pharmacokinetics includes the study of bodily absorption, distribution, metabolism, and excretion of drugs via mathematical modeling.
- Volume of distribution, clearance, and elimination half-life are 3 dose-independent pharmacokinetic parameters that can be used for interspecies comparison.
- Pharmacodynamics is the study of the effects of a drug on the body and depends on the dose-response curve.
- Clinically relevant parameters include bioavailability, maximum concentration, time to maximum concentration, and half-life.
- The presence of plasma drug concentrations does not automatically correlate to a pharmacodynamic response.

INTRODUCTION

A variety of studies can aid the clinician in selecting drug doses and appropriate dosing intervals. A combination of pharmacokinetic (PK) and pharmacodynamic (PD) studies can be used to formulate an effective dose within a species. PKs can be defined as the modeling of the time course of a drug in the body.[1] These studies seek to generate mathematical models to quantify physiologic processes in the body, tailoring a dose for a given population and optimizing therapeutic effectiveness while minimizing toxicity. A PK study measures the concentration of a given drug or its metabolites in blood, tissue, feces, or urine over a set period of time.[2] The most common and accessible site is blood, leading to most PK studies reporting this compartment. However, presence of drug within the plasma does not equate to therapeutic drug concentrations at the targeted site. For example, if the target is the brain, inferences can be made regarding the ability of a drug to cross the blood-brain barrier;

Disclosure Statement: The author has no conflict of interest.
Anatomy, Physiology and Pharmacology, Auburn University, Auburn, AL, USA
* 137 North Park Street Upper, Kalamazoo, MI 49007.
E-mail address: visserm0512@gmail.com

however, unless the concentration within the brain tissue is measured, there is no 100% certainty. Also, if a drug is given orally to treat a pyoderma, efficacy cannot be guaranteed unless the drug concentration is quantified in the skin.[3] Establishing therapeutic efficacy of a drug warrants the use of PD studies, which evaluate the effect of the drug on the body at a given dose, including effects at the molecular level, the clinical response, and potential adverse events (AEs). Using the measured plasma (or serum) drug concentration (PDC), mathematical modeling can be used to calculate PK parameters and, when integrated with PD, provides the dose-response relationship. This relationship is best described as

$$Dose = \frac{Cl \times ED_{50}}{F} \tag{1}$$

In which Cl is overall clearance, ED_{50} is the therapeutic effective PDC in 50% of the population, and F is the bioavailability of the drug given by a specific route.[2,3] Both PK and PD studies depend on the PDC; the former to calculate parameters for dosing and dosing interval, the latter to determine a therapeutically effective dose and minimize the risk of toxicity.

BUILDING CONFIDENCE IN INTERPRETING PHARMACOKINETIC OR PHARMACODYNAMIC PAPERS

Before examining the results of a PK or PD study, the study design should be critically evaluated. There are 5 central questions that the clinician should always ask and be able to answer, using a journal article to build confidence.

What Was the Number, Gender, and Age of Animals Used in the Study?

Because PK and PD studies are based on a calculation of averages, a higher number of animals ensures that the individual variation in overall clearance and drug metabolism will have less impact on the final parameters. On average, most exotic PK studies involve a limited number of animals and only a limited number of samples can be collected due to their size. By having a large population size, the influence of a single individual does not skew the results. It is also vital to include gender whenever possible because there are reported gender differences in the rate of metabolism in some species.[4] Species with reported gender PK differences include paroxetine in parrots[5] and meloxicam in ferrets.[4] However, these studies included a very small number of animals and the clinical impact of these differences has yet to be determined. The same challenges occur when considering age. Young animals have less fat and more water compared with healthy adult animals. As the animal ages, there is a loss of lean body mass, a decrease in renal function, and an increase in fat. Therefore, drugs with significant renal excretion (eg, aminoglycosides) require a prolonged dosing interval and drugs with significant fat distribution (eg, diazepam, hormones) will have lower PDC and prolonged elimination half-lives.[6] PK comparisons between different age groups are limited, and the use of therapeutic drug monitoring (TDM) is recommended.

Is the Study Designed as a Cross-Over, Parallel, or Single-Route Study?

In a cross-over study, the same animals are given 2 or more formulations, routes, or doses of a drug (eg, intravenous [IV] vs oral meloxicam).[7] This removes individual variability when comparing parameters such as area under the curve and bioavailability. In a parallel study, animals are divided into groups depending on the number of routes being tested but each will have only a single route or dose tested, thereby increasing the variation. If 2 routes are being compared, the study design should ideally describe a cross-over study with an appropriate washout period.

Is the Washout Period Long Enough?

A washout period is required for all animals in a cross-over study. This period is the time when the animal receives no drug, allowing the body to clear all drug before the administered route is changed. This washout time depends on the half-life of the drug, with some drugs only requiring a washout period of 1 to 2 days, whereas others may need weeks. If a drug is given while part of the previous dose is present, this will not only interfere with quantification of the drug but may also, in case of a PD study, lead to misleading results because the remaining drug will also exert an effect. To determine an appropriate washout period, the elimination half-life can be used. In general, 5 half-lives must have passed for a drug to be completely eliminated.[8]

Was the Study Randomized and Blinded?

To prevent bias and proper evaluation of the drug's effects, a PD study should include a placebo group and a proper randomization procedure. Randomization removes the bias of selecting individuals that the researcher suspects will prove their hypothesis. In addition, bias can be prevented by ensuring that the researcher collecting the data is blinded to the treatment received by each individual.[1] For most PD studies, a randomized clinical trial is used to determine the effectiveness of a drug. This involves the enrollment of subjects to compare 1 drug to another or a drug to a placebo. In a well-designed clinical trial, the participants, clinicians, and data collectors are blinded to the groups. Four types of blinding have been described: unblinded, single-blinded, doubled-blinded, and triple-blinded. In an unblinded study, all participants are aware of the group assignments, increasing bias of both the researchers and participants. In a single-blinded study, the clinician may know the groups or only the data collector is blinded. This method allows for bias to skew the results of the study. A trial in which the clinician, the data-collector, and the participant are unaware of group assignments is known as double-blind or triple-blind studies. These can be difficult to develop but they reduce the risk of bias within the study.[9]

Was the Drug Used in the Study an Approved Formulation or a Compounded Product?

Drug compounding can lead to completely different PK parameters owing to differences in drug absorption. Thus, if possible, an approved product should be used.[10] If a compounded product is used, the investigator should report the concentration of the compounded formulation to verify that targeted concentrations are reached. (See Lauren V. Powers and Gigi Davidson's article, "Compounding and Extralabel Use of Drugs in Exotic Animal Medicine," in this issue.)

DETERMINANTS OF PLASMA DRUG CONCENTRATION

When the clinician is satisfied with the underlying methodology, the reported PK parameters can be evaluated. All PK parameters are determined by plotting the PDC versus time. Certain parameters can be identified by visually examining the plot, including the maximum concentration (C_{max}) and time to C_{max} (T_{max}) (**Fig. 1**). The area underneath the graph is called the area the curve and serves as the basis for additional PK modeling. Two basic graphs can be generated based on the route of administration: 1 for the IV (**Fig. 2**) and 1 for the extravascular route (**Fig. 3**).[1] The decision between routes of administration depends on physiochemical properties of the drug, physiologic impact on the drug, and the goals of treatment (**Table 1**).

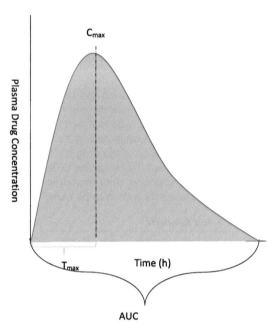

Fig. 1. PK parameters that can be visually identified. AUC, area under the curve.

PK parameters are used to mathematically describe the 4 components of drug movement throughout the body: absorption, distribution, metabolism, and elimination. It is important to recognize that each component has its challenges for drug movement and these problems will vary by species (**Table 2**).

Absorption

Only IV administration does not require an absorption phase. All other routes necessitate movement of the drug from the site of administration, through a barrier such as intestinal or lung epithelium, to the bloodstream. Depending on the site of administration, the drug particle has to traverse a variety of barriers and can undergo

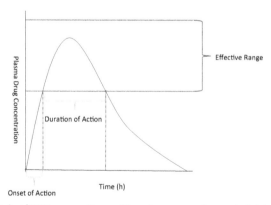

Fig. 2. Typical graph of PDC versus time with extravenous drug administration. This differs from IV administration due to the time lag before the onset of action.

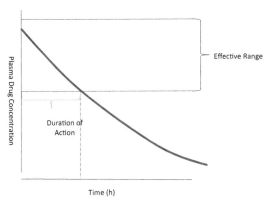

Fig. 3. Plot of PDC versus time when a drug is administered IV.

metabolism before distribution throughout the body. Absorption can also be delayed by drug formulation to create depots that allow the drug to slowly be released into systemic circulation, such as subcutaneous deslorelin[11–13] or ceftiofur crystalline-free acid.[14,15] The T_{max} depends on the route of administration and the rate of absorption. Depending on the route, both T_{max} and C_{max} can have significant variation, and should be a factor in deciding the most suitable route of administration.

$$F = \frac{AUC_{EXV}}{AUC_{IV}} \times \frac{Dose_{IV}}{Dose_{EXV}} \times 100 \tag{2}$$

In which differences in drug absorption due to differences in routes of administration are described as relative or absolute bioavailability (*F*), and are expressed as a percentage (Equation 2). Absolute *F* compares IV administration to any other route of administration, such as extravascular (*EXV*). The area under the curve is given as *AUC*. The relative bioavailability (*F*) compares any 2 extravascular routes to each other.[16]

A clinician may be tempted to try and increase the dose if the bioavailability is very low. For example, if bioavailability is 25%, why not merely quadruple the dose? However, in many cases, a mere increase of the dose will not solve the problem because bioavailability accounts not only for absorption but also for any metabolism the drug undergoes before systemic distribution, referred to as first-pass metabolism.[17] When referring to the first-pass effect, absorption from the gastrointestinal (GI) tract and metabolism via the liver is the most common example. However, the lung can also have a first-pass effect, as in the case of prostaglandin $F_{2\alpha}$, for which a

Table 1
Variation between the routes of administration

Intravascular	Extravascular
• No absorption phase	• Absorption phase always present
• Onset of action is immediate	• Onset of action depends on the drug formulation, route of administration, first-pass effect
• The entire dose is given with no influence first-pass metabolism	
• Provides the quickest onset of action	• First-pass effect can decrease the amount of drug that reaches circulation
• AEs are challenging to control, requires accurate doses calculation	

Table 2
Sites of action for each phase of drug movement through the body, including challenges faced at each site

	Administration	Distribution	Metabolism	Elimination
Sites	• Cornea • GI tract • Lung • Intraperitoneal or intracoelomic • Mucosal (buccal, nasal) • Muscle • Skin or subcutis	• Blood • Bone • Fat • Interstitial • Lymphatics	• Hepatic • Intestinal • Renal	• Eggs • Hepatic • Lactation • Renal • Respiratory
Challenges	• Drug size • First-pass metabolism • Ionization • Metabolizing enzymes • Microbial degradation	• Drug lipid solubility • Membrane barriers • Plasma protein binding • Transport proteins	• Enzymatic activity • Hepatic blood flow	• Enterohepatic recirculation • Renal portal system

Data from Refs.[1–6]

90% first-pass metabolism via lungs is reported.[16,18] Research has shown that, when bioavailability is very low, variation in PK will often be extreme, thereby rendering it likely that the patient may be overdosed or underdosed.[16] Although there is no set limit, the author recommends that clinicians select another route if the bioavailability is less than 50% due to individual variation.

Bioavailability differs from bioequivalence, which compares 2 products with the same active pharmaceutical ingredient in different formulations and administered via the same route.[10] Bioequivalence can vary significantly between 2 products, especially for products requiring the formation of micelles to improve absorption across the GI tract.[19] Differences in bioequivalence between pilot versus compounded products include cyclosporine in dogs,[20] itraconazole in penguins and dogs,[10,21] and paroxetine[5] and pimobendan[22] in parrots.

The following PK parameters can be used to examine absorption (**Box 1**):

- C_{max}: peak plasma concentration at a given dose, which reflects the rate of absorption compared with the rate of elimination
- C_0: peak plasma concentration when the drug is given IV, which will be at time 0

Box 1
Rule of thumb for absorption in exotics

- Do not assume bioequivalence of products. Several studies have shown marked variation between approved products, generics, and compounded formulations.
- Bioavailability varies between species and route of administration.
- If bioavailability is less than 50%, requiring a doubling of the dose, this route should not be used.
- PK studies are performed in healthy animals and there may be changes in the rate of absorption with illness (intestinal or hepatic), particularly if the drug is given orally.

- T_{max}: time needed to reach C_{max} following administration of the drug
- Bioavailability: the percentage of a drug that appears in the bloodstream and depends on the route of administration and the impact of first-pass metabolism (Equation 2)
- Bioequivalence: determines whether 2 products with the same active pharmaceutical ingredient and administered via the same route reach the same therapeutic PDC.

Distribution

Distribution moves the drug from the central compartment to the peripheral tissues, depots, and the site of action. The volume of distribution (V_d) is a mathematical concept, usually reported in liters per kilogram, giving an estimation of the amount of distribution.[23] The V_d is constant for a particular drug regardless of dose, until dose saturation is reached, and can be used for comparison between species. Clinically, the V_d is relevant when the drug has a high V_d, indicating that the drug is lipophilic (fat-loving) or a low V_d and, therefore, remains in the plasma compartment. Drugs that have a large V_d will have a low concentration in the plasma but a high tissue distribution and a prolonged elimination (eg, propofol, phenobarbital, enrofloxacin). Patients that are obese can be expected to have lower than usual PDC due to drug parking in the fat.[23] Drugs with a low V_d (aminoglycosides) can have high plasma concentrations and, therefore, high clearance, increasing the risk of AEs. Little research in the veterinary field has been completed to compare changes in the V_d due to age; however, some rule-of-thumb guidance (**Box 2**) is provided based on reviews in human medicine.[24,25]

Plasma protein binding occurs across a wide variety of drugs, and albumin is the predominant protein necessary for distribution. Protein binding hides the drug from the body, preventing distribution to tissues and clearance. However, if the drug is displaced from the protein (eg, due to disease or competition), it is cleared rapidly following an initial influx of PDC.[27] Therefore, drugs will reach subtherapeutic concentrations faster, requiring a shorter dosing interval. Overall, the plasma protein-binding profile is similar across mammals; however, some studies have reported differences in the protein-binding affinity of drugs in avian and reptile species, resulting in more rapid clearance.[28,29] Examples of drugs with a high protein-binding affinity for which the PK may vary significantly across species include cefovecin, diazepam, maropitant, and meloxicam.[28–33]

Box 2
Rule of thumb for distribution in exotics

- Protein binding is different in reptiles and birds. If possible, avoid drugs that are highly protein-bound due to unpredictable rates of clearance.

- Protein binding greater than 95% can have a significant impact on distribution and clearance of a drug. If hypoalbuminemia is present, consider an alternative drug.[26]

- Drugs with a Vd greater than 27 L will be distributed to fat, and obese patients are likely to have lower PDC and prolonged elimination times

- Drugs with a Vd less than 3 L only remain in the plasma compartment, and patients should be dosed based on lean body mass.

- Elderly patients will have less lean body mass, higher fat content, and decreased renal clearance. Therefore, lower doses and prolonged dosing intervals should be used.

$$Loading\ dose\ \left(\frac{mg}{kg}\right) = \frac{Target\ PDC\ \left(\frac{mg}{L}\right) \times V_d(L/kg)}{F} \qquad (3)$$

In which the following PK parameters can be used to examine distribution:

- V_d can be used clinically to calculate a loading dose
  - V_d reported by an extravenous route must be corrected for bioavailability (F) and is reported as V_d/F.

Metabolism

Most metabolism occurs in the liver, using oxidation and conjugation reactions to produce polar compounds that can be excreted. Metabolism activates prodrug (enrofloxacin to ciprofloxacin), or creates active metabolites (diazepam to nordiazepam). However, these activations require specific enzymes, which may or may not be present in every exotic species.[34] Two of the large enzyme families involved in drug metabolism are cytochrome P450 (CYP450) and UDP-glucuronosyltransferase (UGT), have variation between species. For example, koalas have far more extensive CYP450 meloxicam metabolism compared with dogs,[35] and the UGT enzyme in ferrets are poor metabolizers, placing them at higher risk for acetaminophen toxicity.[36] Metabolism can also vary significantly between individuals' due to genetic variation, leading to therapeutic failure. Therefore, careful monitoring of drug efficacy and toxicity is recommended (**Box 3**).

Several drugs can also inhibit or induce drug metabolizing enzymes. Well-known examples include ketoconazole, phenobarbital, and rifampin. The clinician should be aware of potential drug-drug interactions when combining multiple drugs (polypharmacy). This can be challenging due to the lack of species-specific data; however, charts are available in humans as an initial reference (http://medicine.iupui.edu/clinpharm/ddis/main-table/). (See Marike Visser and Seth C. Oster's article, "The Educated Guess: Determining Drug Doses in Exotic Animals using Evidence-Based Medicine," in this issue.)

Excretion

Two significant sites of drug elimination are the kidneys and liver. Conjugation by the liver allows a drug to be excreted into the bile, where it can either be excreted or unconjugated by GI microbiota and reabsorbed. This reabsorption and distribution phenomena is known as enterohepatic recirculation and can be seen on a PK profile by a second peak during the later stages of a study. Reptiles and birds have an additional challenge due to the renal portal system, which can carry the drugs to the kidneys before systemic distribution, thereby potentially resulting in a rapid renal clearance and/or increasing the risk of (renal) toxicities.[37] As such, convention holds that drugs should be given in the anterior rather than the posterior limbs. However, studies that have evaluated effects of administration site in chelonians and snakes did not report

---

Box 3
Rule of thumb for metabolism in exotics

- Use drugs with caution if there are reported toxicities in that species.
- Drugs extensively metabolized by CYP450 require TDM if the enzyme profile is unknown in the species
- If liver disease is present, drugs metabolized by liver should be used with caution.

changes in the PK parameters, thereby rendering it questionable whether avoiding the hind legs as a route of administration is really necessary.[38–40]

When a PK study reports clearance, this usually comprises all clearance routes, including renal and hepatic, as well as other potential routes, reflecting total clearance from the plasma. Clearance is 1 of the 3 parameters used to calculate doses (Equation 1), and also allows for a calculation of the elimination half-life ($t_{1/2}$ in formulas) and has been used for allometric scaling.[41,42] Half-life reports the time it takes for 50% of the dose to be cleared. It is a generally accepted rule of thumb that 5 half-lives are required to remove 97% of a drug. Alternatively, because 50% of a dose is cleared during 1 half-life period, doubling the dose will add 1 half-life. Half-life is essential when determining steady-state concentrations and the dosing interval, and to minimize the risk of toxicity.[8] The use of half-life can vary from determining the PDC at which a drug may be subtherapeutic (eg, anticonvulsants), limiting toxicity (eg, aminoglycosides), or maintaining PDC to prevent the development of antimicrobial drug resistance. (See Marike Visser and Seth C. Oster's article, "The Educated Guess: Determining Drug Doses in Exotic Animals using Evidence-Based Medicine," in this issue.)

The following PK parameters can be used to evaluate excretion (**Box 4**):

- Clearance (*Cl*), which reflects total clearance from the plasma and is independent parameter that does not depend on the given dose
- Half-life, which reflects the time needed to clear 50% of the dose, and can be calculated using *Cl*.

Steady State Concentrations

Steady state concentrations are reached when there is minimal PDC fluctuation during the dosing interval. This is achieved by decreasing the dosing interval compared with the elimination half-life, allowing for an accumulation of the drug. Preventing wild fluctuations is essential to maintaining therapeutic efficacy (eg, preventing seizures, managing pain). The length of time necessary to reach steady state varies significantly between drugs, and a loading dose can be calculated (Equation 3) to reach an effective PDC quickly. Drugs for which a loading dose is recommended includes phenobarbital, bromide, and opioids (hydromorphone and fentanyl). If a drug is cleared before the dosing interval, no accumulation occurs and steady state is never reached. The use of constant rate infusion or transdermal patch, provides a constant addition of drug and can maintain PDC. Additional options to maintain steady state concentration is the use of tissue depots (ceftiofur crystalline free acid), drugs that are highly protein bound (eg, maropitant), or formulated topicals (eg, selamectin).[43,44]

Pharmacokinetic Parameters: From Paper to Practice

The theory underlying frequently provided PK parameters was previously discussed. Through the use of PK research, a C_{max} for a given dose can be determined. Using

---

Box 4
Rule of thumb for excretion in exotics

- Multiply half-life by 5 to determine when the drug will be 97% cleared from plasma.
- A patient may be subtherapeutic before the drug has been completely cleared, use TDM to determine an appropriate dosing interval.

the half-life, a rough estimate of the dosing interval can be determined. For example, if the C_{max} is 50 μg/mL and the half-life is 2 hours, then 97% of the drug will be eliminated in 10 hours, at which time there will be an estimated PDC of 1.5 μg/mL. Therefore, dosing every 8 to 12 hours is necessary, depending on the drug. A comparison of bioavailability can determine whether a selected route will provide an effective C_{max}, or if the dose needs to be increased. If a loading dose is required, the use of V_d in Equation 3 can provide a dose.

PHARMACODYNAMICS

PK focuses on the movement of a drug through the body; the effect solicited by that drug is the PD. Although the clinician focuses on the clinical response (analgesia, sedation, resolution of infection), it is also important to recall that drugs target receptors and modulate the response of the receptor (ie, activate or inhibit). Correlation of PDC to physiologic effect is known as the dose-response relationship and forms the basis for determining subtherapeutic, therapeutic, and toxic doses. The necessary dose to elicit the needed effect can vary based on the presence of receptors and the binding affinity of these receptors. A comparison of opioid receptors in amphibians, avians, and mammals report differences in binding affinity, altering the effectiveness of various opioids, resulting in different dosing intervals.[45–48] The same drug may require different dosing intervals when used for the treatment of different diseases. Deslorelin implants are used in ferrets to manage adrenocortical disease[13] and in birds for chronic egg laying.[11,12] However, different doses are required for each and the dosing interval must be tailored to the individual patient based on clinical response.

Developing on appropriate model to determine effectiveness can be a challenge, especially when targeting pain or behavioral changes. Numerous pain models, including a decrease in inhalant mean alveolar concentration, thermal nociception, and inducement of inflammatory conditions have been used in rabbits and birds to determine whether PDC provides analgesia.[49] Facial grimace scores have been developed in rabbits, mice, and ferrets and can be applied clinically to help determine the effectiveness of an analgesic.[50–52] Understanding of normal behavior for a particular species combined with pain scores can aid the clinician in evaluating the efficacy of an analgesic and critically evaluate whether dose adjustments are necessary. Monitoring for each disease must be tailored to the disease itself and combined with TDM. For example, seizure management may target a decrease in the frequency of seizures, or the management of diabetes mellitus focuses on maintaining the blood glucose within a range and the resolution of polyuria or polydipsia.

Integrating Pharmacokinetics and Pharmacodynamics for Antimicrobial Selection

Antimicrobials are drugs for which PK and PD modeling is most frequently performed, in which species PK is integrated with the PD of the microbe. The goal is to determine the antimicrobial PDC needed to kill an organism, which depends on the mechanism of action of the antimicrobial and PK within the patient species. Therefore, the clinician must incorporate the culture and susceptibility data with the PK of the antimicrobial to determine the dose, route, dosing interval, and how long to treat the patient. The dose selection, dosing interval, bacteriostatic or bactericidal nature of the drug, and length of treatment determine the risk of drug-resistance development. This is a complex topic, and the reader is referred to several reviews discussing the implication of antimicrobial drug resistance.[53–57]

Table 3
Causes for therapeutic failure

	Factor	Causes of Therapeutic Failure
Patient Factor	Pharmacokinetic	• Inadequate blood supply (dehydration, cardiovascular insufficiency) • Poor penetration to target site (neoplasia or infectious) • Poor absorption, distribution, altered metabolism, increased elimination
	Pharmacodynamic	• Presence of foreign body, abscess, granuloma, biofilm, fluid • Pharmacologic interaction or antagonism
	Etiologic	• Not infectious disease • Underlying chronic disease
	Therapeutic	• Poor owner and patient compliance • Incorrect dose, route, frequency of drug administration • Compounded formulation failure
Organism Factor	Resistance	• Intrinsic resistance factors (efflux pumps, inhibitors) • Development of resistance
	Organism	• Intracellular • Creation of biofilm, keratin
	Isolation, identification, and testing	• Incorrect organism identification • Incorrectly performed or tested • Induced resistance • Poor sample collection

Data from Refs.[58–60]

SUMMARY

This article covers the usefulness of PK and PD studies for species in which there is limited information and no approved drugs. PK and PD studies can offer a tremendous amount of information to incorporate into an evidence-based practice, including differences in bioavailability, the creation of appropriate dosing interval, and integration with microbial PD to achieve therapeutic concentrations. Unfortunately, there is a lack of PK and PD data in exotic species. However, with an understanding of PK and PD concepts the clinician can critically determine causes and remedies for therapeutic failure (**Table 3**). Moreover, the availability of PK data across multiple species continues to expand and, with the incorporation of PD results, safer doses and proper dosing intervals continue to be developed. Nevertheless, although PK and PD data are a pillar in the development of therapeutic interventions for exotic species, each drug requires specialized considerations.

REFERENCES

1. Jambhekar SS, Breen PJ. Basic pharmacokinetics. Philadelphia: Pharmaceutical Press; 2012.
2. Toutain PL. Pharmacokinetic/pharmacodynamic integration in drug development and dosage-regimen optimization for veterinary medicine. AAPS PharmSci 2002; 4(4):E38.
3. Toutain PL, Lees P. Integration and modelling of pharmacokinetic and pharmacodynamic data to optimize dosage regimens in veterinary medicine. J Vet Pharmacol Ther 2004;27(6):467–77.
4. Chinnaduri SK, Messenger KM, Papich MG, et al. Meloxicam pharmacokinetics using nonlinear mixed-effects modeling in ferrets after single subcutaneous administration. J Vet Pharmacol Ther 2014;37(4):382–7.

5. van Zeeland Y, Schoemaker N, Haritova A, et al. Pharmacokinetics of paroxetine, a selective serotonin reuptake inhibitor, in grey parrots (*Psittacus erithacus erithacus*): influence of pharmaceutical formulation and length of dosing. J Vet Pharmacol Ther 2013;36(1):51–8.

6. Boothe DM. Principles of drug therapy. St. Louis (MO): Saunders; 2012.

7. Lacasse C, Gamble KC, Boothe DM. Pharmacokinetics of a single dose of intravenous and oral meloxicam in red-tailed hawks (*Buteo jamaicensis*) and great horned owls (*Bubo virginianus*). J Avian Med Surg 2013;27(3):204–10.

8. Toutain PL, Bousquet-Melou A. Plasma terminal half-life. J Vet Pharmacol Ther 2004;27(6):427–39.

9. Page SJ, Persch AC. Recruitment, retention, and blinding in clinical trials. Am J Occup Ther 2013;67(2):154–61.

10. Smith JA, Papich MG, Russell G, et al. Effects of compounding pharmacokinetics of itraconazole in black-footed penguins (*Sphenicus demersus*). J Zoo Wildl Med 2010;41(3):487–95.

11. Cowan ML, Martin GB, Monks DJ, et al. Inhibition of the reproductive system by deslorelin in male and female pigeons (*Columba livia*). J Avian Med Surg 2014; 28(2):102–8.

12. Petritz OA, Sanchez-Migallon Guzman D, Paul-Murphy J, et al. Evaluation of the efficacy and safety of single administration of 4.7-mg deslorelin acetate implants on egg production and plasma sex hormones in Japanese quail (Coturnix coturnix japonica). Am J Vet Res 2013;74(2):316–23.

13. Wagner RA, Piche CA, Jochle W, et al. Clinical and endocrine responses to treatment with deslorelin acetate implants in ferrets with adrenocortical disease. Am J Vet Res 2005;66(5):910–4.

14. Sadar MJ, Hawkins MG, Byrne BA, et al. Pharmacokinetics of a single intramuscular injection of ceftiofur crystalline-free acid in red-tailed hawks (*Buteo jamaicensis*). Am J Vet Res 2015;76(12):1077–84.

15. Adkesson MJ, Fernandez-Varon E, Cox S, et al. Pharmacokinetics of a long-acting ceftiofur formulation (ceftiofur crystalline free acid) in the ball python (*Python regius*). J Zoo Wildl Med 2011;42(3):444–50.

16. Toutain PL, Bousquet-Melou A. Bioavailability and its assessment. J Vet Pharmacol Ther 2004;27:455–66.

17. Neirinckx E, Vervaet C, De Boever S, et al. Species comparison of oral bioavailability, first-pass metabolism and pharmacokinetics of acetaminophen. Res Vet Sci 2010;89(1):113–9.

18. Roerig DL, Kotrly KJ, Ahlf SB, et al. Effect of propranolol on the first pass uptake of fentanyl in the human and rat lung. Anesthesiology 1989;71(1):62–8.

19. Toutain PL, Koritz GD. Veterinary drug bioequivalence determination. J Vet Pharmacol Ther 1997;20(2):79–90.

20. Jorga A, Holt DW, Johnston A. Therapeutic drug monitoring of cyclosporine. Transplant Proc 2004;36(2 Suppl):396S–403S.

21. Mawby DI, Whittemore JC, Genger S, et al. Bioequivalence of orally administered generic, compounded, and innovator-formulated itraconazole in healthy dogs. J Vet Intern Med 2014;28(1):72–7.

22. Guzman DS-M, Beaufrère H, KuKanich B, et al. Pharmacokinetics of single oral dose of pimobendan In Hispaniolan Amazon parrots (*Amazona ventralis*). J Avian Med Surg 2014;28(2):95–101.

23. Toutain PL, Bousquet-Melou A. Volumes of distribution. J Vet Pharmacol Ther 2004;27(6):441–53.

24. Reeve E, Wiese MD, Mangoni AA. Alterations in drug disposition in older adults. Expert Opin Drug Metab Toxicol 2015;11(4):491–508.
25. Delafuente J. Pharmacokinetic and pharmacodynamic alterations in the geriatric patient. Consult Pharm 2008;23(4):324–34.
26. Roberts JA, Pea F, Lipman J. The clinical relevance of plasma protein binding changes. Clin Pharmacokinet 2013;52(1):1–8.
27. Toutain PL, Buosquet-Melou A. Free drug fraction vs free drug concentration: a matter of frequent confusion. J Vet Pharmacol Ther 2002;25(6):460–3.
28. Nardini G, Barbarossa A, Dall'Occo A, et al. Pharmacokinetics of cefovecin sodium after subcutaneous administration to Hermann's tortoises (*Testudo hermanni*). Am J Vet Res 2014;75(10):918–23.
29. Sypniewski LA, Maxwell LK, Murray JK, et al. Cefovecin pharmacokinetics on the red-eared slider. J Exot Pet Med 2017;26(2):108–13.
30. Stegemann MR, Sherington J, Blanchflower S. Pharmacokinetics and pharmacodynamics of cefovecin in dogs. J Vet Pharmacol Ther 2006;29(6):501–11.
31. Cotler S, Gustafson JH, Colburn WA. Pharmacokinetics of diazepam and nordiazepam in the cat. J Pharm Sci 1984;73(3):348–51.
32. Benchaoui HA, Cox SR, Schneider RP, et al. The pharmacokinetics of maropitant, a novel neurokinin type-1 receptor antagonist, in dogs. J Vet Pharmacol Ther 2007;30(4):336–44.
33. Busch U, Schmid J, Heinzel G, et al. Pharmacokinetics of meloxicam in animals and the relevance to humans. Drug Metab Dispos 1998;26(6):576–84.
34. El-Merhibi A, Ngo SN, Marchant CL, et al. Cytochrome P450 CYP3A in marsupials: cloning and identification of the first CYP3A subfamily member, isoform 3A70 from Eastern gray kangaroo (*Macropus giganteus*). Gene 2012;506(2):423–8.
35. Kimble B, Li KM, Valtchev P, et al. In vitro hepatic microsomal metabolism of meloxicam in koalas (*Phascolarctos cinereus*), brushtail possums (Trichosurus vulpecula), ringtail possums (*Pseudocheirus peregrinus*), rats (*Rattus norvegicus*) and dogs (*Canis lupus familiaris*). Comp Biochem Physiol C Toxicol Pharmacol 2014;161:7–14.
36. Court MH. Acetaminophen UDP-glucuronosyltransferase in ferrets: species and gender differences, and sequence analysis of ferret UGT1A6. J Vet Pharmacol Ther 2001;24(6):415–22.
37. Vermeulen B, De Backer P, Remon JP. Drug administration to poultry. Adv Drug Deliv Rev 2002;54(6):795–803.
38. Holz P, Barker I, Burger JP, et al. The effect of the renal portal system on pharmacokinetic parameters in the red-eared slider (*Trachemys scripta elegans*). J Zoo Wildl Med 1997;28(4):386–93.
39. Beck K, Loomis M, Lewbart G, et al. Preliminary comparison of plasma concentration of gentamicin injected into the cranial and caudal limb musculature of the eastern box turtle. J Zoo Wildl Med 1995;26(2):265–8.
40. Holz PH, Burger JP, Baker R, et al. Effect of injection site on carbenicillin pharmacokinetics in the carpet python, *Morelia spilota*. J Herp Med Surg 2002;12(4):12–6.
41. Riviere JE, Martin-Jimenez T, Sundlof SF, et al. Interspecies allometric analysis of the comparative pharmacokinetics of 44 drugs across veterinary and laboratory animal species. J Vet Pharmacol Ther 1997;20(6):453–63.
42. Hunter RP. Interspecies allometric scaling. In: Comparative and veterinary pharmacology. Springer; 2010. p. 139–57.

43. Sarasola P, Jernigan AD, Walker DK, et al. Pharmacokinetics of selamectin following intravenous, oral and topical administration in cats and dogs. J Vet Pharmacol Ther 2002;25(4):265–72.
44. Toutain P-L, Bousquet-Mélou A. Plasma clearance. J Vet Pharmacol Ther 2004; 27(6):415–25.
45. Stevens CW. The evolution of vertebrate opioid receptors. Front Biosci (Landmark Ed) 2009;14:1247.
46. Hoppes S, Flammer K, Hoersch K, et al. Disposition and analgesic effects of fentanyl in white cockatoos (Cacatua alba). J Avian Med Surg 2003;17(3):124–30.
47. Paul-Murphy JR, Brunson DB, Miletic V. Analgesic effects of butorphanol and buprenorphine in conscious African grey parrots (Psittacus erithacus erithacus and Psittacus erithacus timneh). Am J Vet Res 1999;60(10):1218–21.
48. Paul-Murphy J, Hess JC, Fialkowski BJP. Pharmacokinetic properties of a single intramuscular dose of buprenorphine in African grey parrots (Psittacus erithacus erithacus). J Avian Med Surg 2004;18(4):224–8.
49. Cole GA, Paul-Murphy J, Krugner-Higby L, et al. Analgesic effects of intramuscular administration of meloxicam in Hispaniolan parrots (Amazona ventralis) with experimentally induced arthritis. Am J Vet Res 2009;70(12):1471–6.
50. Matsumiya LC, Sorge RE, Sotocinal SG, et al. Using the Mouse Grimace Scale to reevaluate the efficacy of postoperative analgesics in laboratory mice. J Am Assoc Lab Anim Sci 2012;51(1):42–9.
51. Hampshire V, Robertson S. Using the facial grimace scale to evaluate rabbit wellness in post-procedural monitoring. Lab Anim 2015;44(7):259.
52. Reijgwart ML, Schoemaker NJ, Pascuzzo R, et al. The composition and initial evaluation of a grimace scale in ferrets after surgical implantation of a telemetry probe. PLoS One 2017;12(11):e0187986.
53. Weese JS, Giguere S, Guardabassi L, et al. ACVIM consensus statement on therapeutic antimicrobial use in animals and antimicrobial resistance. J Vet Intern Med 2015;29:487–98.
54. Zhao X, Drlica K. A unified anti-mutant dosing strategy. J Antimicrob Chemother 2008;62(3):434–6.
55. Wise R. Maximizing efficacy and reducing the emergence of resistance. J Antimicrob Chemother 2003;51(Suppl 1):37–42.
56. von Baum H, Marre R. Antimicrobial resistance of Escherichia coli and therapeutic implications. Int J Med Microbiol 2005;295(6–7):503–11.
57. Southwood LL. Principles of antimicrobial therapy: what should we be using? Vet Clin North Am Equine Pract 2006;22(2):279–96, vii.
58. Prescott JF, Dowling PM. Antimicrobial therapy in veterinary medicine. Ames (IO): John Wiley & Sons; 2013.
59. Papich MG. Antimicrobials, susceptibility testing, and minimum inhibitory concentrations (MIC) in veterinary infection treatment. Vet Clin North Am Small Anim Pract 2013;43(5):1079–89.
60. Markey B, Leonard F, Archambault M, et al. Clinical veterinary microbiology. St. Louis (MO): Elsevier Health Sciences; 2013.

The Educated Guess
Determining Drug Doses in Exotic Animals Using Evidence-Based Medicine

Marike Visser, DVM[a],*, Seth C. Oster, DVM[b]

KEYWORDS

- Evidence-based veterinary medicine • Dosing selection • Pharmacokinetics
- Allometric scaling

KEY POINTS

- When determining drug doses, 3 parameters can be used to compare between species: volume of distribution, clearance, and elimination half-life.
- Allometric scaling does not account the physiologic difference between species and can only be used for a limited set of drugs with the availability of specific pharmacokinetic data.
- With empirical drug selection, there is a high risk of adverse events, and patients should be carefully monitored.

EVIDENCE-BASED VETERINARY MEDICINE

Evidence-based veterinary medicine (EBVM) has become a key component in clinical decision making. Several articles and reviews have discussed the use of EBVM in practice.[1] The process follows 5 critical steps:

1. Identify a clinical problem and formulate an answerable question.
2. Search for the best evidence available.
3. Critically appraise the evidence.
4. Integrate the evidence with clinical experience to answer the clinical problem.
5. Evaluate the outcome and determine if any corrective action is necessary.

Incorporation of EBVM in the selection of a dose for a patient can help minimize the risk of adverse events (AEs) and improve therapeutic efficacy. Several reviews have described the use of EBVM in exotic animal medicine, including the critical evaluation

Disclosure Statement: The authors have nothing to disclose.
[a] Department of Anatomy, Physiology and Pharmacology, Auburn University, 1010 Wire Road, Auburn, AL 36849, USA; [b] Department of Clinical Science, Auburn University, 1500 Wire Road, Auburn, AL 36849, USA
* Corresponding author. 137 North Park Street, Kalamazoo, MI 49007.
E-mail address: visserm0512@gmail.com

Vet Clin Exot Anim 21 (2018) 183–194
https://doi.org/10.1016/j.cvex.2018.01.002
1094-9194/18/© 2018 Elsevier Inc. All rights reserved.
vetexotic.theclinics.com

and application of scientific literature. There is a wide variety of research regarding pharmacology in veterinary medicine and exotic medicine, which can be tiered based on the levels of scientific rigor applied (**Fig. 1**). The first tier consists of primary literature sources including case reports of AEs and perceived efficacy of a specific drug, and online forums discussing clinical cases and experiences. Often, these clinical experiences will form the basis for experimentally designed pharmacokinetic (PK) and pharmacodynamic (PD) studies, found throughout journals and conference proceedings.[2,3] For certain diseases, there can be a wide variety of interventions with varying degrees of success. Collections of these reports are used in secondary analysis to compare and contrast the therapeutic interventions, and results are reported as systematic reviews and meta-analyses. These investigations may indicate a single superior treatment, no efficacious treatment, or several potential options. Eventually, this information is reported and distributed via third-tier sources such as textbooks and formularies.

PK articles are among the main sources of first-tier scientific reports. The development of robust search engines such as Google Scholar, Scopus, Web of Science, and PubMed gives the clinician access to primary and secondary tier data in a matter of minutes. Each of these search engines has their strengths and weakness,[4] and the clinician should always critically evaluate journal articles from unknown journals to ensure an adequate peer review process. The influence of pay-to-publish predatory journals continues to be a challenge in the scientific community. Although paying a fee for manuscript submission occurs frequently, predatory journals will accept articles without an appropriate peer review process or with an inadequate period for critical article review. Several articles have been published concerning the identification of predatory journals, detailing red flags for authors.[5,6] Frequently, the article is available to the general public as an open access journal, hoodwinking the scientific community into assuming that the article has undergone peer review. To combat this, open access publishers have developed the Directory of Open Access Journals (http://www.doaj.org), which requires a publisher to fulfill specified criteria before listing their journal. Currently, this directory offers the most efficient method for identifying peer-reviewed open access scientific literature.

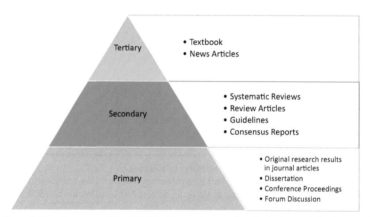

Fig. 1. Tier of literature used in EBVM. The primary tier includes original experimental research, case studies, conference proceedings, and forum discussion. The second tier is based on reviews and analysis of the primary tier to develop consensus statements and guidelines. Based on the primary and secondary, essential research and techniques are reported in the tertiary tier.

FOUR PRINCIPLES OF DRUG MOVEMENT

The number of species-specific PK reports can vary significantly, with much data available on the ferret, rabbit, guinea pig, and other small rodents due to their use as laboratory models in early drug discovery; however, there is little to no information on PK in other mammals (eg, sugar gliders or hedgehogs), birds, or reptiles.[7] (See Marike Visser's article, "Translating Pharmacokinetic and Pharmacodynamic Data into Practice," in this issue.) A broad overview of the concepts is provided here. PK studies develop mathematical models to explain the 4 principles of drug movement: absorption, distribution, metabolism, and excretion (ADME). In some circumstances, this information may be enough to formulate a dosing plan when therapeutic drug concentrations are established, such as antibiotics. All pharmaceuticals administered via an extravenous route undergo an absorption phase, requiring movement through a variety of barriers and metabolizing organs before entering the circulatory system. The circulatory system distributes the drug throughout the body. Distribution of a compound depends on the lipophilicity of the drug, protein binding, and membrane barriers such as the blood-brain barrier. Most metabolism occurs in the liver, via phase I and phase II enzymes, with the presence and efficiency of these proteins changing between species. Metabolism is required to render compounds water-soluble for renal excretion, detoxification of intermediates, and production of active metabolites. Excretion occurs primarily via the kidneys and hepatobiliary system, with the lungs important for elimination of inhalant gases.

Differences in the ADME between species can be seen via comparison of 3 PK parameters: volume of distribution (V_d), clearance (Cl), and elimination half-life ($t_{1/2}$) (**Table 1**).

Table 1
PK variation of meloxicam between species

Species	Dose (mg/kg)	Route	V_d	Cl	$t_{1/2}$
Nile tilapia[8]	1	IV	0.127 L/kg	N/A	1.35 h
Nile tilapia[8]	1	IM (F = 50%)	N/A	N/A	1.8 h
Pigeon[9]	1.1	IV	0.14 L/kg	0.039 L/h/kg	2.4 h
Duck[9]	1.1	IV	0.065 L/kg	0.061 L/h/kg	0.72 h
Turkey[9]	1.1	IV	0.079 L/kg	0.055 L/h/kg	0.99 h
Ostrich[9]	1.1	IV	0.58 L/kg	0.2 L/h/kg	0.5 h
Chicken[9]	1.1	IV	0.058 L/kg	0.013 L/h/kg	3.21 h
Red-tailed hawk[10]	0.5	IV	0.137 L/kg	0.154 L/h/kg	0.78 h
Great horned owl[10]	0.5	IV	0.832 L/kg	1.675 L/h/kg	0.49 h
African gray parrot[11]	1	IV	0.091 L/kg	0.0022 L/h/kg	31.4 h
Hispaniolan Amazon parrot[12]	1	IV	0.232 L/kg	0.122 L/h/kg	15.9 h
Red-eared slider[13]	0.2	IV	0.215 L/kg	0.018 L/h/kg	9.78 h
Green iguana[14]	0.2	IV	0.745 L/kg	0.487 L/h/kg	9.93 h
Loggerhead sea turtle[15]	0.1	IV	0.192 L/kg	0.0052 L/h/kg	38.5 h
Loggerhead sea turtle[15]	0.1	IM (F = 32%)	N/A	N/A	3.26 h
Albino rat (male)[16]	1	IV	0.257 L/kg	0.015 L/h/kg	13.4 h
Albino rat (female)[16]	1	IV	0.244 L/kg	0.005 L/h/kg	36.8 h
Mini-pig[16]	10	IV	2.97 L/kg	0.043 L/h/kg	121h

Abbreviations: F, bioavailability; IM, intramuscular; IV, intravenous; N/A, not applicable.

These parameters are useful for comparison because they are dose-independent and physiologic function–dependent.

As shown in **Table 1**, there are significant differences in the Cl, V_d, and $t_{1/2}$ between species, making dose extrapolation a challenge. The species difference in Cl and V_d is among the reasons for the failure of linear dose extrapolation. Regardless of the route, there is remarkable variation in the $t_{1/2}$ across the various species, which will have a significant impact on the dosing interval. Among the main challenges when using PK studies for dosing determination is the limited data that can be collected if the dose is only administered via an extravenous route. This results in an inaccurate V_d and Cl owing to the influence of absorption, which changes the amount of drug available for systemic distribution. The description of this change compared with the intravenous route is known as bioavailability (F).[17] If information regarding the V_d, Cl, or $t_{1/2}$ is available, it can easily be applied to determine a dose (**Table 2**).

However, if there are no species-specific data available, the aforementioned process cannot be used to establish a dose and dosing interval. As such, clinicians need to revert to other methods to develop a dose and dosing interval in the given species.

ALLOMETRIC SCALING

Allometric scaling is a technique used for interspecies dose scaling based on the whole body metabolic rate and body size of the animal. This equation correlates metabolic rate to not only body size but also to body surface area, organ blood flow, and glomerular filtration rate. The basic equation used for allometric scaling

$$Y = aW_b \tag{6}$$

In which Y is the $t_{1/2}$, Cl, or V_d, a is the y-intercept of the drug, W is the average species body weight, and b is the scaling component based on the drug. The challenge with using Equation 6 is the need for research into individual drugs to verify a correlation to 1 of the 3 Y parameters and determine the a and b covariates. Drugs for which V_d and Cl can be scaled are enrofloxacin, ciprofloxacin,[18] and several aminoglycosides, with differences present between birds and mammals for both gentamicin

Table 2 Equations used in dose calculations	
Calculation	**Restrictions and Suggestions**
Equation 1: Dose $= \frac{C_{max} \times V_d}{F}$	• Must use IV route of administration or correct for F • Make sure all the units are correct
Equation 2: Cl $= V_d \times k_{el}$	• PK data must be from IV administration • The elimination constant (k_{el}) can be used to calculate the half-life
Equation 3: $k_{el} = \ln \frac{\frac{C_{max}}{C_{min}}}{t_2 - t_1}$	• Equation that can be used to determine elimination constant from TDM data
Equation 4: $t_{1/2} = \frac{0.693}{k_{el}}$	• Calculate the half-life based on Equation 3.
Equation 5: Maintenance Dose $= \frac{Cl \times C_{max} \times \tau}{F}$	• Must have intravenous Cl from PK Data • If giving by another route, need F • The dosing interval (τ) must be feasible • Make sure all the units are correct

and apramycin.[19] Therefore, Equation 1 could be used for these specific drugs, with allometric scaling of the V_d to determine a dose. Using this method, a study comparing 44 drugs reported that only 25% of the selected drugs could be allometrically scaled.[20] With all these caveats in place, allometric scaling can only be used in a limited number of drugs, reflecting the physiologic differences between species[21]:

1. Rate of absorption

    The rate and extent of absorption depend on the physiochemical properties of the drug and physiologic factors such as gastrointestinal (GI) transit time, pH, and membrane permeability. The most significant differences can be seen in a drug that is given orally because this must pass through the GI tract and survive metabolism by the liver before systemic distribution. Variation in F has been reported for meloxicam between Amazon parrots (F = 49%–75%)[12] and red-tailed hawks (F = 100%).[10] A recent study also reported on differences in the time to maximum concentration between lions and cheetahs receiving meloxicam, indicating different rates of absorption.[22] Reptile drug absorption can be influenced by the prandial state, especially in species with variable feeding[23] and environmental temperature.[24]

2. Rate of drug distribution

    Drug distribution depends on blood flow and the properties of the drugs. Smaller animals will have a higher rate of blood flow, and the drug will reach the target receptor faster but the drug is cleared faster. Drugs with a high V_d will move from the plasma compartment to fat, decreasing the plasma drug concentration and prolonging the rate of elimination. In contrast, drugs that are limited to the plasma will result in high plasma drug concentration and should be dosed on lean body weight. Another essential factor for distribution is the extent of protein binding, which prevents a drug from being released.[21] There is significant variation in protein binding between mammals, reptiles, and avian species. Bound drug is hidden from the body, unable to distribute beyond the vascular compartment and is not available for metabolism or elimination. Any free drug is rapidly eliminated, leading to a shorter dosing interval. The vast differences in the PK of cefovecin highlight the importance of protein binding, with the drug effective in most mammals but rapidly eliminated in birds and reptiles.[25–27]

3. Metabolism

    Drug metabolism depends on the presence of several enzyme superfamilies, including the cytochrome P450 family (CYP450), which varies significantly between species. After a PK study reported that koalas had significantly different Cl compared with other mammals, researchers developed an in vitro assay to examine the influence CYP450. Using liver microsomes, the rate of intrinsic Cl (Cl_{int}) of meloxicam metabolism of koalas, brushtail opossums, ringtail opossums, rats, and dogs was compared. CYP450 metabolism varied widely between the species, with brushtail opossums having the fastest rate of Cl_{int}, whereas koalas and ringtail opossum had similar rates of Cl_{int}, and the canine had minimal Cl_{int}.[28] Another enzyme family with known species differences is UDP-glucuronosyltransferase (UGT). The domestic feline has 2 nonfunctional UGT enzymes, placing this species at greater risk for acetaminophen toxicity. Unlike the domestic feline, the ferret does have functional UGT. However, in vitro studies report that the ferret enzyme is also slow to glucoronate acetaminophen, increasing the risk of hepatoxcity.[29] In addition to enzyme efficiency, studies in reptiles report that injections into the caudal half of the subjects changes the reported PD effects of hepatically metabolized anesthetics, highlighting a unique difference that is not found in mammalian or avian exotic species.[30,31] These significant differences in drug metabolism can lead to AE or subtherapeutic concentrations. Extensively metabolized drugs should not be scaled owing to vast differences in metabolism in exotic species.

4. Excretion or elimination

Most drugs are eliminated via the renal or hepatobiliary system, and the rate of excretion depends on the rate of blood flow, the physiochemical properties of the drug, and protein binding. Transporters in both the biliary and renal tissues can vary significantly between species; however, these differences have not been teased out. Also, species with prolonged GI transit times can have increased hepatobiliary resorption, as reported with ball pythons receiving azithromycin.[23]

Based on the limitations placed on allometric scaling, this method should be reserved for use in only limited situations and ideally with the consultation of a clinical pharmacologist.

DOSE SELECTION ALGORITHM

With all the caveats placed on the use of allometric scaling, other methods should be considered to help the clinician in the decision-making process regarding the drug dose and dosing interval to be used. Similar to the concepts described for the initial search for PK and PD data, the use of EBVM becomes vital. The authors recommend that clinicians use the described drug algorithm (**Fig. 2**) to select a dose when no PK data in the species of interest are available, followed by therapeutic drug monitoring (TDM) and dose adjustments as necessary.

Pharmacokinetic Data in a Related Species

When no PK data are available within the species, the use of a closely related species provides a platform to design an appropriate dose and dosing interval. With the development of mitochondrial genotyping, taxonomic reorganization has improved the understanding of the evolutionary relationship between species. The comparison between 2 different species goes beyond class and order. Although hawks and owls are both considered birds of prey and part of the Aves class, owls are part of the Strigiformes order and hawks are part of the Accipitriformes order.[32] A PK comparison of meloxicam between red-tailed hawks and great horned owls reports almost a 2-fold difference in the Cl and $t_{1/2}$ (see **Table 1**), suggesting differences in metabolism and the rate of excretion. Therefore, the clinician should aim to find a species that has a similar diet and is as evolutionary close as possible.

Plasma Protein Binding

Plasma protein binding can have a significant impact on the rate of Cl. Changes in a disease state or competitive binding can alter the free plasma drug concentration, which is the only drug available for metabolism and Cl.[33] This means that drugs that are highly protein bound will have a prolonged Cl, prolonging the dosing interval. Although there is debate regarding the clinical effect of changes in plasma protein binding,[34] rapid changes can increase Cl, thereby shortening the dosing interval. Drugs that are highly protein bound includes examples such as cefovecin, meloxicam, maropitant, and doxycycline. Although protein binding appears to be consistent in most mammal species, there are significant differences when compared with reptile and avian species. Cefovecin was reported to be 98% protein bound in canine[25]

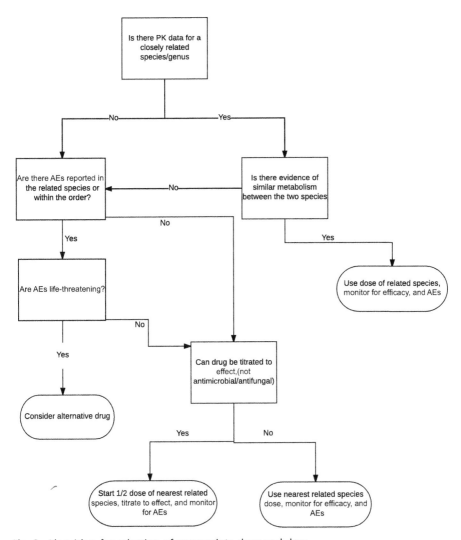

Fig. 2. Algorithm for selection of appropriate drug and dose.

but less than 50% is protein bound in Hermann's tortoise.[26] PK in other avian and reptile species also report a rapid Cl, suggesting poor protein binding.[27] Therefore, if possible, drugs with high protein-binding affinity should be avoided in avian and reptile species unless in vitro protein binding assays or PK data are available.

Evaluating the Risk of Adverse Events

A drug AE is defined as any unanticipated or negative event that occurs after the administration of a pharmaceutical and suspected to be due to the pharmaceutical. The event can range from mild (itchiness, nausea) to life-threatening anaphylaxis and death. Some monotherapy AEs are well recognized, such as the risk of GI ulceration and renal toxicity with nonsteroidal antiinflammatories (NSAIDs), the risk of acute renal failure with the use of aminoglycosides, or dose-dependent hepatotoxicity with phenobarbital.[35] Some AEs are more species-specific, such as the use of penicillin orally in rabbits causing a fatal enterotoxaemia.[36] (See Olivia A. Petritz and Sue Chen's article, "Therapeutic Contraindications in Exotic Pets," in this issue.)

Toxicities due to overdosing are frequently reported and are a challenge in exotic species in which empirical use can result in an AE. Cases series of overdosing resulting in AEs have been reported in penguins receiving voriconazole[37] and vitamin B6 in gyrfalcons and peregrine falcons.[38] Case series can be beneficial in identifying doses causing AEs. However, this does not necessarily imply that the drug should not be used at all in the species. Instead, it emphasizes that a lower dose should be considered and the patient carefully monitored.

Beyond the risk within the species, an individual patient may be at higher risk depending on age, gender, or disease state. There are very few studies comparing PK between ages or in disease states. Several in vitro studies have reported differences between male and female enzyme efficiency; however, the clinical implications have not been explored.[29,39] Disease states, especially renal or hepatic, can significantly increase the risk of an AE. Drugs that require close TDM in the presence of renal insufficiency include the aminoglycosides, digoxins, and NSAIDs. (See Marike Visser's article, "Techniques for Monitoring Drug Efficacy," in this issue.)

Challenges of Polypharmacy

The combination of multiple drugs, polypharmacy, can have unpredictable effects and increase the risk of AEs. Toxicity can occur due to competition for metabolism, increasing the plasma drug concentration of certain drugs or targeting the same receptor, causing an overdose. The risks of polypharmacy are difficult to predict without knowledge of drug metabolizing enzymes and PK within the individual species. Certain drugs should never be used in combination, such as an NSAID and a glucocorticoid, or an aminoglycoside and an NSAID, without the initiation of TDM. Drugs that are known to change the PK of drugs include phenobarbital, ketoconazole, clarithromycin, and rifampin. These inhibitors depend on the presence of certain enzymes, and the extent of the impact can vary by species.[40,41] The clinician should use their own experience combined with all available literature to develop a safe and effective dose.

The use of herbal supplements, used as either monotherapy or in polypharmacy, with or without veterinary oversight can also lead to AEs. These not only include overdosing on certain vitamins, the potential for pesticide, and heavy metal contamination but also interactions with other medications[42] (**Table 3**). For example, a patient may be receiving an NSAID from their veterinarian, and the owner can add on willow bark (aspirin), leading to an increased risk of GI ulceration and bleeding. Similarly, many of the herbs are inhibitors of metabolizing enzymes, such as CYP450 (goldenseal and St. John's Wort) or P-glycoprotein transporters (St. John's Wort), increasing the risk of high plasma drug concentration and an AE.[43] Unfortunately, for many herbs, there are little to no data regarding their safety and efficacy. Nevertheless, clinicians should always investigate whether a patient is receiving any supplements and consider their use when determining the risk of an AE.

Titrating a Drug

When selecting a dose, it is always safer to start low and increase the dose to effect. This allows the clinician to monitor for any AE with an increase in dose. Drugs with a narrow therapeutic index (TI), the range between the dose that is effective and the dose that can result in an AE, require careful monitoring. Any dose with less than 2-fold difference in the TI should be used with caution and careful monitoring. TI can also vary by species, such as the case of fenbendazole. This drug is considered

Table 3
Examples of commonly used herbal supplements and their interactions with pharmaceutical drugs

Herb	Drugs
St. John's wort	Serotonin reuptake inhibitors, tricyclic antidepressants, digoxin, cyclosporine, azathioprine, methotrexate, mycophenolate, tacrolimus, barbiturates, benzodiazepines, theophylline, warfarin, antifungals, calcium channel blockers
Ginger	Warfarin
Gingko	NSAIDs, anticoagulants, tricyclic antidepressants
Ginseng	Warfarin, heparin, aspirin, NSAIDs, glucocorticoids
Valerian	Barbiturates
Kava kava	Buprenorphine

Data from Miller LG. Herbal Medicinal: selected clinical considerations focusing on known or potential drug-herb interactions. Arch Intern Med 1998;158:2200–11; and Joshi A, Halquist M, Konsoula Z, et al. Improving the oral bioavailability of buprenorphine: an in-vivo proof of concept. J Pharm Pharmacol 2017;69(1):23–31.

to have a wide TI and to be very safe; however, cases of fenbendazole toxicity have been reported in pelicans and storks.[44,45] The safety of any given drug should not be assumed in a given species. TDM should start soon after dose administration, first to monitor for any AEs and then to monitor for efficacy. A thorough knowledge of the PK behavior of the drug and the anticipated effect will help the clinician anticipate any potential AEs. (See Marike Visser's article, "Techniques for Monitoring Drug Efficacy," in this issue.)

There are 2 groups of pharmaceuticals that are an exception to drug titration: antimicrobials and antifungals. Due to the ever-present risk of developing drug resistance, treating at high doses for short periods of time or the use of synergistic antimicrobial combinations are recommended if an acute infection is present. An acute infection should resolve within 2 to 3 days of therapy, and it is recommended to treat for 2 days following the resolution of clinical signs. If a chronic infection is present, then culture and susceptibility (C&S) is recommended.[46–48] For an uncomplicated infection, a first-tier antimicrobial should be selected. First-tier antimicrobials are older classes with a narrow spectrum, including trimethoprim sulfamethoxazole, first-generation and second-generation cephalosporin, extended spectrum ß-lactamases, tetracycline, and metronidazole. If higher tier drugs, such as aminoglycosides, vancomycin, or enrofloxacin, are required, then C&S should be used to select an antimicrobial and determine the appropriate dose required.[49,50] (See Marike Visser's article, "Translating Pharmacokinetic and Pharmacodynamic Data into Practice," in this issue.) If no PK data are available, the use of previously reported AE in other species should be taken into account and TDM techniques applied. (See Marike Visser's article, "Techniques for Monitoring Drug Efficacy," in this issue.)

SUMMARY

Currently, there is no single effective method for determining a dose in the wide variety of exotic species. This is due to the physiologic differences between species, ranging from the rate of absorption to the extent of protein binding, the rate of metabolism, and routes of elimination. Allometric scaling can be used in a small subset of drugs with minimal metabolism and renal excretion; however, the clinician should be very cautious and consult a clinical pharmacologist if unsure. Also, the influence of F can further affect the efficacy of the selected route and varies significantly between species. EBVM can be applied to the described algorithm to develop an initial dose and dosing interval. Using drug monitoring and careful titration, the dose can (gradually) be adjusted based on reported AEs and therapeutic efficacy.

REFERENCE

1. Reynders RM. An introduction to systematic reviews and meta-analyses for exotic animal practitioners. Vet Clin North Am Exot Anim Pract 2017;20(3):973–95.
2. Huntley SJ, Dean RS, Massey A, et al. International evidence-based medicine survey of the veterinary profession: Information sources used by veterinarians. PLoS One 2016;11(7):e0159732.
3. Giuffrida MA. Practical application of evidence-based practice. Vet Clin North Am Exot Anim Pract 2017;20(3):737–48.
4. Falagas ME, Pitsouni EI, Malietzis GA, et al. Comparison of PubMed, Scopus, Web of Science, and Google Scholar: strengths and weaknesses. FASEB J 2008;22(2):338–42.
5. Dadkhah M, Bianciardi G. Ranking predatory journals: solve the problem instead of removing it! Adv Pharm Bull 2016;6(1):1–4.
6. Beall J. Predatory publishers are corrupting open access. Nature 2012; 489(7415):179.
7. Suckow MA, Stevens KA, Wilson RP. The laboratory rabbit, guinea pig, hamster and other rodents. Academic Press; 2011.
8. Fredholm DV, Mylniczenko ND, KuKanich B. Pharmacokinetic evaluation of meloxicam after intravenous and intramuscular administration in Nile Tilapia (*Oreochromis niloticus*). J Zoo Wildl Med 2016;47(3):736–42.
9. Baert K, De Backer P. Comparative pharmacokinetics of three non-steroidal anti-inflammatory drugs in five bird species. Comp Biochem Physiol C Toxicol Pharmacol 2003;134(1):25–33.
10. Lacasse C, Gamble KC, Boothe DM. Pharmacokinetics of a single dose of intravenous and oral meloxicam in red-tailed hawks (*Buteo jamaicensis*) and great horned owls (*Bubo virginianus*). J Avian Med Surg 2013;27(3):204–10.
11. Montesinos A, Ardiaca M, Gilabert JA, et al. Pharmacokinetics of meloxicam after intravenous, intramuscular and oral administration of a single dose to African grey parrots (*Psittacus erithacus*). J Vet Pharmacol Ther 2017;40(3):279–84.
12. Molter CM, Court MH, Cole GA, et al. Pharmacokinetics of meloxicam after intravenous, intramuscular, and oral administration of a single dose to Hispaniolan Amazon parrots (*Amazona ventralis*). Am J Vet Res 2013;74(3):375–80.
13. Uney K, Altan F, Aboubakr M, et al. Pharmacokinetics of meloxicam in red-eared slider turtles (*Trachemys scripta elegans*) after single intravenous and intramuscular injections. Am J Vet Res 2016;77(5):439–44.
14. Divers SJ, Papich M, McBride M, et al. Pharmacokinetics of meloxicam following intravenous and oral administration in green iguanas (*Iguana iguana*). Am J Vet Res 2010;71(11):1277–83.
15. Lai OR, Di Bello A, Soloperto S, et al. Pharmacokinetic behavior of meloxicam in loggerhead sea turtles (*Caretta caretta*) after intramuscular and intravenous administration. J Wildl Dis 2015;51(2):509–12.
16. Busch U, Schmid J, Heinzel G, et al. Pharmacokinetics of meloxicam in animals and the relevance to humans. Drug Metab Dispos 1998;26(6):576–84.

17. Trepanier LA. Applying pharmacokinetics to veterinary clinical practice. Vet Clin North Am Small Anim Pract 2013;43(5):1013–26.
18. Cox SK, Cottrell MB, Smith L, et al. Allometric analysis of ciprofloxacin and enrofloxacin pharmacokinetics across species. J Vet Pharmacol Ther 2004;27(3): 139–46.
19. Dinev TG. Comparison of the pharmacokinetics of five aminoglycoside and aminocyclitol antibiotics using allometric analysis in mammal and bird species. Res Vet Sci 2008;84:107–18.
20. Riviere JE, Martin-Jimenez T, Sundlof SF, et al. Interspecies allometric analysis of the comparative pharmacokinetics of 44 drugs across veterinary and laboratory animal species. J Vet Pharmacol Ther 1997;20(6):453–63.
21. Sharma V, McNeill JH. To scale or not to scale: the principles of dose extrapolation. Br J Pharmacol 2009;157:907–21.
22. Visser M, Boothe DE, Bronson E. Population pharmacokinetics of meloxicam in lion, tiger and cheetah. Paper presented at: 49th AAZV Annual Conference 2017. Dallas, TX.
23. Coke RL, Hunter RP, Isaza R, et al. Pharmacokinetics and tissue concentrations of azithromycin in ball pythons (*Python regius*). Am J Vet Res 2003;64(2):225–8.
24. Caligiuri R, Kollias GV, Jacobson E, et al. The effects of ambient temperature on amikacin pharmacokinetics in gopher tortoises. J Vet Pharmacol Ther 1990;13(3): 287–91.
25. Stegemann MR, Sherington J, Blanchflower S. Pharmacokinetics and pharmacodynamics of cefovecin in dogs. J Vet Pharmacol Ther 2006;29(6):501–11.
26. Nardini G, Barbarossa A, Dall'Occo A, et al. Pharmacokinetics of cefovecin sodium after subcutaneous administration to Hermann's tortoises (*Testudo hermanni*). Am J Vet Res 2014;75(10):918–23.
27. Thuesen LR, Bertelsen MF, Brimer L, et al. Selected pharmacokinetic parameters for Cefovecin in hens and green iguanas. J Vet Pharmacol Ther 2009;32(6): 613–7.
28. Kimble B, Li KM, Valtchev P, et al. In vitro hepatic microsomal metabolism of meloxicam in koalas (*Phascolarctos cinereus*), brushtail possums (*Trichosurus vulpecula*), ringtail possums (*Pseudocheirus peregrinus*), rats (*Rattus norvegicus*) and dogs (*Canis lupus familiaris*). Comp Biochem Physiol C Toxicol Pharmacol 2014;161:7–14.
29. Court MH. Acetaminophen UDP-glucuronosyltransferase in ferrets: species and gender differences, and sequence analysis of ferret UGT1A6. J Vet Pharmacol Ther 2001;24(6):415–22.
30. Yaw TJ, Mans C, Doss G, et al. Influence of injection site on alfaxalone-induced sedation in ball pythons (*Python regius*). Paper presented at: AEMV and ARAV Annual Conference 2017. Dallas, TX.
31. Mans C, Fink D, Doss G, et al. Effect of injection site on dexmedetomidine-ketamine induced sedation in leopard geckos (Eublepharis macularius). Paper presented at: 2017 AEMV and ARAV Annual Conference 2017. Dallas, TX.
32. Lerner HR, Mindell DP. Phylogeny of eagles, Old World vultures, and other Accipitridae based on nuclear and mitochondrial DNA. Mol Phylogenet Evol 2005; 37(2):327–46.
33. Ascenzi P, Fanalo G, Fasano M, et al. Clinical relevance of drug binding to plasma proteins. J Mol Struct 2014;1077:4–13.
34. Benet LZ, Hoener BA. Changes in plasma protein binding have little clinical relevance. Clin Pharmacol Ther 2002;71(3):115–21.
35. Boothe DM. Principles of drug therapy. Saunders; 2012.

36. Varga M. Textbook of rabbit medicine. 2nd edition. Butterworth-Heinemann; 2013.

37. Hyatt MW, Georoff TA, Nollens HH, et al. Voriconazole toxicity in multiple penguin species. J Zoo Wildl Med 2015;46(4):880–8.

38. Samour J, Perlman J, Kinne J, et al. Vitamine B6 (pyridoxine hydrochloride) toxicosis in falcons. J Zoo Wildl Med 2016;47(2):601–8.

39. van Beusekom CD, Schipper L, Fink-Gremmels J. Cytochrome P450-mediated hepatic metabolism of new fluorescent substrates in cats and dogs. J Vet Pharmacol Ther 2010;33(6):519–27.

40. Sikka R, Magauran B, Ulrich A, et al. Bench to bedside: pharmacogenomics, adverse drug interactions, and the cytochrome P450 system. Acad Emerg Med 2005;12(12):1227–35.

41. Court MH. Canine cytochrome P450 (CYP) pharmacogenetics. Vet Clin North Am Small Anim Pract 2013;43(5):1027–38.

42. Miller LG. Herbal medicinal: selected clinical considerations focusing on known or potential drug-herb interactions. Arch Intern Med 1998;158:2200–11.

43. NCCIH Clinical Digest. In:2015.

44. Lindemann DM, Eshar D, Nietfeld JC, et al. Suspected fenbendazole toxicity in an American White Pelican (Pelecanus erythrorhynchos). J Zoo Wildl Med 2016; 47(2):681–5.

45. Weber MA, Terrell SP, Neiffer DL, et al. Bone marrow hypoplasia and intestinal crypt cell necrosis associated with fenbendazole administration in five painted storks. J Am Vet Med Assoc 2002;221(3):417–9, 369.

46. Toutain PL, Bousquet-Melou A, Martinez M. AUC/MIC: a PK/PD index for antibiotics with a time dimension or simply a dimensionless scoring factor? J Antimicrob Chemother 2007;60(6):1185–8.

47. Zhao X, Drlica K. A unified anti-mutant dosing strategy. J Antimicrob Chemother 2008;62(3):434–6.

48. Reynolds R, Potz N, Colman M, et al. Antimicrobial susceptibility of the pathogens of bacteraemia in the UK and Ireland 2001-2002: the BSAC Bacteraemia resistance surveillance programme. J Antimicrob Chemother 2004;53(6):1018–32.

49. Weese JS, Giguere S, Guardabassi L, et al. ACVIM consensus statement on therapeutic antimicrobial use in animals and antimicrobial resistance. J Vet Intern Med 2015;29:487–98.

50. Southwood LL. Principles of antimicrobial therapy: what should we be using? Vet Clin North Am Equine Pract 2006;22(2):279–96, vii.

Compounding and Extralabel Use of Drugs in Exotic Animal Medicine

Lauren V. Powers, DVM, DABVP(Avian Practice), DABVP(Exotic Companion Mammal Practice)[a,*],
Gigi Davidson, BS Pharm, DICVP[b]

KEYWORDS

- Avian • Compounding pharmacy • Exotic animals • Extralabel drug use (ELDU)
- Extemporaneous compounding • United States Pharmacopeia (USP)

KEY POINTS

- Extralabel drug use (ELDU) is the use of a Food and Drug Administration–approved drug in a manner different from what is indicated on the approved label.
- Drug compounding is the process by which a veterinarian or pharmacist prepares a medication in a manner not stipulated on the label to create a compound specifically tailored to the needs of an individual patient. Drug compounding is one type of ELDU.
- A common reason for drug compounding in exotic animal practice is to create a formulation in a vehicle, strength, and flavor suitable for oral drug delivery to exotic animals.
- The compounding pharmacist and pharmacy are invaluable partners in maintaining a high standard of care for safe and effective drug preparation for exotic patients.
- All pertinent federal and state pharmacy and veterinary medicine laws and regulations must be strictly followed when compounding medications in the veterinary hospital and when working with compounding pharmacies.

INTRODUCTION

Extralabel drug use (ELDU) and drug compounding are vital aspects of safe and effective drug delivery to patients in exotic animal practice.[1] Drug compounding is the process by which a veterinarian or pharmacist prepares a medication in a manner not stipulated in the product labeling to create a compound specifically tailored to the needs of an individual patient. Compared with the number of drugs approved by the US Food and Drug Administration (FDA) for use in humans, the number of drugs

Disclosure Statement: The authors declare no conflicts of interest.
[a] Avian and Exotic Pet Service, Carolina Veterinary Specialists, 12117 Statesville Road, Huntersville, NC 28078, USA; [b] College of Veterinary Medicine, North Carolina State University, 1060 William Moore Drive, Raleigh, NC 27607, USA
* Corresponding author.
E-mail address: lvpowers@carolinavet.com

Vet Clin Exot Anim 21 (2018) 195–214
https://doi.org/10.1016/j.cvex.2018.01.005
1094-9194/18/© 2018 Elsevier Inc. All rights reserved.

approved for use in veterinary species is low.[1] Within this subset of approved veterinary medications, there is only a tiny handful of FDA-approved drugs for use in birds and other exotic animals. Even though current federal law permits veterinarians to use and prescribe drugs that are FDA-approved for human use in an extralabel fashion, most medications are only available in formulations impractical or unsafe for use in exotic pets. Compounding also allows access to medications that are not currently commercially available, such as drugs discontinued by pharmaceutical companies for economic reasons or as a result of voluntarily or federally mandated withdrawals and drugs unavailable for use due to temporary shortages.[1]

WHAT IS EXTRALABEL DRUG USE?

ELDU is the use of an FDA-approved drug in any manner different from what is indicated on the approved label. The US Animal Medicinal Drug Use Clarification Act of 1994 (AMDUCA), an amendment to the US Federal Food, Drug, and Cosmetic Act of 1938, allows veterinarians to legally use and prescribe FDA-approved human and veterinary drugs in an extralabel fashion with certain important exceptions, some of which are discussed later. EDLU includes the use of the drug in a different species from that stipulated on the approved label or any changes in the dose or dosage, frequency, duration of therapy, or route of delivery as well as any manipulation of the drug itself not described in the product labeling (compounding). As an example, some avian practitioners dispense injectable formulations of enrofloxacin to be given orally to birds. This is ELDU not only because there are no FDA-approved injectable solutions of enrofloxacin for use in avian species but also because oral use is not a labeled route of delivery for injectable formulations. FDA regulations limit ELDU in veterinary medicine to situations where an animal's health is threatened or where the animal may suffer or die without treatment. A decision tree is assigned by AMDUCA for prioritizing ELDU in animal patients as follows: (1) use an FDA animal drug approved for use in the target species, (2) use an FDA animal drug approved for use in another species, (3) use an FDA-approved human drug, and (4) use a compounded preparation. A decision tree diagram for compounded preparations can be found in **Fig. 1**.

WHAT IS DRUG COMPOUNDING?

Any manipulation of a drug not described on the FDA-approved product labeling is considered compounding. Types of drug manipulation include (but are not limited to) changes to the concentration of a liquid medication (eg, diluting and concentrating), flavoring, mixing of 2 or more drugs together, and the creation of a liquid formulation for oral administration from tablets, capsules, injectable solutions, or bulk substances (active pharmaceutical ingredients [APIs]). In veterinary drug law, compounding is considered 1 type of ELDU.

INDICATIONS FOR DRUG COMPOUNDING IN VETERINARY MEDICINE

In companion animal practice, the most common reason why veterinarians use and prescribe compounded medications is the lack of availability of an approved drug that is practical and safe for administration to a patient. Another common reason for prescribing compounds for companion animals is due to drug shortages or market withdrawals of an approved product.[1] Novel, voluntarily accepted dosage forms, such as medicated treats, as well as long-acting implants and compounded topical transdermal gels, are also popular in companion animal veterinary practice.[1]

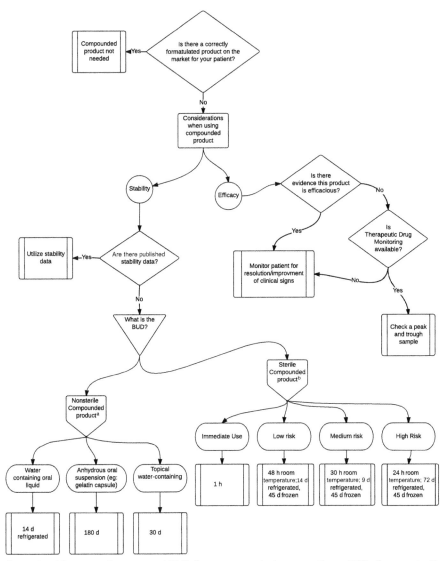

Fig. 1. Decision tree diagram and BUD for compounded preparations. BUDs for nonsterile compounded preparations ([a]) are published in USP-NF <795> and for sterile compounded preparations ([b]) in USP-NF <797>, United States Pharmacopeia National Formulary 2017: USP 40–NF 35, United States Pharmacopeial Convention, Rockville, MD, 2016. Note that all BUDs are subject to change pending scheduled revision of the USP General Chapters in December 2019. (*Courtesy of* Marike Visser, DVM, Auburn University College of Veterinary Medicine, Auburn, Alabama.)

In addition to providing medical therapy to suit the needs of an individual animal patient, compounded preparations also provide benefit when there is no approved product available (either for humans or animals) containing the desired active ingredients. For example, cisapride was withdrawn from the US human market for safety reasons in 2000 but is the only known safe and effective therapy to treat chronic constipation (or megacolon) in cats[2] and has also been used to treat ileus in rabbits.[3] No veterinary drug companies have yet elected to submit applications for cisapride approval for animals, so compounding remains the only option for veterinarians to obtain cisapride for animals in need of this particular prokinetic drug therapy.

Economic reasons are also often cited by veterinarians as a benefit of using compounded drug therapies. Regulatory agencies and professional veterinary organizations have stated that using a compounded preparation over an approved product strictly for economic reasons is inappropriate; however, many veterinarians care for animals owned by persons who are either unable or unwilling to pay for expensive approved therapy. Regardless of initial cost savings, the risk of poor drug quality, lack of bioavailability, and subsequent therapeutic failure from these compounded mimic therapies is significant and predictably may increase overall cost due to lack of clinical response.

INDICATIONS FOR DRUG COMPOUNDING IN EXOTIC ANIMAL MEDICINE

In exotic animal medicine, a common indication for drug compounding is the lack of FDA-approved formulations suitable for safe and practical delivery to exotic patients (see **Fig. 1**). Birds, reptiles, and many exotic companion mammals generally do not accept or tolerate tablets or capsules delivered directly by the oral route. Although some exotic companion animals self-medicate by accepting a medicated treat or by drinking medicated water, many do not. The most practical dosage form for individual dosing in exotic animal patients is often an oral liquid. Many FDA-approved drugs for use in humans and other animal species, however, are not available in a liquid dosage form. Many FDA-approved formulations are also not available in the small doses (strength or size) required for the generally smaller exotic animals. Another commonly requested compound in exotic animal practice is the addition of a flavoring agent to an approved product to improve palatability and patient acceptance, thereby increasing compliance with the prescribed therapy. Without a safe and palatable formulation for drug delivery, client and patient compliance is low and the likelihood of therapeutic failure is high.

STANDARDS AND REGULATIONS FOR EXTRALABEL DRUG USE AND DRUG COMPOUNDING
United States Pharmacopeia Standards

The United States Pharmacopeia (USP) is a nongovernment, private, standards-setting organization that publishes official drug-quality standards. The USP writes General Chapters addressing quality-assurance practices and monographs that provide standards for drug quality, purity, identity, and strength for drug ingredients and for verified recipes for compounded formulations.[4,5] USP General Chapters numbered under 1000 are considered enforceable by law when adopted by either federal or state regulatory agencies and are called out in US federal compounding law for humans (US Drug Quality and Security Act [DQSA] of 2013).[6] The USP publishes of its official compounding standards in the *USP Compounding Compendium,* available for download from the USP Web site for a fee.[5] The *USP Compounding Compendium* is a comprehensive compounding resource essential for any health care practitioner who prescribes or prepares compounds. In addition to general practice standards for compounding, USP also publishes default standard discard times, or beyond-use-dates (BUDs), for preparing compounds in the absence of any long-term stability or sterility data. For example, in the absence of stability studies, the BUD for nonsterile, water-containing oral liquids is 14 days stored in a refrigerator.[5] The BUD for nonaqueous formulations (eg, oil suspensions and gelatin capsules) is "not later than the time remaining until the earliest expiration date of any API or six months, whichever is earlier."[5] USP standards are statutorily recognized in various provisions of the US Federal, Food, Drug, and Cosmetic Act and in laws, regulations, and policies promulgated by states. These standards are enforced by the FDA, states, and other oversight organizations. Almost all states have laws, regulations, or policies specific to compounding. In addition to recognition in US law, USP standards are also recognized and enforced globally in more than 140 countries.

Drug Compounding Laws and Regulations

Regulatory oversight for compounded veterinary therapies varies widely from country to country. The Parsemus Foundation, a small private foundation interested in compounded contraceptive therapies, recently surveyed the veterinary drug regulatory landscape of various countries. In their report surveying legal use for a compounded injectable chemical neutering agent for male dogs,[7] Parsemus characterized countries as those "with a strong veterinary regulatory culture" (European Union, Canada, China, South Africa, Australia, and Japan), those "without a strong veterinary regulatory culture" (Nigeria, Trinidad and Tobago, Bangladesh, Fiji, Ghana, Iraq, Kenya, Nepal, Tanzania, and Sierra Leone), and those "with a special situation" regarding veterinary regulatory culture (Mexico, Bolivia, Panama, Colombia, and the United States). Parsemus stated that the United States generally falls into the "with a strong veterinary regulatory culture" but that "great ambiguity exists around compounding in the U.S., with nearly all small animal veterinarians ordering drugs compounded from bulk substances in situations that are technically contrary to FDA regulations." Although the Parsemus survey was not validated or analyzed for statistical significance, its conclusions seem representative of opinions widely held by relevant stakeholders for veterinary compounding in the United States.

Although veterinarians may legally prepare compounds for animal patients, compounding practice is primarily performed by pharmacists. In most countries, pharmacy practice is regulated by provincial or national boards of pharmacy, and compounding activities are tightly regulated. In the United States, pharmacies are solely regulated by state boards of pharmacy, and, unless pharmacies are engaging in behavior that more closely resembles manufacturing, the FDA has little jurisdiction over compounding pharmacies. Consequently, surveillance and compliance for veterinary compounding varies widely from state to state, and because pharmacies may register with multiple state boards of pharmacy and engage in interstate commerce of veterinary compounds, regulatory action has historically been extremely difficult to accomplish. The magnitude of veterinary compounding in the United States and the lack of regulatory consistency confirm the Parsemus assessment that much ambiguity exists and that veterinarians are able to order and dispense compounds that are technically at odds with FDA regulations. Compounding pharmacies may easily prepare quantities of compounds for sale to veterinary practices in which boards of pharmacy do not have jurisdiction. Veterinarians subsequently dispense these compounds as if they were approved products, and the extent of this activity drops, for the most part, beneath the regulatory radar. To further complicate matters, sweeping reform and enforcement of compounding through the DQSA dramatically increased the regulatory oversight of compounding for humans but was written to specifically exclude regulation of compounding for animals.[6] The resultant regulatory void for veterinary compounding has further contributed to great ambiguity in surveillance and determination of compliance in the United States.

AMDUCA codified the extralabel use of drugs, including compounds, in animal patients. AMDUCA mandated that drug compounding must be done within the context of a valid veterinarian/patient/pharmacist relationship and that drug compounding must be initiated by a valid veterinarian prescription drug order.[1] AMDUCA also mandated that starting ingredients for veterinary compounds must be from FDA-approved products (for humans or animals) only and that nothing in the regulation "shall be construed as permitting compounding from bulk drugs." No other countries seem to have mandated a prohibition on the use of bulk drug substances for compounding. From 1996 to 2015, the FDA practiced regulatory discretion toward compounding with bulk drug substances through internal compliance policy guide (CPG) 608.400.[8] In an attempt to harmonize enforcement with the DQSA, however, the FDA rescinded CPG 608.400 in May 2015 and proposed a new draft Guidance for Industry (GFI) #230 for public comment regarding use of bulk drug substances for animal compounding.[9] On November 7, 2017, the FDA announced withdrawal of GFI #230 after reviewing the comments submitted to the docket. The FDA stated in this announcement that it intends to issue new draft guidance for the compounding of animal drugs from bulk substances in 2018. Until the FDA reveals its regulatory intention in a finalized GFI, it is important to realize after comparison of the CPG and the GFI that the FDA's primary concerns regarding compounding with bulk drug substances are copies of FDA-approved drugs (mimic drugs), resale of office stock compounds, and use of bulk drug substances to compound for food-producing animals.

The FDA has inspected some compounding pharmacies on a for-cause basis and has consequently issued warning letters to pharmacies found to be not in compliance. Unfortunately, a September 2015 audit by the US General Accountability Office[10] found that the FDA had not consistently documented the basis for citing these veterinary compounding infractions and the warning letters had little effect on improving the quality of compounds provided for veterinary patients.

Another unfortunate regulatory void in the United States is the FDA's lack of statutory authority to mandate drug recalls, including recalls for compounds found of unacceptable quality during inspections. Consequently, when the FDA discovers compounds that may potentially cause harm, suffering, or death to animal patients, they must rely on the willingness of the compounding pharmacy to issue a voluntary recall. Regulatory oversight is less for compounded medications than that required for FDA-approved drugs.[11] FDA-approved drugs are manufactured and tested in accordance with good manufacturing practice regulations, which are federal statutes. Compounded drugs are exempt from these regulations.[11]

EXTRALABEL DRUG USE AND DRUG COMPOUNDING LAWS AND REGULATIONS FOR SPECIAL CIRCUMSTANCES
Extralabel Drug Use and Drug Compounding in Food Animal Species

The FDA has clear rules for ELDU and drug compounding for food-producing animal species, regardless of their intended use. For example, chickens, turkeys, and pigs are considered major food-producing animal species even if an owner keeps the animals strictly as pets and does not intend to eat, sell, or give away their meat or eggs. Certain drugs are prohibited from ELDU in any food animal species, such as fluoroquinolones (eg, enrofloxacin) and nitroimidazoles (eg, metronidazole). Extralabel use of cephalosporins is prohibited in major-use food animal species, such as chickens and turkeys.

The Food Animal Residue Avoidance Databank (FARAD) is a risk-management program supported by the US Department of Agriculture to facilitate scientifically derived withdrawal times to prevent violative drug residues in animal tissues used for human consumption. FARAD is an excellent online resource for veterinarians to help determine withdrawal periods after drug use in food-producing animal species. In addition to providing instant access to established drug withdrawal times for certain drugs, FARAD also provides lists of prohibited and restricted drugs in food animal species and information regarding the Veterinary Feed Directive, a regulation governed by the FDA that requires supervision by a licensed veterinarian for the labeled use of Veterinary Feed Directive antimicrobial drugs in medicated feed and drinking water for food animal species. Veterinarians from the United States can submit individual requests for case-specific drug withdrawal times for meat, milk, eggs, and honey on the FARAD Web site.[12]

Compounding of Controlled Substances

Although compounding of controlled substances is generally permitted under federal compounding law, there are additional federal requirements that must be followed. In addition to FDA regulations, prescriptions must comply with US Drug Enforcement Administration (DEA) rules and regulations and comply with all pertinent state-controlled substances laws. Pharmacies compounding controlled substances must register with the DEA as a controlled substance manufacturer. Pharmacies compounding controlled substances for patients must dispense the product directly to the client and may not send them to a veterinary practice for dispensing. If the compounded medication enters a practice or is prepared in a practice, it must be logged into an appropriate controlled substance inventory and dispositioned from receipt to administration in accordance with DEA law for noncompounded controlled substances.

Compounded Medications Prepared for Office Use in the Veterinary Practice

Although the DQSA strictly limits the pharmacy preparation of compounds for use by physicians in the office, DQSA does not apply to compounding for animal patients. As a result, state pharmacy practice laws vary with regard to the preparation of compounded drugs for use in a veterinarian's office. For example, some states (eg, Florida) allow preparation of compounds for administration and dispensing by veterinarians in their practices with no restrictions, treated just as if they were FDA-approved products; some states (eg, New York) prohibit preparation of compounds for office use by veterinarians entirely, and all compounded preparations must be prepared for an individual patient at the time of compounding. Practitioners should be familiar with pertinent state laws and regulations. A helpful state summary report for compounding rules is available through the American Veterinary Medical Association.[13]

RISKS AND ADVERSE EVENTS ASSOCIATED WITH EXTRALABEL DRUG USE AND DRUG COMPOUNDING
Risks Associated with Compounded Therapies for Animals

Although the benefits of compounded therapies for animals are well established,[14,15] the risks of serious harm and therapeutic failure from compounded preparations are significant and also well established. The deaths of 64 humans (at time of writing mortality is 77 deaths) from contaminated sterile compounds in the United States in 2012[16] caused sweeping regulatory oversight for compounds prepared for humans[6]; however, little regulatory attention has been paid to minimize risks posed by compounds to animal patients. Headlines of animal deaths resulting from compounds have become more common in the world media. The deaths of 21 polo ponies in Florida from a 10-fold overdose of a selenium compound,[17] the deaths of 4 horses and permanent injury to 6 others in Florida and Kentucky from superpotent concentrations of compounded pyrimethamine,[18] and the deaths of 3 horses from a 70-fold superpotent clenbuterol compound[19] gained wide attention and prescriber concern, but little has been accomplished on the US regulatory front to reduce the risk of harm from compounded preparations for animals.

Animal suffering and death from compounded therapies can be attributed to many factors, including preparation errors, contamination, chemical and physical instability, and lack of bioavailability in the target patient. Poor quality due to compounding error has been widely investigated and reported for compounds prepared for animals.[20–23] Although no distinction was made between compounds prepared for humans and animals, the Missouri Board of Pharmacy recently found that as many as one-fifth of randomly selected compounds from Missouri licensed pharmacies did not contain the amount of active ingredient (range 0%–450%) indicated on the prescription label.[24] At time of writing, no legal requirements exist in any country that require testing to demonstrate that compounded preparations meet the strength as indicated on the prescription labeling.

Although extensive studies have been conducted to prove safety, efficacy, and bioavailability for drugs FDA approved for animal use, there are no equivalent assurances for these attributes in compounded preparations. Ample evidence exists, however, proving that many compounded preparations are not bioequivalent to approved products in animal patients and that even when administered by the same route are not bioavailable compared with approved products. Although some may ultimately achieve effective blood levels, drugs administered by the transdermal route are consistently less bioavailable than their oral equivalents.[25–29] Compounds prepared from APIs (eg, itraconazole) have also been proved less (or not at all) bioavailable compared with the approved products when given at the same dose by the same route.[30,31] Other studies have demonstrated a significant increase in oral bioavailability of approved drugs when compounded into different dosage forms. For example, the bioavailability of intact mitotane tablets in beagles was shown to increase 38-fold when crushed and suspended in an oil vehicle,[32] posing a significant risk for life-threatening adrenal damage in dogs switched from tablets to compounded oral suspensions.

Humans may also face risk from compounds prepared for use in animals. Drug depletion profiles from tissues of treated food-producing animals have not been determined for compounds, and humans may be exposed to drug residues when eating these patients or their byproducts (eg, meat, milk, eggs. and honey). Veterinarians often fail to consider the risk of human exposure to compounded medications. Compounded formulations of drugs that were removed from the human market for safety reasons (eg, cisapride, bromides, diethylstilbestrol, and trilostane) can cause serious adverse events in humans if exposed.

Adverse Event Reporting for Veterinary Compounds

The extent of adverse events in animals caused by compounds is unknown. There are no mandatory requirements for reporting adverse drug events in animals; any adverse event reporting is voluntary. The FDA's voluntary adverse event reporting form, the Veterinary Adverse Drug Reaction, Lack of Effectiveness, Product Defect Report (form FDA 1932a) is a complex 5-page report designed for adverse event reporting for manufactured products. The 1932a form also does not include a prompt to determine if the adverse drug event was due to a compounded preparation, and the form is too sophisticated for most pet owners to be able to complete. The FDA's adverse drug event reporting system for animals is also not aggregated or comprehensive and is currently being revised. Since 2001, only 62 compound-related adverse events in animals have been reported to the FDA. The wealth of information regarding reported adverse events from veterinary compounds is likely with state boards of pharmacy.

Various privacy and confidentiality laws in the states, however, prevent boards of pharmacy from sharing this information even if they collect adverse events from compounds in animal patients.

CHEMICAL CONSIDERATIONS FOR DRUGS AND COMPOUNDED FORMULATIONS
Effects of Chemical Composition and Chemical Interactions

Drug stability in compounded preparations can be affected by numerous influencing factors, including the presence of excipients or diluents, drug concentration, and storage conditions.[1] Chemical reactions can be facilitated by changes in humidity, light, pH, presence of oxidizing trace metals, and temperature, among other factors.[1] For example, when fluoroquinolones, such as orbifloxacin, are combined with liquids that contain metal ions, such as Lixotinic (Zoetis, Parsippany, New Jersey), a vitamin and mineral supplement that contains iron at 2.5 mg/mL, in vitro stability is greatly reduced due to chelation of the drug.[15] Simple syrups, such as those commonly used as aqueous compounding agents, tend to be acidic and can alter the pH and affect drug stability.[1] Combining drugs may alter the pH and result in an increased risk of drug interactions. Weak acids and weak bases, when combined, may inactivate each other chemically.[1] Excipients can lead to drug instability by altering the pH or by introducing disintegrating agents.[1]

The salt form of a medication may affect absorption and delivery due to differences in stability, pH, and bioavailability of the active drug. For example, metronidazole benzoate is often preferred for oral use in veterinary medicine because it has much better palatability compared with metronidazole hydrochloride. Metronidazole benzoate, however, contains less active drug on a milligram per milligram basis than metronidazole hydrochloride. The dosage of the benzoate salt should be increased by 1.6 from the hydrochloride salt. If a formulary calls for metronidazole hydrochloride to be dosed at 10 mg/kg, then 16 mg/kg of the benzoate salt should be used.[1]

Doxycycline is often used in an extralabel fashion to treat psittacosis (infection with *Chlamydia psittaci*) in companion birds. Dosages for drinking water are published elsewhere.[33,34] Doxycycline hyclate is highly water soluble (50 mg/mL) but doxycycline monohydrate is only slightly soluble in water.[34] Both doxycycline hyclate and doxycycline monohydrate are available in capsules and tablet. Only doxycycline hyclate should be used for medicating drinking water for the treatment of psittacosis in birds.

In black-footed penguins (*Spheniscus demersus*), a commercially available 10-mg/mL solution of itraconazole (Sporanox, Janssen Pharmaceuticals, Titusville, New Jersey) had significantly greater oral absorption than a 10-mg/mL compounded solution of micronized itraconazole powder in a diethylene glycol monoethyl ether mixture, likely due to the presence of hydroxypropyl-β-cyclodextrin, a carrier molecule previously shown to improve oral absorption, in the commercially available solution.[30] Oral administration of a pimobendan solution compounded from commercially available tablets (Vetmedin, Boehringer Ingelheim, St. Joseph, Missouri) into aqueous solution (Ora-Plus, Perrigo, Dublin, Ireland) resulted in greater plasma concentrations and area under the curve than a pimobendan solution compounded from bulk chemical into aqueous solution (Ora-Plus).[35] This effect may have been associated with the presence of a citric acid excipient in the tablet, which likely affected the pH of the solution and resulted in increased oral absorption.[35] Paroxetine hydrochloride compounded to 2 mg/mL in water was found significantly more bioavailable in gray parrots (*Psittacus erithacus*) compared with a paroxetine oral suspension approved for human use (Seroxat, 2 mg/mL, GlaxoSmithKline, Zeist, the Netherlands).[36]

Drug Stability Over Time

One of the most important elements of compounded preparation performance is assurance that the drug concentration at the time of compounding remains at not less than 90% of the labeled concentration throughout its BUD and that no potentially harmful degradants form. Accurate BUDs are only determined by use of stability-indicating assay tests and cannot be determined by potency-over-time tests. USP defines stability as "the extent to which a preparation retains, within specified limits, and throughout its period of storage and use, the same properties and characteristics that it possessed at the time of compounding."[37] Stability testing involves assay method development, validation, forced degradation of the study compound to determine degradants, and a series of at least triplicate samples over time to determine concentrations of remaining parent drug versus accumulating degradants. Assessing drug concentration over time without a validated method can overestimate remaining parent drug because potency studies do not separate parent (biologically active) drug from degradants in the results.

Some drugs are not suitable for compounding into certain formulation due to rapid inactivation and loss of potency or lack of systemic absorption. An excellent example is a comparison of 2 of the most common antibiotics used in exotic animal medicine. Aqueous formulations of enrofloxacin compounded from commercially available 68-mg tablets and a 22.7-mg/mL injectable solution into a commercial liquid sweetener or into corn or cherry syrup maintained drug stability in amber-colored vials at room temperature for 56 days.[38] The stability of doxycycline hyclate, however, compounded from 100-mg tablets into aqueous solution using syrup and commercial liquid sweetener cannot be assured beyond 7 days.[39] Any compounded preparations that demonstrate significant visible changes over time, such as changes in color, odor, and consistency, or appear contaminated should be discarded.

ACTIVE PHARMACEUTICAL INGREDIENTS

Bulk substances (bulk drugs) are the APIs powders that most compounding pharmacists prefer to use to create finished compounded formulations. Bulk drugs are pure drug substances (usually with a $\pm$ 1.5% of label strength) with known quality and purity documented through Certificates of Analysis. They lack excipients often found in manufactured, drugs such as preservatives, stabilizers, fillers, and buffers. Excipients may detrimentally affect the final compounded drug formulation depending on the vehicle used. Currently, the FDA considers APIs unapproved new drugs and only considers compounding from FDA-approved drugs as legal based on its interpretation of AMDUCA.

WORKING WITH THE COMPOUNDING PHARMACIST AND PHARMACY

Historically, most drug compounding has been performed by veterinarians in private practice. Over the past few decades, however, compounding of animal drugs by pharmacists has dramatically increased.[1] There are currently several nationally advertising pharmacies that exclusively compound medications for veterinary patients.[1] Veterinarians rely on compounding pharmacies for many reasons, including a desire and standard of care to provide safe and effective drug delivery to their patients and a lack of training in drug compounding in the veterinary curriculum.[1] Veterinary practices are often busy and drug compounding takes valuable time and resources to be done properly.

Pharmacists are the only health care professionals that are formally trained in the art and science of drug compounding.[1] Compounding pharmacies have access to essential equipment, supplies, and resources to help prepare high-quality compounded drug formulations that meet USP standards and comply with federal and state laws and regulations. For example, compounding pharmacies must be licensed in not only their resident state but also in any other states to which prescriptions are filled. Compounding pharmacies generally prefer to use APIs over manufactured, FDA-approved medications in their formulations in part to avoid the potentially detrimental effects of excipients, such as fillers and preservatives.

Exotic animal practitioners can benefit greatly from establishing close relationships with local and national compounding pharmacies. Visiting local compounding pharmacies is encouraged. Compounding pharmacists can be an integral part of the veterinary team to best meet the medication needs of individual exotic animal patients. It is the veterinarian's responsibility to ensure that the compounding pharmacy is familiar with veterinary prescriptions, strives to meet the highest professional standards, and complies with all pertinent federal and state regulations. The compounding pharmacy should meet minimum standards and ideally be accredited by a compounding accreditation organization (**Box 1**).

DRUG COMPOUNDING IN THE VETERINARY HOSPITAL

Advantages of preparing compounds within a veterinary practice include being able to immediately dispense a tailored medication for an individual patient for use within a prescribed therapeutic period and maximal use of the BUD assigned to the compound. Waiting times for pharmacies to prepare and ship compounds to pet owners can result in worsening of disease or clinical signs, and delays in implementing compounded therapy can often be avoided by veterinarians performing compounding within their veterinary practice. ELDU and extemporaneous drug compounding for in-hospital use and dispensing for veterinary patients is permitted by federal law under AMDUCA provided that a valid veterinarian-client-patient relationship exists. Practitioners must also comply with state pharmacy and veterinary medicine laws and regulations that may or may not include compliance with USP compounding standards.

Box 1
Minimum and ideal criteria for selecting a compounding pharmacist or pharmacy

Minimum legal requirements

Must possess license or registration to practice pharmacy in all applicable states (including resident state and state of dispensing, if not the same). Check with state board of pharmacy [National Association of Boards of Pharmacy, www.nabp.net] to determine if the pharmacy is licensed and in good standing.

Must be fully compliant with USP Chapters <795> and <797>.

Must be aware of and adhere to criteria for animal compounding as delineated in AMDUCA.

Accreditation and professional memberships

Accreditation by the Pharmacy Compounding Accreditation Board is preferable.

Membership in the International Academy of Compounding Pharmacists and/or American Society of Health-System Pharmacists is ideal.

Drug sources

All APIs must be obtained from FDA-registered and DEA-registered suppliers.

All APIs should be substances of USP or USP-NF grade.

All APIs must be accompanied by a valid certificate of analysis.

The most commonly prepared compounds in the exotic animal practice are preparations of aqueous liquid formulations for oral administration from approved tablets, capsules, or injectable solutions. One example used by 1 of this article's authors (Powers) for preparing 10 mL of enrofloxacin suspension at 20 mg/mL is discussed (**Box 2**). Minimum supplies for extemporaneous drug compounding include mortars and pestles; volumetric liquid measuring devices, such as graduated cylinders; aqueous suspending vehicles (eg, Ora-Plus and Ora-Sweet and Syrpalta syrup vehicle [Humco, Austin, Texas]); and liquid dispensing bottles. Flavoring agents (eg, LorAnn Oils [Lansing, Michigan]; FLAVORx [Columbia, Maryland]), rubber spatulas, and a digital gram scale or milligram precision balance can also be useful. In the event that commercially formulated compounding liquids are unavailable or are unsuitable (eg, may contain toxic preservatives or flavors), thickening and sweetening agents, such as corn syrup, cherry syrup, and lactulose, can also be used for many compounded formulations. Commercially available kits with supplies and recipes for flavoring and compounding drugs are available from many vendors (eg, FLAVORx Veterinary Flavoring System [Columbia, Maryland]; Medisca [Plattsburgh, New York]) (**Table 1**). Some of these kits have BUDs supported by stability-indicating assays; however, many do not and should be used within conservatively assigned USP default BUDs. Supporting evidence for any vendor-assigned BUD should always be available on request. Veterinary personnel preparing compounds from these kits or any starting ingredients should use appropriate garbing and personal protective equipment to avoid exposure to manipulated drugs.

Compounding Formulas and Component Selection

Although many verified and peer-reviewed compounding formulas are available for compounded dosage forms intended for human use,[3] these formulas may or may not be appropriate for use in nonhuman species. The USP has developed dozens of verified compounded preparation formulas specifically for veterinary use. USP nomenclature identifies these formulas in its compendia by the following format: drug generic name, compounded, dosage form, and veterinary (eg, enrofloxacin, compounded, oral suspension, and veterinary). USP veterinary compounded preparation monographs have been stability tested to the BUDs or discard dates published in their corresponding

---

Box 2
Instructions for preparing a 10-mL enrofloxacin suspension at a calculated concentration of 20 mg/mL.[a]

Instructions
   Crush three 68-mg coated enrofloxacin tablets in a mortar with a pestle.
   Add 4.0 mL of Ora-Plus oral suspending vehicle.
   Mix thoroughly.
   Allow to sit for 3 minutes to 5 minutes.
   Mix thoroughly again until the suspension is a homogenous purple color.
   Add 4.0 mL of Ora-Sweet oral suspending vehicle.
   Mix thoroughly again.
   Makes a measured 10 mL-volume of enrofloxacin suspension; the calculated drug concentration is 20 mg/mL (68 mg $\times$ 3 = 204 mg; 204 mg/10 mL = 20.4 mg/mL).

Ingredients
   Baytril Purple Tabs (enrofloxacin), 68.0 mg (Bayer Healthcare, Animal Health, Shawnee, Kansas).
   Ora-Plus (Perrigo, Dublin, Ireland) aqueous oral suspending vehicle.
   Ora-Sweet (Perrigo, Dublin, Ireland) flavored syrup vehicle.

[a]A beyond-use date (BUD) of 14 days refrigerated should be used for this preparation.

Table 1
Some supplies useful for in-hospital extemporaneous drug compounding

Item	Example Source(s)
Mortar(s) and pestle(s) of various sizes, preferably ceramic or glass	
Aqueous compounding vehicles	Ora-Plus, Ora-Sweet, Ora-Blend (Perrigo, Dublin, Ireland) Oral Blend, Oral Syrup, Oral Mix (Medisca, Plattsburgh, NY) Syrpalta Syrup Vehicle (Humco, Austin, TX)
Graduated cylinder(s) or other volumetric liquid measuring devices	
Liquid-dispensing bottles	8-dram (30-mL) threaded vials with child-resistant caps and 28-mm bottle inserts (other sizes also available) (Pharmacy-Lite Packaging, Elyria, OH) ORAPAC 1-oz dispensing kit (1-oz PET (polyethylene terephthalate) Boston round bottle, 1-mL oral dispenser, and open orifice bottle adapter); 2-oz kit also available (Viapac Enterprises, Cedar Park, TX)
Flavoring agents	LorAnn Oils (Lansing, MI) FLAVORx (Columbia, MD)
Rubber spatulas	
Digital gram scale and/or precision balance	Precision balances with 0.01-g, 0.1-g, 0.5-g, and 1-g graduations, 120-g to 10-kg capacity (Mars Scales, North York, Ontario, Canada) Medisca (Plattsburgh, NY)
Compounding and flavoring supply companies	FLAVORx Veterinary Flavoring System (FLAVORx, Columbia, MD) Medisca (Plattsburgh, NY)

monographs and contain specific instructions for how to prepare, package, test, store, and label each compound. Many of the approximately 200 USP compounded preparations that are not specified for veterinary use may also be used in animal patients if species-specific toxicity and pharmacodynamics concerns are considered.

When a USP formula monograph is not available, drug manufacturers may sometimes provide extemporaneous compounding information for their products; however, this information is rarely available, and manufacturers often are not willing to share this information due to concerns about liability. Other compounding formula evidence can be located by searching secondary source collections of published peer-reviewed compounded preparation stability studies,[3] again with the caveat that species-specific considerations should be applied to each component used in a published compounded preparation formula. If peer-reviewed evidence cannot be located in secondary resources, a search of primary peer-reviewed literature may reveal a stability-tested formula that is suitable for use in animal patients. The *International Journal of Pharmaceutical Compounding* is a bimonthly scientific and professional journal that frequently features stability-tested formulas for veterinary compounds. When no evidence is available to support stability and ingredient compatibility for a compounded preparation, USP or other compendial compounding defaults should be applied after careful consideration of the inherent stability of the active drug, suitability of components for the target patient/species, and concerns for adverse effects if the compound is not stable throughout the labeled BUD and intended therapy period (see **Fig. 1**). Other resources for compounding formulas include compounding excipient suppliers.[40,41] For example, Perrigo provides formulas for use with Ora-Plus, such as enalapril maleate, 1-mg/mL oral suspension.[40] Other stability studies for drugs commonly used in exotic animal practice have been published, including meloxicam and carprofen,[42] voriconazole,[43] and enalapril, among others (**Table 2**).[44]

IN-HOUSE COMPOUNDED DRUG PRESCRIPTION LABELING

Prescription labels should feature only the most important patient information needed for safe and effective understanding and use (**Fig. 2**). Labels must comply

Table 2
Beyond-use dates for common medications used in exotic animal medicine compounded into water-containing (aqueous) solution.[a]

Drug	Formula	Beyond-Use Date	Reference
Allopurinol	20 mg/mL in OP:OS 1:1	60 d at 5°C and 25°C	51
Amlodipine	1 mg/mL in OP:OS 1:1	90 d at 4°C	52
Amphotericin B	100 mg/mL in methylcellulose, glycerin and cherry flavor	93 d at 25°C	53
Carprofen	5 mg/mL in OP:OS 1:1	21 d at 4°C	42
Celecoxib	10 mg/mL in OP:OS 1:1	93 d at 5°C and 23°C	54
Ciprofloxacin	50 mg/mL in OP:OS 1:1	56 d at 5°C and 25°C	55
Cisapride	1 mg/mL in OP:OS 1:1	60 d at 5°C and 25°C	44
Doxycycline hyclate	33.3 mg/mL and 166.7 mg/mL in OP:OS 1:1	7 d at 2° to 8°C and 22° to 26°C	39
Enalapril	1 mg/mL in OP:OS 1:1	60 d at 5°C and 25°C	44
Enrofloxacin	22.95 mg/mL in water and corn syrup or cherry syrup (from tablets)	56 d at 22°C	38
	11.35 mg/mL in Ora-Sweet (from 22.7-mg/mL injectable solution)	56 d at 22°C	38
Famotidine	8 mg/mL in OP:OS 1:1	95 d at 25°C	56
Gabapentin	100 mg/mL in OP:OS 1:1	91 d at 5°C 56 d at 25°C	57
Ketoconazole	20 mg/mL in OP:OS 1:1	60 d at 5°C and 25°C	58
Levothyroxine	25 mg/mL in deionized water	8 d at 4°C	59
Meloxicam	0.50 mg/mL in methylcellulose 1% gel	28 d at 4°C and at 22°C	42
Metronidazole benzoate	50 mg/mL in OP:OS 1:1	60 d at 5°C and 25°C	58
Phenobarbital	10 mg/mL in OP:OS 1:1	115 d at 25°C	60
Piroxicam	2 mg/mL in potassium sorbate, citric acid and methylcellulose vehicle	6 d at 4°C	4
Terbinafine	25 mg/mL in OP:OS 1:1	42 d at 5°C and 25°C	4
Tramadol	5 mg/mL in OP:OS 1:1	90 d at 5°C and 25°C	61
Ursodiol	50 mg/mL in simple syrup	35 d at 4°C	62
Voriconazole	40 mg/mL in OP:OS 1:1	30 d at 5°C and 21°C	43

[a] A temperature of 2C to 8C is generally considered controlled cold temperature (ie, refrigeration), and room temperature is generally considered 21C to 26C. Most formulations in this table were prepared using commercially available tablets or capsules in a cellulose and carboxymethylcellulose oral suspending vehicle (Ora-Plus [OP]) and a flavored sucrose syrup vehicle (Ora-Sweet [OS]) in a 1:1 mixture (OP:OS 1:1).

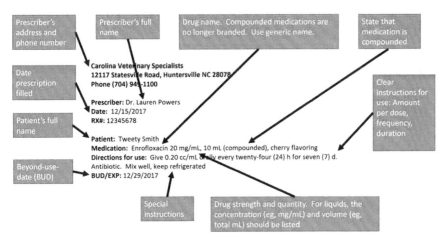

Fig. 2. Example prescription label for an extemporaneously compounded medication.

with USP Chapter <17> (Prescription Container Labeling) guidelines and applicable federal and state pharmacy and veterinary medicine laws and regulations. In addition to basic information regarding the veterinary practice and patient, a few additional items should be included on the label, such as the fact that the preparation was compounded (**Table 3**). Manufactured drugs are given expiration dates. Compounded drugs are assigned BUDs. In the absence of published stability studies to support BUDs, default BUDs are provided in the USP-National Formulary (NF) General Chapters for Compounding (USP-NF <795>) (see **Fig. 1**).[4] As discussed previously, in the absence of stability studies, the USP BUD for nonsterile, water-containing oral liquids is 14 days when refrigerated. Finally, veterinarians should assign a unique identifying number to each compound prepared (ie, lot number) and should keep detailed compounding records of how, when, and by whom the compound was prepared so that the compound may be recalled in the event of a problem with the compound or any of the ingredients.

NOVEL DRUG DELIVERY METHODS FOR EXOTIC ANIMALS

Novel drug delivery systems are particularly attractive for exotic animal patients because they are generally noninvasive or are long acting to minimize forced administration of medications. Prior to use, a compounded novel drug delivery system should be demonstrated to be of sufficient quality and to be safe and effective. This information is often not available, however, for novel compounded dosage forms.[1] Transdermal gels are popular in companion canine and feline practice and allow delivery of small amounts of drugs directly into the capillary blood system via topical application.[1] Evidence for efficacy of transdermal gels is largely lacking in companion animal therapy, and disposition and efficacy have not been evaluated at all for transdermal gels in exotic animal patients. Compounded novel dosage forms that have been used in exotic patients include medicated treats, antibiotic-impregnated polymethylmethacrylate[45] or calcium sulfate hemihydrate (plaster of Paris)[46–48] beads, and drug-impregnated poloxamer gels,[49,50] although use is based primarily on clinical impression, and evidence is lacking to support efficacy of these dosage forms.

Table 3
Minimum requirements for prescription labels for compounded drug preparations

Label Item	Comments
Pharmacy name, address, and phone number	If using a compounding pharmacy
Prescriber name, address, and phone number	If compounded in veterinary practice
Patient's full name	Name or identification of animal and client or owner's last name
Fill date	Date the medication was dispensed
Drug name	Compounded medications are not branded products and, therefore, only the generic name should be listed (eg, enrofloxacin instead of Baytril)
Drug strength and quantity	For compounded liquid formulations, the concentration (eg, milligrams/milliliters) and volume (eg, total milliliters in bottle) should be listed
Quantity dispensed	Total number of milliliters, tablets, capsules, or other dosage units dispensed
Statement that the formulation is compounded	Often placed at the end of the drug description
Explicit clear instructions on use	Volume per dose, frequency, route, and duration of treatment
Special instructions (if any)	For example: keep refrigerated, do not shake, wear gloves
BUD	Manufactured drugs are given expiration dates, compounded formulations are given BUDs
Identifying lot number	Every compound should be assigned a unique identifying number to enable recall in the event that a problem is discovered with the compound or any ingredients.

SUMMARY

Compounding is a critical component of providing veterinary medical therapy. The global animal pharmaceutical industry and approval agencies have provided few approved products for exotic animal species and cannot be expected to keep up with demand for new medical therapies. Consequently, compounding will continue to bridge therapeutic gaps in exotic animal medicine. Because compounds for companion animals are most commonly prepared by pharmacists, state and provincial boards of pharmacy have the primary responsibility for regulating this practice but little ability to do so because most of these compounds end up in veterinary practices as office stock. Until such surveillance is in place, exotic animal veterinarians must self-educate to become aware of relevant compounding laws and regulations and acquire the skills and equipment necessary to perform simple, nonsterile compounding in the veterinary practice.

ACKNOWLEDGMENTS

The authors are grateful to Marike Visser, DVM, for providing the decision tree diagram in **Fig. 1**.

REFERENCES

1. Boothe DM. Veterinary compounding in small animals: a clinical pharmacologist's perspective. Vet Clin North Am Small Anim Pract 2006;36(5):1129–73.

2. Washabau R, Holt D. Pathogenesis, diagnosis, and therapy of feline idiopathic megacolon. Vet Clin North Am Small Anim Pract 1999;29(2):589–603.
3. Wangen K. Therapeutic review: cisapride. J Exot Pet Med 2013;22(3):301–4.
4. Trissel LA. Trissel's stability of compounded formulations. 5th edition. Washington, DC: Amer Pharm Assoc; 2012.
5. USP Compounding Compendium. Rockville (MD): United States Pharmacopeial Convention; 2017.
6. Drug Quality and Security Act, US Public Law 113-54; U.S. Government Printing Office: Washington, DC, 2013.
7. Regulatory status of compounded treatments, by country. The Parsemus Foundation; 2016. Available at: https://www.parsemusfoundation.org/wp-content/uploads/2015/03/CaCl2_Regulatory_Status_Opinion_10-14-2016.pdf. Accessed November 1, 2017.
8. Manual of compliance policy guides. U.S. Food and Drug Administration. Available at: http://www.fda.gov/ICECI/ComplianceManuals/CompliancePolicyGuidanceManual/. Accessed November 1, 2017.
9. Guidance for industry: compounding animal drugs from bulk drug substances. Center for Veterinary Medicine, U.S. Food and Drug Administration; 2015. Available at: https://www.fda.gov/downloads/AnimalVeterinary/GuidanceComplianceEnforcement/GuidanceforIndustry/UCM446862.pdf. Accessed November 1, 2017.
10. Drug compounding for animals. Report to congressional committees. U.S. Government Accountability Office; 2015. Available at: http://www.gao.gov/assets/680/672748.pdf. Accessed November 1, 2017.
11. Gudeman J, Jozwiakowski M, Chollet J, et al. Potential risks of pharmacy compounding. Drugs R D 2013;13(1):1–8.
12. Food Animal Residue Avoidance Databank (FARAD) online request system. Available at: http://cafarad.ucdavis.edu/farmweb/index.aspx. Accessed October 29, 2017.
13. Administration and dispensing of compounded veterinary drugs. State summary report. Amer Vet Med Assoc; 2017. Available at: https://www.avma.org/Advocacy/StateAndLocal/Pages/compoundinglaws.aspx. Accessed October 29, 2017.
14. Frank H. Compounding in the exotic practice. J Exot Pet Med 2006;15(2):116–21.
15. Papich MG. Drug compounding for veterinary patients. AAPS J 2005;7:E281–7.
16. Centers for Disease Control and Prevention (CDC). Multistate outbreak of fungal infection associated with injection of methylprednisolone acetate solution from a single compounding pharmacy-United States, 2012. MMWR Morb Mortal Wkly Rep 2012;61:839–42.
17. Belainesh D, Maldonado G, Reid H. Acute selenium toxicosis in polo ponies. J Vet Diagn Invest 2011;23(3):623–8.
18. Four horses die after receiving compounded EPM drug. Vet Pract News 2014. Available at: http://www.veterinarypracticenews.com/May-2014/4-Horses-Die-After-Receiving-Compounded-EPM-Drug/. Accessed November 1, 2017.
19. Thompson JA, Mirza MH, Barker SA, et al. Clenbuterol toxicosis in three quarter horse racehorses after administration of a compounded product. J Am Vet Med Assoc 2011;239(6):842–9.
20. Cook AK, Nieuwoudt CD, Longhofer SL. Pharmaceutical evaluation of compounded trilostane products. J Am Anim Hosp Assoc 2012;48(4):228–33.

21. Scott-Moncrief JC, Moore GE, Coe J, et al. Characteristics of commercially manufactured and compounded protamine zinc insulin. J Am Vet Med Assoc 2012; 240(5):600–5.

22. Stanley SD, Thomas SM, Skinner W. Comparison for pharmaceutical equivalence of FDA-approved products and compounded preparations of ketoprofen, amikacin, and boldenone. In: Proceedings of the 49th Annual Convention of the American Association of Equine Practitioners, New Orleans, LA, November 21–25, 2003.

23. Umstead ME, Boothe DM, Cruz-Espindola C, et al. Accuracy and precision of compounded ciclosporin capsules and solution. Vet Dermatol 2012;23(5):431.

24. Board of Pharmacy, Missouri Division of Professional Regulation. Annual Reports from 2003–2016. Available at: http://pr.mo.gov/pharmacists-annual-reports.asp. Accessed November 1, 2017.

25. Bennett N, Papich MG, Hoenig M, et al. Evaluation of transdermal application of glipizide in a pluronic lecithin gel to healthy cats. Am J Vet Res 2005;66(4):581–8.

26. Ciribassi J, Luescher A, Pasloske KS, et al. Comparative bioavailability of fluoxetine after transdermal and oral administration to healthy cats. Am J Vet Res 2003;64(8):994–8.

27. Krotscheck U, Boothe DM, Boothe H. Evaluation of transdermal morphine and fentanyl pluronic lecithin organogel administration in dogs. Vet Ther 2004;5(3): 202–11.

28. MacGregor JM, Rush JE, Rozanski EA, et al. Comparison of pharmacodynamic variables following oral versus transdermal administration of atenolol to healthy cats. Am J Vet Res 2008;69(1):39–44.

29. Mealey KL, Peck KE, Bennett BS, et al. Systemic absorption of amitriptyline and buspirone after oral and transdermal administration to healthy cats. J Vet Intern Med 2004;18(1):43–6.

30. Smith JA, Papich MG, Russell G, et al. Effects of compounding on pharmacokinetics of itraconazole in black-footed penguins (Spheniscus demersus). J Zoo Wildl Med 2010;41(3):487–95.

31. Mawby DI, Whittemore JC, Genger S, et al. Bioequivalence of orally administered generic, compounded, and innovator-formulated itraconazole in healthy dogs. J Vet Intern Med 2014;28(1):72–7.

32. Watson ADJ, Rijnberk A, Moolenaar AJ. Systemic availability of o,p'-DDD in normal dogs, fasted and fed, and in dogs with hyperadrenocorticism. Res Vet Sci 1987;43(2):160–5.

33. Carpenter J. Exotic animal formulary. 4th edition. St Louis (MO): Elsevier Saunders; 2013.

34. Plumb PC. Plumb's veterinary drug handbook. 8th edition. Ames (IA): Wiley-Blackwell; 2015.

35. Guzman DS, Beaufrère H, KuKanich B, et al. Pharmacokinetics of single oral dose of pimobendan in Hispaniolan Amazon parrots (Amazona ventralis). J Avian Med Surg 2014;28(2):95–101.

36. van Zeeland YRA, Schoemaker NJ, Haritova A, et al. Pharmacokinetics of paroxetine, a selective serotonin reuptake inhibitor, in grey parrots (Psittacus erithacus erithacus): Influence of pharmaceutical formulation and length of dosing. J Vet Pharmacol Ther 2013;36(1):51–8.

37. United States Pharmacopeial Convention, Inc. United States Pharmacopeia 27-National Formulary 25. Rockville (MD): US Pharmacopeial Convention, Inc; 2007. p. 334, 511. 2nd Suppl.

38. Petritz OA, Guzman DS, Wiebe VJ, et al. Stability of three commonly compounded extemporaneous enrofloxacin suspensions for oral administration to exotic animals. J Am Vet Med Assoc 2013;243(1):85–90.
39. Papich MG, Davidson GS, Fortier LA. Doxycycline concentration over time after storage in a compounded veterinary preparation. J Am Vet Med Assoc 2013; 242(12):1674–8.
40. Ora-Plus Oral Suspending Vehicle [Package insert]. Dublin, Ireland: Perrigo; 2010. Available at: https://www.perrigo.com/files/rx/pdfs/pds173-Ora-Plus%20Sell%20Sheet.pdf. Accessed October 25, 2017.
41. Beyond-use date databank for oral bases. Medisca Network. Available at: https://www.medisca.com/NDC_SPECS/MUS/2511/Downloads/BUD%20Databank%20-%20Oral%20Bases%20-%20MUS%20AUG2016.pdf. Accessed November 1, 2017.
42. Hawkins MG, Karriker MJ, Wiebe V, et al. Drug distribution and stability in extemporaneous preparations of meloxicam and carprofen after dilution and suspension at two storage temperatures. J Am Vet Med Assoc 2006;229(6):968–74.
43. Nguyen KQ, Hawkins MG, Taylor IT, et al. Stability and uniformity of extemporaneous preparations of voriconazole in two liquid suspension vehicles at two storage temperatures. Am J Vet Res 2009;70(7):908–14.
44. Allen LV, Erickson MA. Stability of alprazolam, chloroquine phosphate, cisapride, enalapril maleate, and hydralazine hydrochloride in extemporaneously compounded oral liquids. Am J Health Syst Pharm 1998;55(18):1915–20.
45. Seligson D, Mehta S, Voos K, et al. The use of antibiotic-impregnated polymethylmethacrylate beads to prevent the evolution of localized infection. J Orthop Trauma 1992;6(4):401–6.
46. Phillips H, Boothe DM, Bennett RA. Elution of clindamycin and enrofloxacin from calcium sulfate hemihydrate beads in vitro. Vet Surg 2015;44(8):1003–11.
47. Udomkusonsri P, Kaewmokul S, Arthitvong S, et al. Use of enrofloxacin in calcium beads for local infection therapy in animals. Kasetsart J (Nat Sci) 2010;44(5): 1115–20.
48. Santschi EM, McGarvey L. In vitro elution of gentamicin from plaster of Paris beads. Vet Surg 2003;32(2):128–33.
49. Laniesse D, Guzman DS, Knych HK, et al. Pharmacokinetics of butorphanol tartrate in a long-acting poloxamer 407 gel formulation administered to Hispaniolan Amazon parrots (Amazona ventralis). Am J Vet Res 2017;78(6):688–94.
50. Laniesse D, Smith DA, Knych HK, et al. In vitro characterization of a formulation of butorphanol tartrate in a poloxamer 407 base intended for use as a parenterally administered slow-release analgesic agent. Am J Vet Res 2017;78(6):677–87.
51. Allen LV, Erickson MA. Stability of acetazolamide, allopurinol, azathioprine, clonazepam, and flucytosine in extemporaneously compounded oral liquids. Am J Health Syst Pharm 1996;53(16):1944–9.
52. Nahata MC, Morosco RS, Hipple TF. Stability of amlodipine besylate in two liquid dosage forms. J Am Pharm Assoc 1999;39(3):375–7.
53. Dentinger PJ, Swenson CF, Anaizi NH. Stability of amphotericin B in an extemporaneously compounded oral suspension. Am J Health Syst Pharm 2001;58(11): 1021–4.
54. Donnelly RF. Stability of celecoxib oral suspension. Can J Hosp Pharm 2009; 62(6):464–8.
55. Johnson CE, Wong DV, Hoppe HL, et al. Stability of ciprofloxacin in extemporaneous oral liquid dosage form. Int J Pharm Compd 1998;4:314–7.

56. Dentinger PJ, Swenson CF, Anaizi NH. Stability of famotidine in an extemporaneously compounded oral liquid. Am J Health Syst Pharm 2000;57(14):1340–2.
57. Nahata MC. Development of two stable oral suspensions for gabapentin. Pediatr Neurol 1999;20(3):195–7.
58. Allen LV, Erickson MA. Stability of ketoconazole, metolazone, metronidazole, procainamide hydrochloride, and spironolactone in extemporaneously compounded oral liquids. Am J Health Syst Pharm 1996;53(17):2073–8.
59. Boulton DW, Fawcett JP, Woods DJ. Stability of an extemporaneously compounded levothyroxine sodium oral liquid. Am J Health Syst Pharm 1996; 53(10):1157–61.
60. Cober MP, Johnson CE. Stability of an extemporaneously prepared alcohol-free phenobarbital suspension. Am J Health Syst Pharm 2007;64(6):644–6.
61. Wagner DS, Johnson CE, Cichon-Hensley BK, et al. Stability of oral liquid preparations of tramadol in strawberry syrup and a sugar-free vehicle. Am J Health Syst Pharm 2003;60(12):1268–70.
62. Johnson CE, Nesbitt J. Stability of ursodiol in an extemporaneously compounded oral liquid. Am J Health Syst Pharm 1995;52(16):1798–800.

Overview of Drug Delivery Methods in Exotics, Including Their Anatomic and Physiologic Considerations

Thomas Coutant, Dr med vet, IPSAV (Zoological Medicine),
Claire Vergneau-Grosset, Dr med vet, IPSAV (Zoological Medicine),
CES (Avian Pathol), DACZM, Isabelle Langlois, DMV, DABVP-Avian*

KEYWORDS

- Anatomic differences • Drug delivery • Injectable route • Oral route • Transmucosal
- Topical • Transcutaneous • Nebulization

KEY POINTS

- Drug delivery to exotic animals can usually be extrapolated from small animal medicine.
- Specific techniques may be required owing to physiologic and anatomic differences.
- Drug administration techniques for each species should be chosen accordingly to avoid iatrogenic complications.

INTRODUCTION

To a certain extent, drug delivery to exotic animals follows similar guidelines as those for other domestic animals. However, difference in species' physiology and anatomy may hinder extrapolation and complicate straightforward treatment administration. Knowing these differences is warranted to deliver treatment through the most appropriate routes while ensuring the technique is executed properly. The aim of this review is to provide practitioners with a guide for drug delivery methods and to summarize exotic animal peculiarities that are relevant for drug administration. This article reviews drug delivery methods using injectable routes, the digestive and the respiratory systems, as well as topical, cutaneous, and mucosal dispensing methods. Whenever possible, clinicians should consider operant conditioning for nonstressful administration of drugs (see Brian L Speer and colleagues' article, "Low Stress Medication Techniques in Birds and Small Mammals," in this issue).

The authors have nothing to disclose.
Zoological Medicine Service, Department of Clinical Sciences, CHUV (Centre Hospitalier Universitaire), Faculté de Médecine Vétérinaire, Université de Montréal, 3200 rue Sicotte, Saint-Hyacinthe, Québec J2S2M2, Canada
* Corresponding author.
E-mail address: isabelle.langlois@umontreal.ca

DRUG ADMINISTRATION VIA INJECTABLE ROUTES
Intramuscular, Subcutaneous, Intraperitoneal, and Intracoelomic Drug Administration

Although the general principles of nonvascular parenteral drug administration are very similar between domestic animals and exotic species, some specificities remain, owing to differences in the anatomy and physiology of some species. Parenteral injection sites excluding intravascular injections, are summarized in **Table 1** and illustrated in **Figs. 1** and **2**. As a general rule, for most parenteral injection of hydrosoluble solutions, needle diameter should not exceed a 25-G diameter in the most commonly seen species.[1,2]

Subcutaneous route

In small mammals, the loose skin can easily accommodate large volume of fluid administration. Subcutaneous (SC) fluids are easily delivered using a butterfly needle, which allows the animal to move without the needle being pulled out.[3] In an attempt to reduce the pain associated with this procedure, a larger needle diameter may be chosen, resulting in fluids being pushed out with less force. Some practitioners also noted that the use of a drip system in SC fluids administration resulted in animals being less tensed during the procedure, especially rabbits (Y. van Zeeland, personal communication, 2017). In birds, large volumes can also be administered SC in specific areas despite the overall low elasticity of the avian skin.[10] Proper technique to avoid repeated punctures and subsequent leakage, or prevent inadvertent intracoelomic/intraabdominal injection, is essential. Irritant drugs, such as enrofloxacin, should be diluted to limit the risk of associated pain, skin necrosis, ulceration, depigmentation, and sterile abscess formation.[9,15] Finally, the SC route has been controversial in reptiles owing to the suspected low and variable drug absorption, because reptile skin is poorly vascularized and less elastic than mammalian skin, resulting in undesired leakage of the drug.[1,4,15,16] However, recent studies have shown an adequate therapeutic effect and less variability using the SC route rather than in the intramuscular (IM) route in reptiles.[17,23]

SC access port systems (Skin Button, Norfolk Vet Products, Skokie, IL) may be considered for the long-term delivery of SC drugs and fluids. This technique has been used by the authors in the management of rabbits with chronic renal failure for the long-term administration of fluids at home by the owner. In addition, the technique has also been described in hedgehogs to facilitate administration of fluids and drugs as the injection port remains accessible even when the animal curls.[3]

Intramuscular route

Many popular companion exotic animals including birds and reptiles have a small size and thus small muscle mass. As a consequence, repeated IM injections or use of irritant drugs can cause local pain and muscle necrosis.[1,2,24] Some authors recommend to avoid injection sites such as the muscles of caudal or lateral thigh in small mammals to prevent damage to the sciatic nerve, which could result in lameness or self-mutilation.[2,3,25] Given the high metabolic rate of many small mammals and birds,[26] large volumes may be injected proportionally to the body weight. Therefore, practitioners should fraction injected volumes in multiple injection sites. For example, some authors suggested that IM injection volume should not exceed 0.5 mL/kg by injection sites in rabbits and 1 mL/kg in birds.[9,27] Although empirical, this recommendation can be extrapolated to other exotic species.[5]

Portal systems in nonmammalian species

Regarding at the different injection routes in nonmammalian vertebrates, veterinarians may encounter the recurrent and controversial question of the influence of the renal and hepatic portal systems on clearance of drugs from the system after the use of caudal injection sites. In avian and fish species, the evidence is very scarce regarding the clinical significance of the portal systems, whereas more data are available in nonavian reptiles.

Table 1

Parenteral injection sites for various exotic species, excluding intravascular injection sites

Species/Group	IM	SC	Intraperitoneal/Intracoelomique[a]	Other Routes	Comments	Reference(s)
Ferret (*Mustela putorius furo*)	• Quadriceps muscle • Lumbar muscles (superficial and lateral to the spine to avoid trauma to the spinal cord)	Loose skin over the: • Caudal part of the neck • Interscapular area • Thoracolumbar area	• Generally not recommended for pet animals. Should be performed only under general anesthesia. Performed in the right abdominal quadrant following a line drawn from the right leg held extended with the animal in dorsal recumbency and the body tilted to the left side. Always aspirate before injection		• Thick skin, particularly in the cranial neck area • Caution to avoid giving SC injections into the SC fat tissues because it can significantly lower the absorption • IP injection is mostly a laboratory practice • Make sure to inject subdermally rather than intradermally	1-5
Rabbit (*Oryctolagus cuniculus*)	• Epaxial muscles (just cranial to the pelvis) • Quadriceps muscle	• Interscapular area • Flank • Loose skin over the dorsum			• Thick skin, especially in intact males	
Guinea pig (*Cavia porcellus*)	• Epaxial muscles • Quadriceps muscle	• Cranial dorsal thorax • Dorsal thoracolumbar area			• Thick fur (avoid intrafur injection) • Caution while handling to avoid fur slip	
Chinchilla (*Chinchilla lanigera*)	• Quadriceps muscle	• Cranial dorsal thorax • Flank area				
Small rodents	• Quadriceps muscles • Epaxial muscles	• Scruff of the neck • Skinfold along the back		• Intrahepatic injection has been studied for euthanasia	• Small muscle mass increases the risk of muscle necrosis after IM injection	
Hedgehog (*Atelerix albiventris*)	• Orbicularis muscle of the mantle • Quadriceps muscle (under general anesthesia)	• At the junction of the furred skin and mantle in the flank area: locate the small accessible window in			• IM injection in the orbicularis muscle is easier if the animal is rolled into a ball • Quadriceps muscles can also be accessed in moribund,	

(continued on next page)

Table 1
(continued)

Species/Group	IM	SC	Intraperitoneal/Intracoelomique[a]	Other Routes	Comments	Reference(s)
		the flank area and use a needle long enough to enter deep past the spines			• obese, or very tame individuals • Dermis under the spiny skin poorly vascularized and large amount of subdermal fat tissue present; therefore, it is preferably avoided for injections • Furred skin more elastic and vascular, but not accessible in balled up hedgehogs • Avoid administering fluids laterally into the patagium	
Sugar glider (*Petaurus breviceps*)	• Quadriceps muscle • Biceps femoris muscle • Triceps muscle • Biceps muscle • Epaxial muscles	• Scapular area • Dorsal midline of the thorax				
Pot-bellied pig (*Sus scrofa domesticus*)	• Quadriceps muscle • Semimembranous/semitendinosous muscles (preferred in the unrestrained pig) • Triceps muscle • Neck muscle just caudal to the ear	• Just caudal to the base of the ear (less SC fat) • In a skin fold of the limbs			• Will struggle and vocalize loudly if restrained • Requires a needle long enough to inject deeper than the SC fat layer for IM injections • No need to preserve the limbs for meat quality as in food-producing pigs	1,2,6–8

| Bird | • Pectoral muscles
• Iliotibialis muscles | • Inguinal skin fold
• Axillary skin fold
• Interscapular area
• Pectoral area
• Propatagium
• Dorsal caudal neck area | • Contraindicated because of the close anatomic association with the air sacs (high risk for aspiration) | • Pectoral muscles are sometimes advocated as preferable to bypass renal portal system, even though it is still controversial (cf section on portal renal system in non-mammalian species)
• Avoid pectoral muscles in racing pigeons/birds of prey and pelvic limbs in terrestrial birds to minimize the impact of muscular lesions
• In terrestrial birds, injection in the pectoral muscles may result in slow absorption because of the presence of white muscle with poorer vascularization
• Alternate IM injections between the right and left muscles
• Avoid the neck area for SC in colombiformes because of the risk of fatal hemorrhage from the cervical vascular plexus
• Caution with SC injections in species with SC air sacs (turkey vultures, pelicans)
• SC injections should be performed with a shallow angle to avoid penetrating to deep tissue because the SC space is very limited in birds [1,4,9–14] |

(continued on next page)

Table 1
(continued)

Species/Group	IM	SC	Intraperitoneal/Intracoelomique[a]	Other Routes	Comments	Reference(s)
Chelonian	• Biceps muscle • Quadriceps muscles • Pectoral muscle	• Cervicobrachial area • Prefemoral fossa	• Cranial part of the prefemoral fossa where the skin attaches to the bridge with the animal in dorsal recumbency or tilted • Beware of intravesical injection, urinary bladder trauma, or coelomitis after follicle or ova penetration in reproductively active females	• Epicoelomic route through the cranial plastronal inlet immediately dorsal to the plastron, lateroventral to the head and neck and dorsal to the pectoral muscles	• Avoid injecting in the caudal one-half of the body (renal and hepatic portal system) • Avoid the IM route in animals with reduced muscle mass • Insert the needle between scales	1,2,4,15–17
Lizard	• Biceps muscle • Quadriceps muscles • Epaxial muscles	• Lateral flank (with shallow angle to avoid penetration in the coelomic cavity) • Between scapulae	• Right caudal one-third of the abdomen paramedially (to avoid abdominal vein) with the animal in dorsal recumbency and tilted on its left			
Snake	• Paravertebral muscles	• Laterally to the dorsal spinous processes • Lateral body wall	• Caudal fourth of the body between the first 2 rows of lateral scales just dorsal to the ventral scales			

Amphibian	• Biceps muscle • Quadriceps muscles	• In a skin fold	• Right caudal one-third of the abdomen paramedially (to avoid abdominal vein) with the animal in dorsal recumbency and with caudal end slightly elevated	• Dorsal lymphatic sac in anurans just lateral and cranial to the urostyle	• Topical administration is preferred • Avoid injected in the caudal one-half of the body (renal and hepatic portal system) • SC route can be used only in anurans because of the lack of SC space in other species	1,2,4,18
Fish	• Epaxial muscles • Muscles ventral to the pectoral fins (sometimes preferred for esthetic reasons)	• Not recommended because of the inelasticity of the skin resulting in high risk of drug leakage	• With the fish in dorsal recumbency, lateral to ventral midline between the vent and the pelvic fins		• Insert the needle between scales • Drug leakage after IM injection is very common, even with small volumes • Drugs may be absorbed more quickly if injected in the red lateral muscles than in white poorly vascularized muscles	1,2,19–22

Abbreviations: IC, intracoelomic; IM, intramuscular; SC, subcutaneous.
[a] This route is not recommended if other routes are accessible.

222

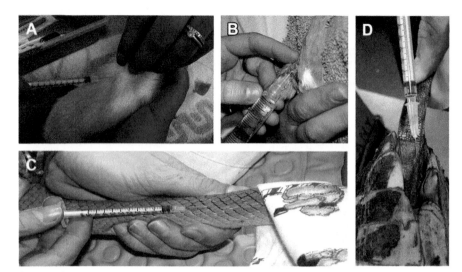

Fig. 1. Subcutaneous injection in the interscapular area of a rat (*Rattus norvegicus*) (*A*), the inguinal fold of a cockatiel (*Nymphicus hollandicus*) (*B*), the paravertebral area in a green palm snake (*Phylodrias viridissimus*) (*C*), and the prefemoral fossa of a Hermann tortoise (*Testudo hermanni*) (*D*). (*Courtesy of* [A] the University of California, Davis; [B, C] Zoological Medicine Service, Université de Montréal, Saint-Hyacinthe, Canada; and [D] CHV Fregis, Thomas Coutant.)

Anatomists have defined 8 anatomic patterns of blood flow in the caudal region of fish, which can be further classified into 4 clinically relevant categories.[28] In most fish, the renal portal system receives blood not only from the caudal part of the body, but also from the segmental veins from the flanks. In cyprinidae, including the goldfish, only some of the blood returning from the caudal part of the body is directed toward the portal system and the rest of the blood is shunted toward the hepatic portal system.[28] In the group including the salmon, lumpfish, and tuna, the blood originating from the tail does not go through the portal system, whereas the blood coming from the segmental veins is directed toward the portal system. The last vascular pattern resembles that of cyprinidae, except that the blood diverted from the portal system returns directly to the heart.[28] The great diversity of fish vasculature makes generalizations about effects of the portal system challenging.

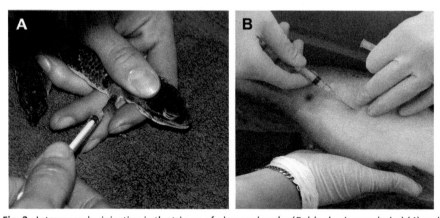

Fig. 2. Intramuscular injection in the triceps of a leopard gecko (*Eublepharis macularius*) (*A*) and intracoelomic injection in an Atlantic cod (*Gadus morhua*) (*B*). (*Courtesy of* [A] Zoological Medicine Service, Université de Montréal, Saint-Hyacinthe, Canada; and [B] Aquarium du Québec, Québec, Claire Vergneau-Grosset.)

In birds, blood flowing from the caudal part of the body through the common iliac vein can participate in the renal perfusion via the renal portal system or bypass the kidneys and directly reach the systemic flow by entering the inferior vena cava.[29] This system is controlled by a valve in the common iliac vein whose opening is under autonomous nervous system regulation, and mainly depends on the vascular resistance of the portal system.[29] This renal portal system anastomoses with capillaries past the renal glomerula at the level of the renal tubules.[29] Consequently, the renal portal system can theoretically impact pharmacokinetic profiles of drugs with a tubular excretion, but not of those with a glomerular filtration. The renal portal system is very similar in birds and in reptiles. However, reptiles also have the particularity to have their abdominal vein, or paired abdominal veins in chelonians and crocodilians, flowing directly through the liver, making a first hepatic passage also possible for drugs injected in the caudal part of their body.[30]

Historically, it has been advocated to avoid injections in the caudal part of the body of nonmammalian vertebrates, especially in reptiles. A theory has been advanced that, because of the renal portal system, a first-pass effect to the kidneys carries a risk of either nephrotoxicity or early clearance of the drug before reaching the target organs. This effect was demonstrated in green iguanas (*Iguana iguana*) by iohexol injection into the ventral coccygeal vein; the contrast medium was drained toward the portal vein and the kidneys. Of note, this was not the case when iohexol was injected into a femoral intraosseous (IO) catheter.[31] It has been shown that the bioavailability of gentamicin, a drug with glomerular filtration, was not affected by the renal portal system in agreement with a previous observation that the renal portal vasculature irrigates the renal tubules.[32,33] Conversely, it has been demonstrated that the blood concentration of carbenicilin, a drug with tubular secretion, was reduced when injected in the hindlimbs compared with the forelimbs.[33] However, this difference was shown to be irrelevant clinically. It is tempting to conclude with the authors of these studies that the renal portal system does not have a clinically relevant effect.[4] In addition, potential adverse effects associated with the renal portal system have not been documented in reptiles thus far. The same theory has been stated for the hepatic portal system. Conversely, the first hepatic passage has been shown to alter the bioavailability of buprenorphine and alfaxalone injected in the hindlimbs of turtles,[34,35] as well as dexmedetomidine and ketamine association injected in the hindlimbs of leopard geckos.[17] Granted these studies were performed in a few species maintained in controlled environmental conditions, extrapolating their results to all reptile species without considering their physiologic or pathologic status is likely inappropriate. Pending more clinical studies, it is deemed appropriate to perform injections in the cranial part of a reptile's body whenever possible.[15] This recommendation is also valid for birds, amphibians, and most fish. Further studies documenting drugs pharmacokinetics after hindlimb injections in these vertebrate classes are required.[1,13,35,36]

Intraperitoneal/intracoelomic route
With the exception of fish, this intraperitoneal or intracoelomic (IC) route is generally not advised for the administration of fluids or drugs in exotic species, because of the associated risk of viscera perforation, injection into the gastrointestinal tract, urinary bladders in chelonians or other intracoelomic organs, and resulting coelomitis.[1–3] Furthermore, the IC route seems to be associated with high interindividual variability and delayed onset of action compared with the intravenous (IV) route, as shown in a study on the IC administration of fospropofol to red-eared sliders (*Trachemys scripta elegans*).[37] This route should, therefore, be reserved for euthanasia when no other route is available.[3,4] In fish, the placement of an IC catheter has been described and was shown to be easier to maintain than an IV catheter.[22] The procedure for IC catheter

placement in fish species is described in **Box 1**.[38] However, similar to other animals, greater interindividual variability has also been noted in fish after IC antibiotic administration. Therefore, other administration routes should be favored when possible, provided that injected volumes do not cause drug leakage after IM injection.[39]

Comparison of the different routes of injection

In rabbits, similar pharmacokinetic profiles or action of drugs have been described after IM or SC administration.[40–42] However, a pharmacokinetic study of penicillin in pigs showed longer half-lives with an SC route compared with the IM route.[43] It is difficult to extrapolate these results to other species of small mammals. Nevertheless, when no pharmacokinetic data are available, it is generally recommended to use to SC route rather than IM route as this route is probably the least painful and results in less resistance of the animal.[40] In birds, some studies have shown similar pharmacokinetic profiles with SC or IM administration, for instance, with enrofloxacin in ostriches (*Struthio camelus*) and buprenorphine in American kestrels (*Falco sparverius*).[44,45] However, in chickens (*Gallus gallus domesticus*), SC gentamicin was associated with a better bioavailability than IM administration of the same drug.[46] In reptiles, similar pharmacokinetic profiles or action of drugs have been described with IM or SC injection route for ceftiofur in green iguanas and bearded dragons (*Pogona vitticeps*) and with danofloxacin in loggerhead turtles (*Caretta caretta*), among others.[23,47,48] Conversely, the effects of a dexmedetomidine-ketamine combination was shown to be both quicker and more consistent after IM injection compared with SC injection in red-eared sliders.[49] In fish, when comparing IM or IC administration, similar pharmacokinetic profiles have been described with cefquinome in tilapia (*Oreochromis niloticus*),[50] whereas ceftiofur has shown different pharmacokinetic profile in koi (*Cyprinus carpio*).[39] Overall, absorption is generally quicker when using the IM route, but the route should always be chosen in the light of available pharmacokinetic studies and potential stress and pain caused to the animal.

Intravenous, Intraosseous, and Intracardiac Drug Administration

Many exotic species display a smaller patient size than domestic carnivores, making IV catheterization more challenging. IO catheterization may be used as an alternative, but certain anatomic specificities, such as pneumatized bones in birds, may preclude this route (discussed elsewhere in this article). In addition, IO catheters are contraindicated in patients presented with osseous lesions, such as hyperparathyroidism or polyostotic hyperostosis. Vascular and IO injection sites for each species (including their particularities) are summarized in **Table 2** and illustrated in **Figs. 3–5**.

Box 1
Placement of an intracoelomic catheter in a fish

- Place the anesthetized fish in right lateral recumbency (anesthesia may be performed by immersion in MS-222 or alfaxalone bath).

- Insert a 23G butterfly catheter of which the plastic wings have been cut between the scales at a 20° angle to the body wall, in the area just dorsal to the caudal edge of the left pelvic fin with the dorsal aspect of the left pectoral fin used as landmark.

- Secure the plastic hub of the catheter with a single suture.

- Place a second skin suture to secure the looped catheter cranially above the left dorsal epaxial muscles.

- Place the injection port at the end of the catheter.

- Flush daily and after each drug injection.

- Can be used for up to 6 days.

Table 2
Vascular and IO routes of injection according to the treated species

Species/Group	IV[a]	IO (Performed Under General or Local Anesthesia with Aseptic Technique)	Intracardiac (Usually Contraindicated Except for Euthanasia Procedure and in Snakes)	Comment	Reference(s)
Ferret	• Cephalic vein[a] • Saphenous vein[a] • Jugular vein • Lateral tail vein • Cranial vena cava	• Proximal tibia in the tibial crest • Proximal femur in the greater trochanter • Proximal humerus	• Between the third and sixth ribs near the elbow (more caudally in ferrets between the sixth and eighth ribs) where the heart beat can be felt or heard using a Doppler probe	• Cranial vena cava is safer to use in ferrets compared with other species owing to the caudal anatomic position of the heart. Generally performed with the ferret under general anesthesia in dorsal recumbency with the needle pointing toward the opposite knee inserted into the thoracic inlet between the manubrium sternum and the first rib	1,3,4,25,27,51–53
Rabbit	• Marginal ear vein (lateral or medial)[a] • Lateral saphenous vein[a] • Cephalic vein[a] • Jugular vein • Femoral vein			• Risk of phlebitis, vascular necrosis, and sloughing when catheterizing the marginal ear vein	1,3,4,51,53,54
Rodents	• Lateral coccygeal vein[a] • Medial and lateral saphenous veins[a] • Femoral vein • Cephalic vein[a] • Jugular vein • Cranial vena cava			• Lateral tail vein is not accessible in hamsters and guinea pigs • Use of the lateral tail vein is contraindicated in gerbils owing to the risk of tail slip • Warming the tail in hot water/with a warm pad or infrared light for 15 minutes can help to visualize the lateral coccygeal vein • The smaller the rodent species, the more difficult IV access	

(continued on next page)

Table 2
(continued)

Species/Group	IV[a]	IO (Performed Under General or Local Anesthesia with Aseptic Technique)	Intracardiac (Usually Contraindicated Except for Euthanasia Procedure and in Snakes)	Comment	Reference(s)
Hedgehog	• Cephalic vein[a] • Lateral saphenous vein[a] • Femoral vein • Jugular vein			• Catheter is virtually impossible to maintain in conscious nonobese hedgehogs owing to their curling behavior • Proximal tibia can be accessible even when the animal is in a curled position • Some hedgehogs have died from hemorrhage after cranial vena cava venipuncture; this technique should only be used as a last resort owing to the risk of cardiac venipuncture and laceration	1,3,4,51–55
Sugar glider	• Saphenous vein[a] • Cephalic vein[a] • Lateral ear vein[a] • Femoral vein • Ventral coccygeal vein • Subcutaneous abdominal vein[a]				1,3,4,51,53
Pot-bellied pig	• Cephalic vein[a] • Lateral saphenous vein[a] • Jugular vein			• Cut down techniques may be required for catheterization of the cephalic, saphenous, or jugular vein in adult animals because of the thick skin and SC fat tissue • Sedation is usually required for catheter placement in nonobtunded animals	2,6,53,56

| Bird | • Basilic vein[a]
• Medial metatarsal vein (medial aspect of the tibiotarso-tarsometatarsal joint)[a]
• Jugular vein (right jugular usually more developed than the left) | • Proximal tibiotarsus
• Distal ulna (just distal to the dorsal ulnar condyle with the manus slightly pronated)
• Proximal ulna | • Just cranial to the sternum in the midline between the clavicular bones | • Wing veins are prone to hematoma formation
• In columbiformes, the jugular vein can be hidden by the neck venous plexus, making it difficult to reach
• Maintenance of IV catheters in psittaciformes usually requires placement of an Elizabethan collar and suturing the catheter in place in the ulnar vein; IO catheters are generally not associated with hemorrhage if removed by the bird
• Avoid ulnar IO catheterization in species with pneumatized ulna such as Cathartiformes and some Gruiformes
• Correct placement of IO catheter in the distal ulna can be verified either radiographically or by injecting a small bolus of fluids and observing it flowing proximally in the ulnar vein
• The jugular vein is lying in the cervical apterigium on the ventrolateral aspect of the neck in psittacines and raptor; there is no apterigium in some species of galliforms, columbiforms and anseriforms; injection into the caudal jugular vein in columbiformes | 1,4,9,10,31,51,53,57,58 |

(continued on next page)

Table 2
(continued)

Species/Group	IV[a]	IO (Performed Under General or Local Anesthesia with Aseptic Technique)	Intracardiac (Usually Contraindicated Except for Euthanasia Procedure and in Snakes)	Comment	Reference(s)
Chelonian	• Jugular vein (on the lateroodorsal surface of the neck on a line drawn from the tympanic membrane to the thoracic inlet; right jugular usually larger)[a] • Dorsal coccygeal vein • Brachial vein • Subcarapacial sinus (dorsal to the cervical neck directly on the midline just ventral to the carapace); should be reserved for euthanasia or used as last resort, owing to the risk of subsequent spinal trauma and Hind-limb and tail paralysis	• Bridge • Carapace • Gular scute • Distal ulna • Distal femur • Proximal tibia	• Midline between humeral and abdominal scute in ventral recumbency (not practical in big specimens)	• Jugular vein is the most common vascular access for catheterization (sedation or anesthesia often required with or without cut down) • Maintaining IO catheter in the limbs is very difficult because of the capacity to withdraw the limbs into the carapace • Passage in vascular compartment is less efficient via the shell (IO catheter) compared with a long bone	1,2,4,15,16,51,59,60
Lizard	• Ventral coccygeal vein (caudal to the hemipenes) • Ventral abdominal vein • Brachial vein[a] • Jugular vein • Cranial vena cava (with a very large angle in the thoracic inlet to avoid puncturing the heart) • Axillary venous plexus caudal to the humerus near the shoulder joint	• Distal femur • Proximal tibia • Proximal humerus	• Use Doppler imaging or palpation to locate the heart and puncture via the thoracic inlet just above the symphysis of the clavicles	• The needle should be inserted between scales	1,2,4,15,51,53

Species					
Snake	Not applicable	• Ventral coccygeal vein (caudal to the hemipenes and scent glands) • Jugular vein (left jugular located to the right of midline in the ball python; the jugular lies medially to the ribs, 9 or 10 ventral scales cranial to where the heart beat is visible; cut down is required for catheter placement)[a] • Palatine vein	• Locate the heart at one-fourth to one-third the distance from the snout while the animal is placed in dorsal recumbency • After palpation of the heart, orient the needle toward the cranial end of the snake • Direct beat visualization may sometimes be possible to confirm correct localization • Cardiac laceration is a potential risk	• The needle should be inserted between scales • Intracardiac administration of propofol was shown to be safe but intracardiac injections are used as a last resort for other drugs in the absence of safety studies	1,2,4,51,61,62
Amphibian		• Saphenous vein • Femoral vein • Ventral coccygeal vein (in caudates only) • Ventral abdominal vein (very superficial, risk of extravascular drug injection) • Lingual venous plexus (at the base of the tongue) • Facial vein in ranidae • Plexus caudal to the stifle in toads	• Proximal tibiofibula	• Midline in the pectoral region (visualization, palpation or Doppler imaging)	• Do not use chlorhexidine, povidone-iodine, or alcohol to prepare injection sites because of potential toxicity; use sterile saline for skin preparation to avoid mucus layer disruption
					1,2,4,18,63

(continued on next page)

Table 2
(continued)

Species/Group	IV[a]	IO (Performed Under General or Local Anesthesia with Aseptic Technique)	Intracardiac (Usually Contraindicated Except for Euthanasia Procedure and in Snakes)	Comment	Reference(s)
Fish	• Ventral coccygeal vein • Dorsal or ventral aorta (catheterization described) • Branchial vein	Not applicable	• Impractical • Catheterization of the sinus venosus has been described using 18-gauge 3.8-cm intravascular needles in free-swimming fish for 2 wk without major complications in striped bass (*Morone saxatilis*)	• Use sterile saline for skin preparation to avoid mucus layer disruption	2,4,22,64,65

Abbreviations: IO, intraosseous; IV, intravenous.
[a] Access also commonly used for long-term catheter placement.

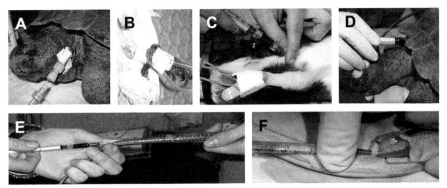

Fig. 3. Intravenous catheterization of the jugular vein of a Desert tortoise (*Gopherus agassizii*) (*A*) and of the medial metatarsal vein in a white cockatoo (*Cacatua alba*) (*B*). Intravenous injection in the cranial vena cava of a guinea pig (*Cavia porcellus*) (*C*), the subcarapacial sinus of a Desert tortoise (*G agassizii*) (*D*), the ventral tail vein of a common garter snake (*Thamnophis sirtalis*) (*E*), and the jugular vein of a Burmese python (*Python molurus bivittatus*) using a cutdown technique (*F*). (*Courtesy of* [*A, C, D*] the University of California, Davis; and [*B, E, F*] Zoological Medicine Service, Université de Montréal, Saint-Hyacinthe, Canada.)

Intravenous route

As in domestic mammals, IV drug administration usually results in a faster onset of action compared with other parenteral routes.[66] Except for collapsed patients, general anesthesia or at least sedation is usually required for catheter placement owing to the stress associated with the procedure in nondomestic animals. In very docile rabbits, IV catheter placement can be tried without sedation after the application of a topical anesthetic (lidocaine and/or prilocaine cream).[3,27] Maintaining IV catheters in exotic animals can be very challenging because they may chew the tubulure or the catheter. Elizabethan collars may be used, but their maintenance can be challenging and they often cause stress-related anorexia in rodents, rabbits, and psittacines. In small mammals, alternate options to prevent access to the catheter include maintaining the limb in extension, protecting the tubulure using syringe cases, and putting distasteful substances on the bandage.[2–4] Hedgehogs can retract their limbs under the mantle, which commonly extracts the IV catheter; thus, IO catheter placement may be preferred. Similarly, chelonians can pull back their head and limbs in their shell, although a technique has been described to maintain long-term jugular polyurethane central venous catheters.[3,4,67] An indwelling time of 4 months maximum has been described with this technique.

Similar as for the routes described previously, the renal and hepatic portal systems should be taken into consideration when deciding on a location for IV catheter placement. For instance, when IV contrast is administered, such as for angiography or glomerular filtration rate measurement, it is advisable to place a catheter in the cranial part of the body, as exemplified in bearded dragons.[68]

Intraosseous route

IO catheters are usually easier to place than IV catheters in hypovolemic/hypotensive patients.[4] Contraindications include dermatitis at the site of insertion and pneumatized long bones in birds, such as the humerus, femur, and ulna in certain species (eg, turkey vultures [*Cathartes aura*], gruiformes). Immature bones with active growth plates, hyperostotic bones in avian reproductive females, or diseased bones are not suitable for IO catheter placement.[27] Drugs delivered through the IV and IO routes are considered to have a similar onset of action and peak blood levels.[69–73] Unless

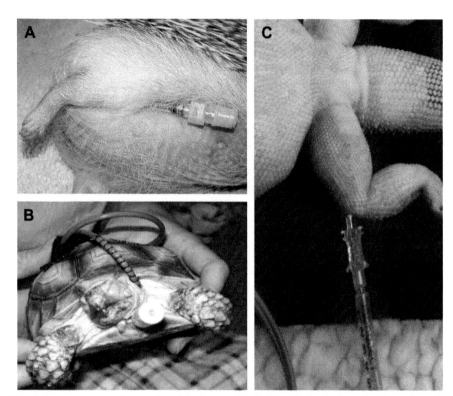

Fig. 4. Intraosseous catheter placed in the proximal tibia of a hedgehog (*Atelerix frontalis*) (*A*), in the gular scute of an African spurred tortoise (*Centrochelys sulcata*) (an oesophagostomy red-rubber tube can also be noted dorsally) (*B*), and the distal femur of a bearded dragon (*Pogona vitticeps*) (*C*). (*Courtesy of* [A, C] Zoological Medicine Service, Université de Montréal, Saint-Hyacinthe, Canada; and [B] the University of California, Davis.)

immediate access is required for cardiopulmonary resuscitation, the IO catheter site preparation and placement should be performed under aseptic conditions to minimize the risk of osteomyelitis.[1,4] IO catheter placement is performed under sedation in noncritical patients. In debilitated patients, IO catheters may be placed with local anesthesia, such injection of 2 mg/kg lidocaine or lidocaine/prilocaine cream

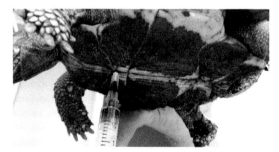

Fig. 5. Intracardiac injection in a Hermann tortoise (*Testudo hermanni*). (*Courtesy of* CHV Fregis, Thomas Coutant.)

application 10 minutes prior.[2,4] Spinal needles containing a stylet are ideal to limit the risk of coring the needle with a bone plug. Correct placement of the catheter may be verified by orthogonal radiographic projections. As a general rule, the catheter should occupy 33% to 67% of the bone marrow cavity at its smallest diameter. When the catheter is managed to be placed parallel to the bone marrow cavity, it may be advanced to the full length of the needle (making sure that it is not longer than the bone itself). If the catheter is placed with an angle or in a curved bone, it can be advanced until resistance of the opposite cortical is felt. The delivery of the drug will be efficient as long as the tip of the catheter is fully seated in the bone cavity.[53] As in human medicine, serious complications after IO catheter placement are rarely observed in veterinary medicine.[53,74]

Intracardiac route
This route of drug administration is mostly accepted for euthanasia under anesthesia.[75] In all other situations, even in case of cardiac arrest, other routes should be preferred because intracardiac injection carries risks of myocardial damage, cardiac tamponade, and ultimately death.[1,2] However, it has been shown in ball pythons (*Python regius*) that intracardiac injection of propofol was a safe and effective method of induction with only mild cardiac lesions that resolved over a period of 14 days.[61]

Vascular access ports
Vascular access ports consist of an indwelling IV catheter with an SC injection port (**Fig. 6**). Such ports allow for long-term catheterization with a reduced risk of removal or infection, because the device is surgically implanted under the skin of the animal. Techniques to implant vascular access ports in small mammals have been widely described and used in laboratory settings (**Box 2**).[76] The jugular vein is generally used to implant the vascular access port in mammals. This technique is also described for long-term chemotherapy[2,3,77] and for long-term antibiotic therapy (5 months) in a chicken with pododermatitis.[78] Of note, a vascular access port has maintained patency for up to 18 months in a green iguana receiving chemotherapy.[79]

Extended Release Devices and Intralesional Drug Administration

In nontrained, nondomestic animals, the physical restraint needed for medication is stressful and can both negatively impact healing and deteriorate the relationship with the caregiver. Drug administration may also be difficult for inexperienced owners.

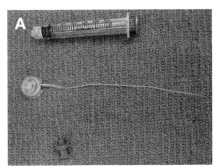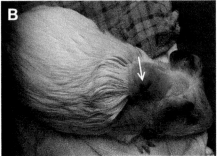

Fig. 6. Vascular access port pieces (*A*) and guinea pig (*Cavia porcellus*) after the placement of a jugular vascular access port (*white arrow*) (*B*). (*Courtesy of* Miranda Sadar, DVM, DACZM, University of California, Davis.)

> **Box 2**
> **Placement of a vascular access port**
>
> - Make a curvilinear incision slightly larger than the body of the port in the selected area.
> - Bluntly dissect the subcutaneous tissues to create a pocket slightly larger than the body of the port and the insertion point of the catheter.
> - Maintain this site moist by placing saline-impregnated gauzes in the pocket while the other surgical steps are performed.
> - Make an incision over the vessel of interest and isolate it with blunt dissection.
> - Place elastic vessel loops around the vessel proximally and distally to the venotomy site.
> - Pass a tunneling rod subcutaneously from the vessel to the port pocket to place the catheter through the rod and fix it to the body of the port.
> - Preplace retention beads to fix the catheter when removing the rod and prevent postoperative movement of the catheter.
> - Perform the venotomy after tightening the vessel loops previously preplaced and leaving the blood vessel filled.
> - Place the catheter through the venotomy site.
> - Suture the catheter into place between suture beads (1 or 2 beads into the lumen of the vessel and another outside the venotomy site).
> - Place the coil of the catheter in the tissue surrounding the vessel to relieve tension on the catheter during postural changes.
> - Suture the vessel site.
> - Suture the port in place in the pocket, beginning with 1 deep suture in the pocket to pull the port into the deepest part of it. The sutures should anchor the port on the muscular layer.
> - Close the port incision, while ensuring that the dead space is eliminated.
> - The port can be used for more than 1 month.

Therefore, extended release formulations and devices are particularly useful in exotic pet medicine. Several antibiotics in the β-lactam and tetracyclin families, antiparasitic agents such as ivermectin, and analgesics such as butorphanol and buprenorphine have been used as long-acting depot formulations in exotic species.[80–89] Several gonadotropin-releasing hormone agonists, such as leuprolide acetate extended release formulation, or deslorelin acetate implants, have been used in ferrets,[90–95] other small mammals,[96] birds[97–102] (**Fig. 7**), reptiles,[103,104] and fish[105] with varying success. Self-removal has been reported in psittacines; thus, the implant site should be monitored after implantation. The lasting effect of these gonadotropin-releasing hormone agonists is well-known in some small mammals such as ferrets, and in cockatiels (*Nymphicus hollandicus*), pigeons (*Columba livia*), Hispaniolan Amazon parrots (*Amazona ventralis*), chickens, and Japanese quails (*Coturnix coturnix japonica*) among birds (see Nico J. Schoemaker's article, "GnRH Agonists and Other Contraceptive Medications in Exotic Companion Animals," in this issue.) However, more studies are needed in other species to assess intraspecies and interspecies differences in durations of action.[98,106] Another extended release device that has received increasing attention is the osmotic pump, which consists of an SC implant containing a reservoir filled with the drug of interest. After implantation, the device is progressively compressed in a constant manner by osmotic pressure, creating an SC constant rate infusion of the drug. Osmotic pumps have demonstrated promising

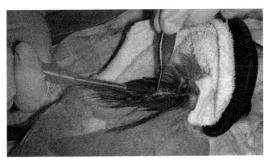

Fig. 7. Placement of a deslorelin implant in the intrascapular area of a rose-ringed parakeet (*Psittacula krameri*). (*Courtesy of* the University of California, Davis.)

results in managing individual cases and pharmacokinetics studies have been performed for various molecules in rodents, birds, and reptiles.[107–109] The use of long-lasting intralesional chemotherapy, electrochemotherapy, and photodynamic therapy for curative or adjunct tumor treatment in association with surgery or radiation therapy have also been described in rodents and birds.[79,110–115] In the absence of clinical studies for these therapeutic alternatives in exotic species, techniques are generally extrapolated from domestic animals.[3] Discussing these techniques specifically is beyond the scope of this review; for this purpose, readers may refer to other texts.[116,117]

DRUG ADMINISTRATION IN THE DIGESTIVE AND RESPIRATORY SYSTEMS
Oral Drug Administration

The oral route is usually readily accessible for owners to medicate their pet at home, except in chelonians and some lizard species. Alternate options to facilitate oral medication in chelonians are discussed elsewhere in this article. This route should not be used in case of vomiting, regurgitation or ileus, because drug absorption may be impaired. In addition, in amphibians, the enteral administration of certain drugs may be less efficient than topical administration.[118] Oral drug administration may be accomplished through the food and drinking water, directly in the oral cavity by syringe or using a gavage tube, with patient restraint or operant conditioning, or via a feeding tube.

Oral drug administration via food or drinking water
Oral drug administration through the drinking water is the least technical.[1] However, this method comes with serious limitations that render it unadvised in most situations. The real dose ingested by the animal is undefined, resulting into a risk of underdosing or overdosing.[1,10,27,119] Improper homogenization also carries a risk of improper dosing. Furthermore, adding medication to the drinking water may alter the taste, thus, having a deleterious effect on water intake in species distrusting unfamiliar tastes.[3,27] One way to partially overcome the risk of underdosing because of improper consumption of water is to remove all other sources of water, including fluid-rich foods such as vegetables and fruits. In chelonians, the delivery of medications through the drinking water is of no use owing to the unpredictable nature of their drinking behavior.[16] There is also experimental evidence that antibiotics administered in water are ineffective in rabbits, except for enrofloxacin.[120] Nevertheless, medicating in the water is sometimes the only option for people unable to give medication otherwise (especially in birds) or for group treatment such as in breeding facilities and aviaries.

For instance, oral treatment through the water has proven efficient in cockatiels administered fluconazole 100 mg/L for 8 days and doxycycline 400 mg/L for 21 days. When administering tetracycline or fluoroquinolone treatment, calcium supplementation should be stopped for the duration of the treatment owing to antibiotic chelation by divalent cations.[121,122] Whenever medicating the water, any other water sources should be removed to ensure proper intake.

Medication can also be incorporated into the food, through medicated feed or by mixing it with a treat, provided that the patient is not anorexic. Each species and patient has its own preferences when it comes to which item is best accepted. It may be in a grape in chinchillas, oral supplements in ferrets, mealworms in hedgehogs, fruits in pot-bellied pigs, fresh preys in carnivorous birds and reptiles, or gut-loaded *Artemia* or a special mix in gelatin cubes for fishes.[1,3,4,9,15,22,123] Hand feeding will ensure the animal ingests the exact drug dose. When medicated feed are used, clinicians should comply with regulations of their area regarding food animal species, such as for chickens, pigs, and fishes.

Intraoral administration by syringe and gavage feeding

For better dosage precision, the drug can be delivered directly into the oral cavity, esophagus, or stomach of the animal. Small drug volumes may be delivered directly into the oral cavity, making sure the animal swallows progressively to avoid aspiration (**Fig. 8**).[2] As in domestic animals, oral administration should be avoided if the patient is too debilitated to swallow or stand upright, because of the risk of aspiration.[2–4] In rodents and lagomorphs, syringe administration of drugs may be easily achieved by inserting the syringe's tip within the interdental space located between the incisors and the jugal teeth.[1–4] To increase acceptance, drugs can be mixed with a small amount of food or formulated with an appreciated flavor.[3,4] There are some limitations to the oral medication in psittacine birds owing to their particular digestive anatomy, especially when considering tablets and pills. First, capsules and tablets are difficult to give to psittacines owing to their beak shape. Next, their crop acts as a storage compartment with a higher pH than mammals' stomach pH. Therefore, it is expected that the pharmacokinetics of the drugs contained in tablets and capsules will be affected. This problem may be overcome by crushing tablets for dilution in liquid

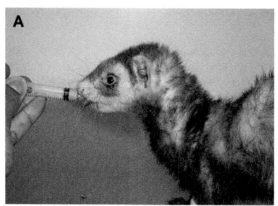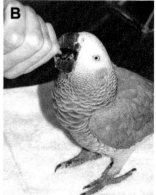

Fig. 8. Syringe feeding in a ferret (*Mustela putorius furo*) (*A*) and an African gray parrot (*Psittacus erithacus*) (*B*). (*Courtesy of* [A] Claire Grosset, med vet, IPSAV, CES, DACZM, Clinique vétérinaire de la Gare, Taverny, France; and [B] Zoological Medicine Service, Université de Montréal, Saint-Hyacinthe, Canada.)

form, but the vehicle and initial formulation may affect the pharmacokinetic parameters as well.[124] The effect of coated tablets is questionable in birds because the coating may be destroyed by the muscular gizzard.[10] As a general rule, for any species, a pharmacist should always be consulted if the original formulation of a medication needs to be altered for animal delivery (see Lauren V. Powers and Gigi Davidson's article, "Compounding and Extralabel Use of Drugs in Exotic Animal Medicine," in this issue). In ferrets and hedgehogs, the administration of bitter or unpalatable liquids can be difficult because they usually hypersalivate.[25] In hedgehogs, anointing behavior will result in drug spreading onto the spines.[3,4] Fruit-flavored medications may be more readily accepted in this species; thus, mixing the drug with fruit-flavored liquids such as grape juice may be considered. For ferrets, acceptance may generally be increased by adding beef, chicken and sweet flavors.[3,4] Certain drugs may cause dysbiosis when administered orally to hindgut fermenters, such as rabbits and myomorph rodents (eg, chinchillas and guinea pigs). This is the case for β-lactam antibiotics, clindamycin, erythromycin, and lincosamide (see Olivia A. Petritz and Sue Chen's article, "Therapeutic Contraindications in Exotic Pets," in this issue).[3] In pot-bellied pigs, forceful administration of drugs in the mouth may be complicated owing to poor animal compliance and sharp canines. However, the delivery of medication using apple sauce or fruit juices will generally be well-accepted.

In birds, drug delivery directly in the crop and, less commonly, the proventriculus may be indicated when a large volume needs to be administered or for specific drug administration such as amphotericin B in cases of *Macrorhabdus ornithogaster*.[125] The technique for gavage feeding in birds is presented in **Box 3** and illustrated in **Fig. 9**A.[1,10,126] Gastric gavage is rarely performed in small mammals. If needed for a single administration, gastric intubation techniques have been described using a red rubber or polyethylene catheter with a small mouth gag to prevent the animal from chewing the tube in most small mammals species.[1,27] A nasogastric tube may also be placed to deliver oral treatments in small mammals (discussed elsewhere in this article). Choosing a tube with a diameter exceeding the animal's tracheal diameter decreases the likelihood of inserting the tube into the trachea. The tube can be premeasured from the mouth to the last rib. Proper positioning of the tube may be verified by the observation of a negative pressure once the tube is in the esophagus, by palpation of the esophagus, and finally by instilling a few drops of water. If there is any doubt as to the appropriate positioning of the tube, radiographs should be performed. This technique should not be used for repeated dosing because of the associated risk of laryngeal and esophageal trauma.[3,25,119]

Syringe feeding can be performed quite easily in most lizard species. In leopard geckos (*Eublepharis macularius*), spontaneous opening of the oral cavity may be seen after rubbing of the side of the jaw. In certain lizards such as green iguanas, it is possible to elicit a vagal reflex by compressing the globes while pulling gently on the mandibular skin to open the jaw. Syringe feeding is difficult in snakes, which may not swallow, and in chelonians, which can withdraw their head into their carapace.[4,15] To prevent this maneuver, a chelonian's head should be gently grasped at the level of the quadrate bone.[127] The beak may be opened using a speculum of appropriate texture and size. It is sometimes easier to put the tube in the reptile's mouth before grasping its head because it generally has a more relaxed jaw when untouched.[127] The technique for tubing the stomach of reptiles is very similar to what is described in **Box 3** for birds, and is illustrated in **Fig. 9**B. The reptile should be held in an upright position to avoid regurgitation. Care must be taken not to traumatize the tomia of chelonians or the jaws of lizards with suspected secondary nutritional hyperparathyroidism with the tube or speculum.[1,2,4] In snakes, the tube should reach the

---

Box 3
Crop or proventricular gavage feeding in birds

- Calculate the volume of feeding formula to be administered (generally 25–50 mL/kg, with the lower end of this range used in adult large parrots).

- Use a ball-tipped metal feeding tube for psittacine birds (curved ones are generally more practical) or semirigid plastic or red rubber tube in nonpsittacine birds. Choose a large tube to avoid entering the trachea or carefully visualize the glottis.

- Warm up the gavage formula (at 39–40°C [102–105°F]) maximum to avoid crop burn) and palpate the crop to ensure it is empty.

- Estimate the tube's length required by evaluating the distance of the bird ventrum from the bill tip to the crop or proventriculus (depending on the target organ) and lubricate the exterior of tube.

- Extend the neck of the bird to minimize the risk of trauma during tube insertion.

- In psittacine birds, a speculum is not needed when using a metal feeding tube; once the tube is introduced in the pharynx, the bird will keep the beak open. The rhamphotheca of certain birds may be very fragile and tape strips held with tension may be used to open the beak without traumatizing it.

- Pass the tube near the left commissure of the beak toward the right side, laterally and dorsally to the glottis.

- Palpate the tip of the tube in the crop or the esophagus before administration. The trachea may be palpated independently to ensure the feeding tube is not inserted into it.

- If placing the tube directly into the proventriculus (sometimes used in raptors because their crop is less developed than in other bird species, or in case contrast medium is administered to birds with delayed crop emptying and regurgitations), take particular care to gently go through the cardia because the distal esophagus is thin walled and may be prone to perforation. If placing the tube into the crop, take care not to press on the crop while restraining the bird.

- Administer a feeding bolus while watching the inside of the oral cavity for regurgitation. If regurgitation occurs, remove the tube and release the bird to allow it to expel regurgitated formula and avoid aspiration. If the patient is too debilitated, hold the bird with the head down and swab the oral cavity to remove feeding formula.

- After completing administration, pinch the tube (if applicable) and remove it promptly from the oral cavity.

- Place the bird back in its cage or box with no further handling until the food has passed (unless it is really necessary because of a life-threatening situation).

---

stomach or caudal esophagus, which corresponds with the length from the snout to approximately one-third of the body's length.

Long-term oral drug administration: feeding tube placement

Long-term oral drug administration may be facilitated by the placement of a feeding tube directly in the stomach (or more rarely in the duodenum). The most common techniques used in exotic animals are nasogastric, pharyngostomy, and esophagostomy tube placement, although gastrostomy and duodenostomy tube placement have also been anecdotally reported in some species.[3,10] These tubes are typically placed when long-term nutritional support is required, tube feeding is difficult because the animal is not cooperative, when severe oral or pharyngeal pathology results in painful deglutition, or when head lesions prevent jaw movements.[16] The techniques for nasogastric or esophagostomy tube placement are similar to those described in small animals.[128] Nasogastric tube placement is most commonly used in anorectic rabbits

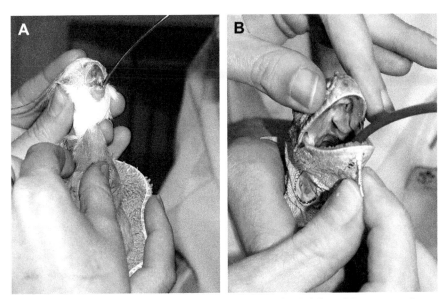

Fig. 9. Tube feeding in a cockatiel (*Nymphicus hollandicus*) (*A*) and in a green iguana (*Iguana iguana*) (*B*). (*Courtesy of* [*A, B*] Zoological Medicine Service, Université de Montréal, Saint-Hyacinthe, Canada.)

and usually requires local anesthesia and/or some form of sedation.[129] This procedure is well-tolerated in rabbits, who can eat with the tube in place. Potential complications include infection owing to nasal mucosa trauma and epistaxis.[27] Some authors discourage nasogastric tube placement because the stress associated with such a procedure may impair gastrointestinal motility, and because the use of an Elizabethan collar may be needed, thereby preventing caecotrophy.[3] Pharyngostomy and esophagostomy tubes have been described in rabbits and ferrets. Potential complications such as abscess formation at the placement site have been reported, particularly in rabbits.[27,52,130,131] In hedgehogs, even though the use of pharyngostomy or esophagostomy tube can seem problematic because of their curling behavior, it has been described with some success in 1 case report.[132] The placement of an esophagostomy tube has also been described in birds.[10,133,134] In reptiles, the technique is by far the most used in chelonians (**Fig. 10**).[1,4,15,79] Esophagostomy tubing is the only method allowing for consistent, long-term drug administration in chelonians owing to their anatomy (very small nostrils and the presence of the shell).[16] It is usually well-tolerated, does not require forceful opening of the beak, and the animal can still eat with the tube in place.[4] This technique can also be used in semiaquatic species if reducing their water exposure to avoid contamination of the tube entry point.[1] Semiaquatic species are typically dry-docked or provided with a low water depth reaching ventral to the tube entry point while the tube remains in place. In an experimental setting, the successful use of a duodenostomy catheter has been described in 5 pigeons, where it was used for 14 days without complications. Nevertheless, this technique should only be considered when upper gastrointestinal tract bypass is required.[135]

Transmucosal Drug Administration

The transmucosal route offers a practical route for drug delivery, thanks to the easy access to some mucosa. It is associated with rapid drug absorption owing to the

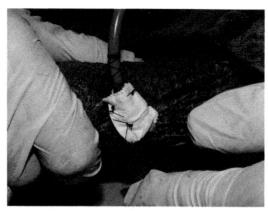

Fig. 10. Esophagostomy tube transcutaneous entrance site in a Desert tortoise (*Gopherus agassizii*). (*Courtesy of* the University of California, Davis.)

mucosal vascularization. The most common of these routes used in exotic veterinary medicine is the intranasal (IN) route followed by the sublingual and the intrarectal or intracloacal routes.

Intranasal route

In exotic medicine, the IN route is mostly used for sedation/anesthesia. In avian medicine, the delivery of small drug volumes directly into the nares is easy, pain free, and leads to rapid drug absorption (**Fig. 11**).[136] Numerous studies have investigated the effects of various sedation protocols using the IN route in avian species, which revealed this route to be as efficient, yielding even faster results than the traditional IM route, although higher dosages are typically required.[137–141] For instance, IN midazolam reversed with IN flumazenil is a commonly used protocol in birds. IN sedation with medetomidine and ketamine has also been studied in rabbits.[2,54] Some sedative effects was obtained, but 2 fatalities occurred in a recent study.[142] IN midazolam has been used by some authors for sedation in pot-bellied pigs with some success.[143] In chelonians, the IN route has also been tested[144,145]; however, there is little evidence that this route of drug administration is efficient in studies including a control group.[146] Of note, IN atipamezole yielded similar to effect as compared with IM and SC administration in red-eared sliders, but no control group was included in this study. The IN route can also be useful in the management of seizures with diazepam or midazolam if venous access is not readily available because IN transmucosal absorption exceeds IM uptake.[3] IN phenylephrine administration has been described to reduce nasal congestion caused by influenza in ferrets used as a model for human influenza.[147,148] Finally, this route was studied for analgesic agents such as tramadol; an injectable formulation has been shown to have increased bioavailability when administered IN compared with oral administration in rats (*Rattus norvegicus*).[149] Nevertheless, the IN delivery of drugs has limitations owing to the necessity to use only small volumes. Therefore, its practicality depends on the drug dose and concentration.[144] Moreover, irritant drugs should be avoided to prevent mucosal damage.[150]

Oral transmucosal route

The sublingual route is an underused route of drug delivery in exotic pet species. It is mostly used for anesthesia and analgesia in veterinary medicine. Buprenorphine is an

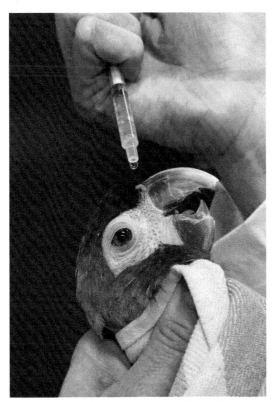

Fig. 11. Intranasal administration of midazolam in a yellow-collared macaw (*Primolius auricollis*). (*Courtesy of* Zoological Medicine Service, Université de Montréal, Saint-Hyacinthe, Canada.)

efficient sedative drug if delivered transmucosally to guinea pigs.[151] An oral transmucosal detomidine gel has also been used for sedation in ferrets and demonstrated some success.[152]

Intrarectal or intracloacal routes

Intrarectal or intracloacal routes can be used in exotic species for diazepam administration in seizure management when IV or IO access is not in place or difficult to establish. As stated, the absorption time is fast using this route.[3] Diazepam has also been used intracloacally in birds by the authors. Of note, use of the intracloacal route in chelonians for anesthesia has also been studied with unpredictable results.[153] Other treatment types, such as the use of benzimidazole intracloacally, is also described in chelonians.[4]

Another indication for this route is rehydration. Passive rehydration by cloacal absorption may be accomplished in chelonians by placing them in a warm bath. Active rehydration using a warm enema directly into the cloaca using a red rubber catheter is reported in chelonians, birds, and sugar gliders.[1–3,154] It is critical to avoid damaging the mucosal tissue during this procedure.

Administration of Medications into the Respiratory Tract

In the case of upper or lower respiratory disease, animals may benefit from drugs being administered directly into the respiratory tract. Three main techniques are used in exotic species that can be used to achieve this goal, namely (1) IN/intrasinusal administration for local action (as opposed to transmucosal administration as discussed elsewhere in this article), (2) direct application of the drug in either the trachea, lungs, or air sacs in birds, and (3) aerosol therapy with nebulization.

Intranasal and intrasinusal routes

In exotic species, nasal flush is mostly used in birds for the management of nasal or choanal infection. A nasal flush can be performed by holding the bird with the head lower than the body and flushing the medication (isotonic solution, drug) directly into the nasal cavity using a syringe with or without an adaptor pressed against each nostril. Fluids should exit through the opposite nare as well as the choana and mouth.[10,153] While flushing, the opposite nare may also be obstructed with a finger, which allows somewhat of a pressure buildup in the nasal cavity before the fluid exits through the choana (**Fig. 12**). In general, 1 to 3 mL per nostril are used for flushing in small birds and up to 10 to 15 mL for large species. One author also mentions the possible use of ophthalmic preparations administered intranasally to treat nasal infections.[155] Sinusal flush is typically performed under sedation holding the bird in an upright position with the head secured.[10] The needle is inserted between the commissure of the beak and the medial canthus of the eye directed with a 45° angle under the zygomatic arch with the beak held open.[10] In small mammals, a sinusal tube may be placed during rhinotomy to allow repeated sinusal flush and drug delivery for managing chronic rhinitis.[156] A ciprofloxacin gel has shown promising pharmacokinetic results when administrated intranasally for the treatment of rhinosinusitis in rats.[157]

Intratracheal route

The intratracheal route is most notably used for the administration of epinephrine, or atropine for cardiorespiratory resuscitation when venous access is difficult or would take too long to obtain.[3,4,18,52,77,103,126] The trachea is visualized and can be entered with an endotracheal tube, an IV catheter, or a small diameter metal feeding needle.[10] In salamanders, the trachea is short, so care should be taken not to insert the administration device too far and damage the pulmonic epithelium.[18] In rats, the most efficient

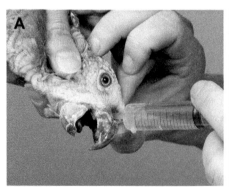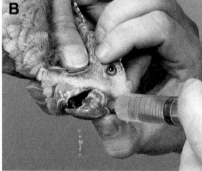

Fig. 12. Nasal flush in a blue fronted Amazon parrot (*Amazona aestiva*). For this procedure, the patient is tilted upside down to prevent water from running into the trachea. After applying a syringe filled with sterile, lukewarm saline in one of the nares, the saline is forcefully flushed into the nasal passage while the other nare simultaneously can be held closed with a finger (*A*). Often, material leaks out of the choanal slit, which may subsequently be collected for further workup (*B*) (eg, cytology, culture, and sensitivity testing). (*Courtesy of* Yvonne van Zeeland, DVM, MVR, PhD, DECZM (Avian, Small mammal), CPBC University of Utrecht.)

and safest method for intratracheal drug administration is high-speed administration with the animal restrained in a head up position.[158] The use of this route has also been described for local antiinfectious treatment, especially in the treatment of tracheal or syringeal aspergillomas in birds. Endoscopically guided administration of the drug directly onto the lesion under anesthesia is optimal, but blind administration is also possible under sedation, especially if an air sac cannula is in place for enhanced safety.[159] A recent study has shown amphotericin B can achieve therapeutic concentration for 9 days in 1 lung lobe, and for 24 hours hours in the contralateral lung lobe after intratracheal administration at 3 mg/kg in mallard ducks (*Anas platyrhynchos*).[160]

Intrapneumonic and air sac delivery routes
In reptiles, techniques have also been described to deliver the drug directly into the lung in case of focal disease via a catheter surgically positioned within the lesion.[1,15] Because nonavian reptiles have no need for negative pressure to enable their lungs to be functional, this procedure is well-tolerated and does not impact their breathing. In chelonians, the procedure requires the drilling of a hole into the shell over the desired location in the lung.[161] For 1-shot therapy in chelonians, injection into the lungs via the inguinal fossa has also been described.[162] The intrapneumonic approach has also been described in sedated amphibians. After checking anatomic landmarks with transillumination or imaging (radiographs or ultrasound examination), treatment may be administered in the lung with a small gauge needle using a caudolateral approach.[4,18] Endoscopically assisted drug administration into the avian lungs and air sacs is also described in case of aspergillomas.[163]

Nebulization
As in domestic animals, nebulization therapy enables drug delivery to the respiratory tissue directly by using a nebulizer to compress air and convert liquid formulations into a fog that is breathed by the animal.[27] This delivery method allows to achieve high local drug concentration for maximal effects while limiting absorption, thus reducing the systemic toxicity of the drug.[1,9,27] The reduced systemic absorption after nebulization has been studied for several drugs in birds through pharmacokinetic studies showing low plasma concentration for small durations.[164–168] Some authors have brought together dosages and frequencies of administration for the main drugs used for nebulization in exotic species, which can also applied for IN route.[10,169,170] Nebulization potentially enables to reach diseased tissue with decreased vascularization or poorly perfused respiratory structures such as the avian air sacs. However, in cases with considerable airway congestion, the drug may not reach the tissues with severe lesions.[10] Another goal of nebulization is to enhance the clearance of exudates and other debris. This maneuver is especially useful in reptiles that lack ciliated epithelial lining and mucociliary escalator in their respiratory tract, thus decreasing their ability to expel foreign material and exudates.[15] In reptiles, the use of acetylcysteine may help mucous to break down and maximize the distribution and epithelial contact of the drug.[15] Nebulizers used in cats may be applied to similar sized exotic species, such as rabbits. Furthermore, nebulization can be performed without handling the patient, thus reducing stress, which is paramount when dealing with fragile exotic patients with respiratory difficulties.[1] In birds, it is also possible to nebulize a drug directly in the air sacs using an air sac cannula, if indicated. Because some nebulized drugs may be irritating and induce bronchospasm, the nebulization chamber should allow for the visualization of the animal during the entire procedure.[9,15,27] Nebulization has also been described in amphibians, but cases of deaths have been reported; it remains unknown whether

the drug dose or the nebulization procedure itself were responsible for the fatal outcome in these cases.[4,18]

The success of nebulization therapy depends on the particle size, with recommendations varying across species. The smaller the nebulized particles, the more likely they will reach the deeper sections of the respiratory tract.[8] In rabbits, a particle size of less than 5 microns has been shown to penetrate the narrow branches of the lower airways.[171,172] Similar recommendations have been made by some authors in reptiles to be able to penetrate the tertiary falveoli/ediculae of their lungs.[15] Studies about the effect of nebulization have been performed in pigeons and chickens.[173–175] For microspheres smaller than 5 μm in diameter, there was a significant increase in lower airway deposition and these particles were able to reach lower respiratory tract in 2- to 4-week-old chickens.[173] Thus, nebulization with a particle size of less than 3 μm was recommended.[173] In contrast, microspheres up to 20 μm in size have been shown to reach the air sacs of 1-day-old chicks, possibly owing to open-beak breathing.[173] When using a nebulizer producing particles measuring 1 μm in diameter (Acorn II, Marquest Medical Products, Inc, Englewood, CO), nebulization had to be performed for at least 2 hours to result in detectable amounts of particles in pigeons' air sacs.[175] The vehicle used for drug administration through nebulization may also be important; in pigeons, saline resulted in greater diffusion into the air sacs than propylene glycol, with some air sac diffusion being detectable after only 30 minutes of nebulization with the saline vehicle.[174] The type of nebulizer used should also be adapted to the nature of the vehicle; compressor nebulizers will have a greater ability to nebulize viscous liquids such as heavy lipidic fluids than ultrasonic nebulizers.[9] There are no well-established protocols for nebulization in exotic animals, but most authors recommend 10 to 30 minutes per session 1 to 3 times a day.[9,10,15,27] However, the duration of the nebulization's session may be underestimated in birds when using lipophilic vehicles, as it is mostly the case for antifungal drugs.[175]

There is a growing interest in veterinary medicine for the use of metered dose inhalers as an alternative to nebulization. This technique proved respiratory tract deposition of inhalant medications in dogs.[176] However, its use in exotic pet medicine remains anecdotical and studies are required before it can be recommended (**Fig. 13**).

DRUG ADMINISTRATION VIA TOPICAL ROUTES
Transcutaneous Absorption

As in companion animals, antiparasitic spot-on can be used in a similar way with the same application method in small mammals.[3,27,177] The exact dosage and toxicity in the target species should always be verified. In birds, spot-on therapies have been

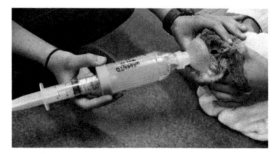

Fig. 13. Use of a metered dose inhaler in a rabbit (*Oryctolagus cuniculus*). (*Courtesy of* the University of California, Davis.)

described for ivermectin and selamectin with the drug being applied over the apteric skin overlying the jugular veins near the thoracic inlet.[1,10,154,178,179] Some spot-on formulations have also been shown to pass the thick skin of several reptile species.[180–183] Transdermal administration through patches has been described in several exotic species, such as rabbits, chicken, prehensile-tailed skinks (*Corucia zebrata*), ball pythons (*P regius*), and terrestrial amphibians, with promising results in terms of analgesia and innocuity.[3,27,103,182–185] In rabbits, the patch showed optimal efficiency when the hair was clipped instead of chemically depilated or left in place. When using this route of administration, the animal should be monitored closely to ensure it does not eat the patch, and maintains body weight, because weight loss was reported after the use of fentanyl patches in rabbits.[3] When using the smallest patch size in very light species, it is possible to remove the patch sticky cover only partially to deliver a partial dose. A patch should never be cut down, because this may result in increased delivery of the drug through the cut surface.

The amphibians constitute a family in which transdermal drug administration has the greatest potential because their skin is highly permeable.[1,18] By this route, all kinds of drugs can be administered, from antimicrobial drugs to anesthetic drugs and fluid therapy. The transdermal administration of drugs in amphibians can be accomplished in 2 ways, that is, either by applying the drug directly onto the skin or by bathing (**Fig. 14**). Some anesthetic gels with isoflurane or sevoflurane as well as some antimicrobial drugs have been successfully and safely used in amphibians through this route.[4,186–188] It should be emphasized that applying nontested drugs directly onto the skin of amphibians is not recommended because several excipients used in other route preparations can be irritating to the amphibian's skin and highly concentrated preparations (eg, ophthalmic drops) may easily result in overdosing. In any case, the amphibian should be monitored closely after application.[1,18] Bathing may be used in amphibians to rehydrate, remove excess fluid, induce anesthesia, or treat infectious diseases.[1,2,189,190] Typically, the ventrum of the animal is immersed in the bath.[18] Because handling of the animal is not required, the technique can be highly advantageous to use. However, the amount of drug absorbed is unclear most of the time.[118] The temperature and pH of the solution should be monitored because brutal changes in these parameters can induce adverse effects and mortality in amphibians and weak animals should be observed closely to prevent drowning.[1,4] In some cases, the drug can be added directly in the tank of aquatic species; however, this approach may damage the biological and chemical filtration system and requires frequent water changes.[18] Transcutaneous drug administration is, therefore, a very useful technique in amphibians, but necessitates close monitoring of the animal and prerequisite innocuity testing of a substance before its use.

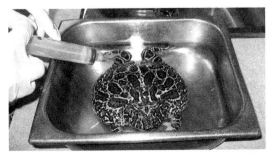

Fig. 14. Medicated bath given to an Argentine horned frog (*Ceratophrys ornata*). (*Courtesy of* Zoological Medicine Service, Université de Montréal, Saint-Hyacinthe, Canada.)

Topical Treatments

The principles, advantages, and disadvantages of topical medication administration in exotic animals can be extrapolated from other species. Topical treatment options include cutaneous, ocular, and intraauricular, as well as intralesional (eg, on wounds or in abscesses).[3,9,103,191] The dose and potential toxicity of the drug need to be evaluated carefully in the target species, especially those in which grooming comprises an important part of their daily routine, such as rabbits, rodents, hedgehogs, and birds, because they can ingest the drug in the process.[3,4,10,192] Potential toxicity is also an issue in species with very thin skin, such as birds, because an undesirable transdermal absorption of drugs may take place. This phenomenon has been described extensively after the use of a topical preparation containing corticosteroids, which led to adverse effects including death.[9,126] It should be noted that, for anatomic reasons, intraauricular treatment cannot be used in reptiles and fish unless myringotomy has been performed beforehand and that intraocular treatment is not possible in sauropsidae with spectacles unless their spectacle has been incised.[4] In fish, topical drug administration is different, given their aquatic environment, which prevents the adherence of topical preparation onto external sites. Topical treatments are most commonly used in fish medicine for external parasites and cutaneous infection.[4,22] It is not of particular use to address internal pathology, because the drug rarely reaches therapeutic levels in targeted tissues.[4,22] Two approaches may be considered: (1) bath treatment by placing the fish in a medicated tank for a short time exposure, and (2) tank/pond treatment by adding the drug directly into the fish's environment (see Claire D. Erlacher-Reid's article, "Considerations for Treatment of Large Zoological Collections: Fish," in this issue).[22] During treatment, the fish should always be monitored closely and placed back in fresh water in case adverse effects or obvious signs of distress are seen.[4,22] Disadvantages of the bath treatment include the added stress of catching the fish and the short time exposure to the treatment. In contrast, drugs introduced in the usual environment can harm the biological filter and increase the risk of environmental pathogens developing resistance to the drug used.[4] Because the efficacy of the treatment can be altered by several water parameters and organic material, the water quality should be monitored.

The topical route is also widely used in wound management in exotic animals. As mentioned, the same rules for wound management in companion animals can be applied to exotic species. The tendency of some species such as rodents, hedgehogs or psittacines to self-investigate wound site complicates management and increases the risk for toxicity owing to oral uptake. Restriction methods such as an Elizabethan collar or stockinette cotton tubular bandage are sometimes needed, but should be used as a last resort and adjunct sedation may be beneficial.[4,10] The veterinarian should ensure that the animal is able to self-feed before being discharged. In reptiles, topical dressing on wounds also can be beneficial. However, a comparative study showed mixed results, that is, some dressings (eg, occlusive polyurethane film) produced good results, whereas some others (eg, antibiotic ointment) were found to be of little value in wound models.[193] In another study in red eared sliders, the application of topical insulin on experimentally created wounds was shown to accelerate wound contraction, and to enhance epithelialization, collagen synthesis, and remodeling of the wound. Topical insulin also downregulated the inflammatory response in this study.[194] However, this last technique cannot be recommended at this time because of the unknown effect of insulin on a potentially contaminated or infected wound, and should be first tested

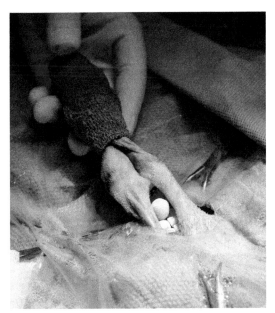

Fig. 15. Antibiotic impregnated polymethylmethacrylate beads in the abscess cavity at the ear base of a rabbit (*Oryctolagus cuniculus*). (*Courtesy of* Zoological Medicine Service, Université de Montréal, Saint-Hyacinthe, Canada.)

on nonexperimental wounds. In turtles, water exposure should be limited during wound management. However, turtles may be left in the water if an occlusive waterproof system is used.[195] In amphibians, bandages or classic topical antibiotics are of little value and can even be toxic given the extreme permeability of the amphibian skin. However, the local application of hypertonic saline or baths in electrolyte solutions offers some kind of wound antiseptic and temporary liquid bandages (such as products used in dentistry) can provide a barrier against osmotic loss and wound protection.[4,15,196] Finally, in fish, a wound should generally be treated open with surgical debridement under anesthesia and can be packed with a protective sealant, because suturing is frequently impractical owing to skin tension. Povidone-iodine or potassium permanganate bath can be used for disinfection.[1,23]

The use of antibiotic-impregnated polymethylmethacrylate beads may be considered, in the management of deeper contaminated wounds, abscesses, pododermatitis, osteomyelitis, otitis media, or arthritis in most exotic species (except fish and amphibians).[1,3,4,15,27,126,154,162,191,197] After wound closure, gradual but continued antibiotic elution may occur for several days up to weeks (**Fig. 15**). Except when used to treat arthritis, the beads usually do not need to be removed unless they serve as a nidus for recurrent infection.[15,126] One of the advantages of this drug delivery method is that it results in high localized concentrations, thereby enabling the use of antibiotics that could be toxic if given systemically. This property is in particular valuable in hindgut fermenters species, provided that the location does not allow the animal to ingest the antibiotic, such as can be the case with dental abscesses.[3,27] In these patients, antimicrobial impregnated gauze packing may be considered as an alternative, as has been described in rabbits.[198]

SUMMARY

Drug delivery in exotic species comes with several challenges for the general practitioner. Knowledge of the basic anatomy and physiology of each treated species is essential to choosing the most appropriate route and technique for treatment delivery. Mastering the manual and chemical restraint techniques is also fundamental to be able to optimally apply these techniques with the least risk of (iatrogenic) complications. Finally, whenever treating an exotic species, practitioners are recommended to review the current literature so that this information can be included in their decision-making process and prioritize treatment options based on the availability of pharmacokinetic, pharmacodynamic, effectiveness, and safety studies in the species of interest.

REFERENCES

1. Meredith A, Redrobe S. BSAVA manual of exotic pets. 4th edition. Gloucester: British Small Animal Veterinary Association; 2002.
2. Longley L. Anaesthesia of exotic pets. 1st edition. St Louis (MO): Saunders Elsevier; 2008.
3. Quesenberry KE, Carpenter JW. Ferrets, rabbits and rodents clinical medicine and surgery. 3rd edition. St Louis (MO): Saunders Elsevier; 2012.
4. Mitchell MA, Tully TN. Manual of exotic pet practice. 1st edition. St Louis (MO): Saunders Elsevier; 2009.
5. Johnson-Delaney CA. Common procedures in hedgehogs, prairie dogs, exotic rodents, and companion marsupials. Vet Clin North Am Exot Anim Pract 2006; 9(2):415–35.
6. Braun WF, Casteel SW. Potbellied pigs miniature porcine pets. Vet Clin North Am Small Anim Pract 1993;23(6):1149–77.
7. Hodgkinson O. Practical sedation and anaesthesia in pigs. Practice 2007;29(1): 34–9.
8. Lisle G. Veterinary management of pot-bellied pigs. 1st edition. Davis (CA): School of Veterinary Medicine University of California; 1998.
9. Beaufrère H, Perlman J, Bailey TA, et al. Medical, nursing, and cosmetic procedures. In: Samour J, editor. Avian medicine. 3rd edition. St Louis (MO): Elsevier; 2016. p. 204–45.
10. Dorrestein GM. Nursing the sick bird. In: Tully TN, Dorrestein GM, Jones AK, editors. Handbook of avian medicine. 2nd edition. Oxford (UK): Butterworth Heinemann Elsevier; 2000. p. 74–111.
11. Curro TG. Anesthesia of pet birds. In: Seminars in avian and exotic pet medicine, vol. 7. St Louis (MO): Elsevier; 1998. p. 10–21.
12. Steinohrt LA. Avian fluid therapy. J Avian Med Surg 1999;13(2):83–91.
13. Ratliff CM, Zaffarano BA. Therapeutic use of regional limb perfusion in a chicken. J Avian Med Surg 2017;31(1):29–32.
14. King AS, McLelland J. Skeletomuscular system. In: King AS, McLelland J, editors. Birds, their structure and function, vol. 1, 2nd edition. Eastbourne (UK): Baillière Tindall; 1984. p. 43–78.
15. Mitchell MA. Therapeutics. In: Divers S, Mader D, editors. Reptile medicine and surgery. 2nd edition. St Louis (MO): Saunders Elsevier; 2006. p. 631–64.
16. Chitty J, Raftery A. Basic techniques. In: Chitty J, Raftery A, editors. Essentials of tortoise medicine and surgery. 1st edition. Oxford (UK): Wiley Blackwell; 2013. p. 80–113.

17. Doss GA, Fink DM, Sladky KK, et al. Comparison of subcutaneous dexmedeto-midine– midazolam versus alfaxalone–midazolam sedation in leopard geckos (Eublepharis macularius). Vet Anaesth Analg 2017;44(5):1175–83.
18. Whitaker BR, Wright KM. Clinical techniques. In: Wright KM, Whitaker BR, editors. Amphibian medicine and captive husbandry. 1st edition. Malabar (FL): Krieger Publishing Company; 2001. p. 89–110.
19. Fredholm DV, Mylniczenko ND, KuKanich B. Pharmacokinetic evaluation of meloxicam after intravenous and intramuscular administration in Nile tilapia (*Oreochromis niloticus*). J Zoo Wildl Med 2016;47(3):736–42.
20. Rigos G, Katharios P, Papandroulakis N. Single intramuscular administration of long-acting oxytetracycline in grouper (*Epinephelus marginatus*). Turk J Vet Anim Sci 2011;34(5):441–5.
21. Ross LG, Ross B. Anaesthesia of fish: III. Parenteral and oral anaesthesia. In: Ross LG, Ross B, editors. Anaesthetic and sedative techniques for aquatic animals. 3rd edition. Oxford (UK): Blackwell Publishing; 2008. p. 137–49.
22. Noga EJ. General concepts in therapy. In: Noga EJ, editor. Fish disease diagnosis and treatment. 2nd edition. Ames (IA): Wiley Blackwell; 2010. p. 347–73.
23. Churgin SM, Musgrave KE, Cox SK, et al. Pharmacokinetics of subcutaneous versus intramuscular administration of ceftiofur crystalline-free acid to bearded dragons (*Pogona vitticeps*). Am J Vet Res 2014;75(5):453–9.
24. Sinclair KM, Church ME, Farver TB, et al. Effects of meloxicam on hematologic and plasma biochemical analysis variables and results of histologic examination of tissue specimens of Japanese quail (*Coturnix japonica*). Am J Vet Res 2012;73(11):1720–7.
25. Williams BH. Therapeutics in ferrets. Vet Clin North Am Exot Anim Pract 2000;3(1):131–53.
26. Sharma V, McNeill JH. To scale or not to scale: the principles of dose extrapolation. Br J Pharmacol 2009;157(6):907–21.
27. Varga M. Rabbit basic science. In: Varga M, editor. Textbook of rabbit medicine. 2nd edition. Oxford (UK): Butterworth Heinemann Elsevier; 2014. p. 3–108.
28. Stoskopf MK. Anatomy. In: Stoskopf MK, editor. Fish medicine, vol. 1, 2nd edition. Baltimore (MD): ART Sciences LLC; 2010. p. 2–30.
29. Dzialowski EM, Crossley DA. The cardiovascular system. In: Scanes C, editor. Sturkie's avian physiology. 6th edition. London: Elsevier; 2015. p. 193–283.
30. Holz P. Renal anatomy and physiology. In: Divers S, Mader D, editors. Reptile medicine and surgery. 2nd edition. St Louis (MO): Saunders Elsevier; 2006. p. 135–44.
31. Benson KG, Forrest L. Characterization of the renal portal system of the common green iguana (*Iguana iguana*) by digital subtraction imaging. J Zoo Wildl Med 1999;30(2):235–41.
32. Beck K, Loomis M, Lewbart G, et al. Preliminary comparison of plasma concentrations of gentamicin injected into the cranial and caudal limb musculature of the eastern box turtle (*Terrapene carolina carolina*). J Zoo Wildl Med 1995;26(2):265–8.
33. Holz P, Barker IK, Burger JP, et al. The effect of the renal portal system on pharmacokinetic parameters in the red-eared slider (*Trachemys scripta elegans*). J Zoo Wildl Med 1997;28:386–93.
34. Kummrow MS, Tseng F, Hesse L, et al. Pharmacokinetics of buprenorphine after single-dose subcutaneous administration in red-eared sliders (*Trachemys scripta elegans*). J Zoo Wildl Med 2008;39(4):590–5.

35. Scheelings TF. Use of intravenous and intramuscular alfaxalone in Macquarie river turtles (*Emydura macquarii*). J Herp Med Surg 2013;23(3–4):91–4.
36. Zimmerman DM, Armstrong DL, Curro TG, et al. Pharmacokinetics of florfenicol after a single intramuscular dose in white-spotted bamboo sharks (*Chiloscyllium plagiosum*). J Zoo Wildl Med 2006;37(2):165–73.
37. Schroeder CA, Johnson RA. The efficacy of intracoelomic fospropofol in red-eared sliders (*Trachemys scripta elegans*). J Zoo Wildl Med 2013;44(4):941–50.
38. Lewbart GA, Butkus DA, Papich MG, et al. Evaluation of a method of intracoelomic catheterization in koi. J Am Vet Med Assoc 2005;226(5):784–8.
39. Grosset C, Weber ES, Gehring R, et al. Evaluation of an extended-release formulation of ceftiofur crystalline-free acid in koi (*Cyprinus carpio*). J Vet Pharmacol Ther 2015;38(6):606–15.
40. Williams AM, Wyatt JD. Comparison of subcutaneous and intramuscular ketamine–medetomidine with and without reversal by atipamezole in Dutch belted rabbits (*Oryctolagus cuniculus*). J Am Assoc Lab Anim Sci 2007;46(6):16–20.
41. Fernandez-Varon E, Marin P, Escudero E, et al. Pharmacokinetic–pharmacodynamic integration of danofloxacin after intravenous, intramuscular and subcutaneous administration to rabbits. J Vet Pharmacol Ther 2007;30(1):18–24.
42. Marín P, Álamo LF, Escudero E, et al. Pharmacokinetics of marbofloxacin in rabbit after intravenous, intramuscular, and subcutaneous administration. Res Vet Sci 2013;94(3):698–700.
43. Ranheim B, Ween H, Egeli AK, et al. Benzathine penicillin G and procaine penicillin G in piglets: comparison of intramuscular and subcutaneous injection. Vet Res Commun 2002;26(6):459–65.
44. De Lucas J, Solano J, González F, et al. Pharmacokinetics of enrofloxacin after multiple subcutaneous and intramuscular administrations in adult ostriches. Br Poult Sci 2013;54(3):391–7.
45. Guzman DS-M, Knych HK, Olsen GH, et al. Pharmacokinetics of a sustained release formulation of buprenorphine after intramuscular and subcutaneous administration to American kestrels (*Falco sparverius*). J Avian Med Surg 2017;31(2):102–7.
46. Abu-Basha EA, Idkaidek NM, Al-Shunnaq AF. Comparative pharmacokinetics of gentamicin after intravenous, intramuscular, subcutaneous and oral administration in broiler chickens. Vet Res Commun 2007;31(6):765–73.
47. Benson KG, Tell LA, Young LA, et al. Pharmacokinetics of ceftiofur sodium after intramuscular or subcutaneous administration in green iguanas (*Iguana iguana*). Am J Vet Res 2003;64(10):1278–82.
48. Marín P, Bayón A, Fernández-Varón E, et al. Pharmacokinetics of danofloxacin after single dose intravenous, intramuscular and subcutaneous administration to loggerhead turtles *Caretta caretta*. Dis Aquat Organ 2008;82:231–6.
49. Lahner LL, Mans C, Sladky KK. Comparison of anesthetic induction and recovery times after intramuscular, subcutaneous or intranasal dexmedetomidineketamine administration in red-eared slider turtles (Trachemys scripta elegans). In: Proceedings of the American Association of Zoo Veterinarians (AAZV). Kansas City (MO): 2011. p. 136–7.
50. Shan Q, Zhu X, Liu S, et al. Pharmacokinetics of cefquinome in tilapia (*Oreochromis niloticus*) after a single intramuscular or intraperitoneal administration. J Vet Pharmacol Ther 2015;38(6):601–5.
51. Briscoe JA, Syring R. Techniques for emergency airway and vascular access in special species. Sem Avian Exotic Pet Med 2004;13(3):118–31.

52. Orcutt CJ. Emergency and critical care of ferrets. Vet Clin North Am Exot Anim Pract 1998;1(1):99–126.
53. Lennox AM. Intraosseous catheterization of exotic animals. J Exotic Pet Med 2008;17(4):300–6.
54. Varga M. Anaesthesia and analgesia. In: Varga M, editor. Textbook of rabbit medicine. 2nd edition. Oxford (UK): Butterworth Heinemann Elsevier; 2014. p. 178–202.
55. Lennox AM. Emergency and critical care procedures in sugar gliders (*Petaurus breviceps*), African hedgehogs (*Atelerix albiventris*), and prairie dogs (*Cynomys spp*). Vet Clin North Am Exot Anim Pract 2007;10(2):533–55.
56. Snook CS. Use of the subcutaneous abdominal vein for blood sampling and intravenous catheterization in potbellied pigs. J Am Vet Med Assoc 2001; 219(6):809–10.
57. O'Malley B. Clinical anatomy and physiology of exotic species. 1st edition. London: Saunders Elsevier; 2005.
58. Stringfield C. The California condor (Gymnogyps californianus) veterinary program: 1997-2000. In: Miller RE, Fowler M, editors. Fowler's zoo and wildlife animal medicine current therapy. 7th edition. St Louis (MO): Saunders Elsevier; 2012. p. 186–96.
59. Andreani G, Carpenè E, Cannavacciuolo A, et al. Reference values for hematology and plasma biochemistry variables, and protein electrophoresis of healthy Hermann's tortoises (*Testudo hermanni ssp.*). Vet Clin Pathol 2014;43(4): 573–83.
60. Young BD, Stegeman N, Norby B, et al. Comparison of intraosseous and peripheral venous fluid dynamics in the desert tortoise (*Gopherus agassizii*). J Zoo Wildl Med 2012;43(1):59–66.
61. McFadden MS, Bennett RA, Reavill DR, et al. Clinical and histologic effects of intracardiac administration of propofol for induction of anesthesia in ball pythons (*Python regius*). J Am Vet Med Assoc 2011;239(6):803–7.
62. Perry SM, Joslyn S, Mitchell MA. Why stick a needle in the heart when a jugular will do? Developing a consistent approach for jugular venipuncture in the snake. In: Proceedings of the American Exotic Mammal Veterinarians (AEMV) and Association of Reptilian and Amphibian Veterinarians (ARAV). Dallas (TX): 2017. p. 89.
63. Forzán MJ, Vanderstichel RV, Ogbuah CT, et al. Blood collection from the facial (maxillary)/musculo-cutaneous vein in true frogs (family Ranidae). J Wildl Dis 2012;48(1):176–80.
64. Bakal RS, Harms CA, Khoo LH, et al. Sinus venosus catheterization for repeated vascular access in the hybrid striped bass. J Aquat Anim Health 1999;11(2): 187–91.
65. Horsberg TE. Experimental methods for pharmacokinetic studies in salmonids. Annu Rev Fish Dis 1994;4:345–58.
66. Di Ianni F, Parmigiani E, Pelizzone I, et al. Comparison between intramuscular and intravenous administration of oxytocin in captive-bred red-eared sliders (*Trachemys scripta elegans*) with nonobstructive egg retention. J Exotic Pet Med 2014;23(1):79–84.
67. Pardo MA, Divers S. Jugular central venous catheter placement through a modified Seldinger technique for long-term venous access in chelonians. J Zoo Wildl Med 2016;47(1):286–90.
68. Bercier M, Giglio RF, Winter MD, et al. Limitations and impacts of the renal portal system on the determination of the glomerular filtration rate using contrast-

enhanced computed tomography and plasma clearance of iohexol in bearded dragons (*Pogona viticeps*). In: Poster at the American Association of Zoo Veterinarians (AAZV). Dallas (TX): 2017.

69. Lamberski N, Daniel GB. Fluid dynamics of intraosseous fluid administration in birds. J Zoo Wildl Med 1992;23(1):47–54.

70. Aguilar RF, Johnston GR, Callfos CJ, et al. Osseous-venous and central circulatory transit times of technetium-99m pertechnetate in anesthetized raptors following intraosseous administration. J Zoo Wildl Med 1993;24(4):488–97.

71. Maxwell LK, Jacobson ER. Allometric scaling of kidney function in green iguanas. Comp Biochem Physiol A Mol Integr Physiol 2004;138(3):383–90.

72. Spivey WH, Lathers CM, Malone DR, et al. Comparison of intraosseous, central, and peripheral routes of sodium bicarbonate administration during CPR in pigs. Ann Emerg Med 1985;14(12):1135–40.

73. Andropoulos DB, Solfer SJ, Schreiber MD. Plasma epinephrine concentrations after intraosseous and central venous injection during cardiopulmonary resuscitation in the lamb. J Pediatr 1990;116(2):312–5.

74. Hallas P, Brabrand M, Folkestad L. Complication with intraosseous access: Scandinavian users' experience. West J Emerg Med 2013;14(5):440–3.

75. American Veterinary Medical Association. AVMA guidelines for the euthanasia of animals. Schaumburg (IL): AVMA; 2013.

76. Swindle MM, Nolan T, Jacobson A, et al. Vascular access port (VAP) usage in large animal species. J Am Assoc Lab Anim Sci 2005;44(3):7–17.

77. Marini RP. Physical examination, preventive medicine, and diagnosis in the ferret. In: Marini RP, Fox JG, editors. Biology and diseases of the ferret. 3rd edition. Oxford (UK): Wiley Blackwell; 2014. p. 235–58.

78. Doneley RJT, Smith BA, Gibson JS. Use of a vascular access port for antibiotic administration in the treatment of pododermatitis in a chicken. J Avian Med Surg 2015;29(2):130–5.

79. Folland DW, Johnston MS, Thamm DH, et al. Diagnosis and management of lymphoma in a green iguana (*Iguana iguana*). J Am Vet Med Assoc 2011;239(7): 985–91.

80. Skeeles JK, Swafford WS, Wages DP, et al. Studies on the use of a long-acting oxytetracycline in turkeys: serum levels and tissue residues following injection. Avian Dis 1985;29(1):145.

81. Helmick KE, Papich MG, Vliet KA, et al. Pharmacokinetic disposition of a long-acting oxytetracycline formulation after single-dose intravenous and intramuscular administration in the American alligator (*Alligator mississippiensis*). J Zoo Wildl Med 2004;35(3):341–6.

82. Flammer K, Aucoin DP, Whitt DA, et al. Potential use of long-acting injectable oxytetracycline for treatment of chlamydiosis in Goffin's cockatoos. Avian Dis 1990;34(1):228.

83. Sladky KK, Krugner-Higby L, Meek-Walker E, et al. Serum concentrations and analgesic effects of liposome-encapsulated and standard butorphanom tartrate in parrots. Am J Vet Res 2006;67(5):775–81.

84. Paul-Murphy J, Sladky KK, Krugner-Higby LA, et al. Analgesic effects of carprofen and liposome-encapsulated butorphanol tartrate in Hispanolian parrots (*Amazona ventralis*) with experimentally induced arthritis. Am J Vet Res 2009;70(10): 1201–10.

85. Wojick KB, Langan JN, Adkesson MJ, et al. Pharmacokinetics of long-acting ceftiofur crystalline-free acid in helmeted guineafowl (*Numida meleagris*) after a single intramuscular injection. Am J Vet Res 2011;72(11):1514–8.

86. Hope KL, Tell LA, Byrne BA, et al. Pharmacokinetics of a single intramuscular injection of ceftiofur crystalline-free acid in American black ducks (*Anas rubripes*). Am J Vet Res 2012;73(5):620–7.

87. Paul-Murphy J, Krugner-Higby LA, Tourdot RL, et al. Evaluation of liposome-encapsulated butorphanol tartrate for alleviation of experimentally induced arthritic pain in green-cheeked conures (*Pyrrhura molinae*). Am J Vet Res 2009;70(10):1211–9.

88. Gleeson MD, Guzman DSM, Knych HK, et al. Pharmacokinetics of a concentrated buprenorphine formulation in red-tailed hawks (*Buteo jamaicensis*). In: Proceedings of the American Association of Zoo Veterinarians (AAZV). Dallas (TX): 2017. p. 24–5.

89. Smith BJ, Wegenast DJ, Hansen RJ, et al. Pharmacokinetics and paw withdrawal pressure in female guinea pigs (*Cavia porcellus*) treated with sustained-release buprenorphine and buprenorphine hydrochloride. J Am Assoc Lab Anim Sci 2016;55(6):789–93.

90. Schoemaker NJ, van Deijk R, Muijlaert B, et al. Use of a gonadotropin releasing hormone agonist implant as an alternative for surgical castration in male ferrets (*Mustela putorius furo*). Theriogenology 2008;70(2):161–7.

91. Johnson-Delaney CA. Medical therapies for ferret adrenal disease. Sem Avian Exotic Pet Med 2004;13(1):3–7.

92. Schoemaker NJ, Kuijten AM, Galac S. Luteinizing hormone-dependent Cushing's syndrome in a pet ferret (*Mustela putorius furo*). Domest Anim Endocrinol 2008;34(3):278–83.

93. Wagner RA, Finkler MR, Fecteau KA, et al. The treatment of adrenal cortical disease in ferrets with 4.7-mg deslorelin acetate implants. J Exotic Pet Med 2009; 18(2):146–52.

94. Wagner RA, Piché CA, Jöchle W, et al. Clinical and endocrine responses to treatment with deslorelin acetate implants in ferrets with adrenocortical disease. Am J Vet Res 2005;66(5):910–4.

95. Wagner RA, Bailey EM, Schneider JF, et al. Leuprolide acetate treatment of adrenocortical disease in ferrets. J Am Vet Med Assoc 2001;218(8):1272–4.

96. Grosset C, Peters S, Peron F, et al. Contraceptive effect and potential side-effects of deslorelin acetate implants in rats (*Rattus norvegicus*): preliminary observations. Can J Vet Res 2012;76(3):209–14.

97. Keller KA, Beaufrère H, Brandão J, et al. Long-term management of ovarian neoplasia in two cockatiels (*Nymphicus hollandicus*). J Avian Med Surg 2013; 27(1):44–52.

98. Mans C, Pilny A. Use of GnRH-agonists for medical management of reproductive disorders in birds. Vet Clin North Am Exot Anim Pract 2014;17(1):23–33.

99. Petritz OA, Guzman DSM, Paul-Murphy J, et al. Evaluation of the efficacy and safety of single administration of 4.7 mg deslorelin acetate implants on egg production and plasma sex hormones in Japanese quail (*Coturnix coturnix japonica*). Am J Vet Res 2013;74(2):316–23.

100. Summa NM, Guzman DSM, Wils-Plotz EL, et al. Evaluation of the effects of a 4.7-mg deslorelin acetate implant on egg laying in cockatiels (*Nymphicus hollandicus*). Am J Vet Res 2017;78(6):745–51.

101. Millam JR, Finney HL. Leuprolide acetate can reversibly prevent egg laying in cockatiels (*Nymphicus hollandicus*). Zoo Biol 1994;13:149–55.

102. Petritz OA, Guzman DS-M, Hawkins MG, et al. Comparison of two 4.7-milligram to one 9.4-milligram Deslorelin acetate implant on egg production and plasma

progesterone concentrations in Japanese quails (*Coturnix coturnix japonica*). J Zoo Wildl Med 2015;46(4):789–97.

103. Gibbons M. Therapeutics. In: Divers S, Mader D, editors. Current therapy in reptile medicine and surgery. 1st edition. St Louis (MO): Saunders Elsevier; 2014. p. 57–69.

104. Johnson JG. Therapeutic review: deslorelin acetate subcutaneous implant. J Exotic Pet Med 2013;22(1):82–4.

105. Hanna J. The effects of deslorelin implantation on the reproductive steroid hormones of females freshwater stingrays. Monterey (CA): Aquatic Workshop; 2015.

106. Cowan ML, Martin GB, Monks DJ, et al. Inhibition of the reproductive system by deslorelin in male and female pigeons (*Columba livia*). J Avian Med Surg 2014; 28(2):102–8.

107. Sykes JM, Ramsay EC, Schumacher J, et al. Evaluation of an implanted osmotic pump for delivery of amikacin to corn snakes (*Elaphe guttata guttata*). J Zoo Wildl Med 2006;37(3):373–80.

108. Moussy Y, Hersh L, Dungel P. Distribution of 3H-dexamethasone in rat subcutaneous tissue after delivery from osmotic pumps. Biotechnol Prog 2006; 22(3):819–24.

109. Clancy MM, KuKanich B, Sykes JM. Pharmacokinetics of butorphanol delivered with an osmotic pump during a seven-day period in common peafowl (*Pavo cristatus*). Am J Vet Res 2015;76(12):1070–6.

110. Ferrell ST, Marlar AB, Garner M, et al. Intralesional cisplatin chemotherapy and topical cryotherapy for the control of choanal squamous cell carcinoma in an African penguin (*Spheniscus demersus*). J Zoo Wildl Med 2006;37(4):539–41.

111. Graham JE, Kent MS, Théon A. Current therapies in exotic animal oncology. Vet Clin North Am Exot Anim Pract 2004;7(3):757–81.

112. Klaphake E, Beazley-Keane SL, Jones M, et al. Multisite integumentary squamous cell carcinoma in an African grey parrot (*Psittacus erithacus erithacus*). Vet Rec 2006;158(17):593.

113. Manucy TK, Bennett RA, Greenacre CB, et al. Squamous cell carcinoma of the mandibular beak in a Buffon's macaw (*Ara ambigua*). J Avian Med Surg 1998; 12(3):158–66.

114. Ramsay EC, Bos JH, McFadden C. Use of intratumoral cisplatin and orthovoltage radiotherapy in treatment of a fibrosarcoma in a macaw. J Assoc Avian Vet 1993;7(2):87.

115. Jaensch SM, Butler R, O'Hara A, et al. Atypical multiple, papilliform, xanthomatous, cutaneous neoplasia in a goose (*Anser anser*). Aust Vet J 2002;80(5): 277–80.

116. Harrison TM, Kitchell BE. Principles and applications of medical oncology in exotic animals. Vet Clin North Am Exot Anim Pract 2017;20(1):209–34.

117. Kent M. Principles and applications of radiation therapy in exotic animals. Vet Clin North Am Exot Anim Pract 2017;20(1):255–70.

118. Sim RR, Sullivan KE, Valdes EV, et al. A comparison of oral and topical vitamin A supplementation in African foam-nesting frogs (*Chiromantis xerampelina*). J Zoo Wildl Med 2010;41(3):456–60.

119. Richardson V. Treatments. In: Richardson V, editor. Diseases of domestic Guinea pigs. 2nd edition. Oxford (UK): Blackwell Science; 2000. p. 104–20.

120. Okerman L, Devriese LA, Gevaert D, et al. In vivo activity of orally administered antibiotics and chemotherapeutics against acute septicaemic pasteurellosis in rabbits. Lab Anim 1990;24(4):341–4.

121. Ratzlaff K, Papich MG, Flammer K. Plasma concentrations of fluconazole after a single oral dose and administration in drinking water in cockatiels (*Nymphicus hollandicus*). J Avian Med Surg 2011;25(1):23–31.

122. Evans EE, Wade LL, Flammer K. Administration of doxycycline in drinking water for treatment of spiral bacterial infection in cockatiels. J Am Vet Med Assoc 2008;232(3):389–93.

123. Simone-Freilicher EA, Hoefer HL. Hedgehog care and husbandry. Vet Clin North Am Exot Anim Pract 2004;7(2):257–67.

124. Guzman DS-M, Beaufrère H, KuKanich B, et al. Pharmacokinetics of single oral dose of pimobendan in Hispaniolan Amazon parrots (*Amazona ventralis*). J Avian Med Surg 2014;28(2):95–101.

125. Phalen DN. Update on the diagnosis and management of *Macrorhabdus ornithogaster* (formerly *Megabacteria*) in avian patients. Vet Clin North Am Exot Anim Pract 2014;17(2):203–10.

126. Doneley B. Clinical techniques. In: Doneley B, editor. Avian medicine and surgery in practice companion and aviary birds. 1st edition. London: Manson Publishing; 2010. p. 55–68.

127. Bonner BB. Chelonian therapeutics. Vet Clin North Am Exot Anim Pract 2000; 3(1):257–332.

128. Marks SL. Nasoesophagal, esophagostomy, gastrostomy, and jejunal tube placement techniques. In: Ettinger SJ, Feldman EC, editors. Textbook of Veterinary Internal Medicine Expert Consult. Volume 1. St Louis (MO): Saunders Elsevier; 2009. p. 1065–9.

129. Paul-Murphy J, Ramer JC. Urgent care of the pet rabbit. Vet Clin North Am Exot Anim Pract 1998;1(1):127–52.

130. Makidon P. Esophagostomy tube placement in the anorectic rabbit. LAB Anim (NY) 2005;34(8):33.

131. Paul-Murphy J. Critical care of the rabbit. Vet Clin North Am Exot Anim Pract 2007;10(2):437–61.

132. Adamovicz L, Bullen L, Saker K, et al. Use of an esophagostomy tube for management of traumatic subtotal glossectomy in an African pygmy hedgehog (*Atelerix albiventris*). J Exotic Pet Med 2016;25(3):231–6.

133. Tully TN. Psittacine therapeutics. Vet Clin North Am Exot Anim Pract 2000;3(1): 59–90.

134. Huynh M, Sabater M, Brandão J, et al. Use of an esophagostomy tube as a method of nutritional management in raptors: a case series. J Avian Med Surg 2014;28(1):24–30.

135. Goring RL, Goldman A, Kaufman KJ, et al. Needle catheter duodenostomy: a technique for duodenal alimentation of birds. J Am Vet Med Assoc 1986; 189(9):1017–9.

136. Mans C. Sedation of pet birds. J Exotic Pet Med 2014;23(2):152–7.

137. Hornak S, Liptak T, Ledecky V, et al. A preliminary trial of the sedation induced by intranasal administration of midazolam alone or in combination with dexmedetomidine and reversal by atipamezole for a short-term immobilization in pigeons. Vet Anaesth Analg 2015;42(2):192–6.

138. Vesal N, Zare P. Clinical evaluation of intranasal benzodiazepines, α2-agonists and their antagonists in canaries. Vet Anaesth Analg 2006;33(3):143–8.

139. Sadegh AB. Comparison of intranasal administration of xylazine, diazepam, and midazolam in budgerigars (*Melopsittacus undulatus*): clinical evaluation. J Zoo Wildl Med 2013;44(2):241–4.

140. Mans C, Guzman DS-M, Lahner LL, et al. Sedation and physiologic response to manual restraint after intranasal administration of midazolam in Hispaniolan Amazon parrots (*Amazona ventralis*). J Avian Med Surg 2012;26(3):130–9.

141. Vesal N, Eskandari MH. Sedative effects of midazolam and xylazine with or without ketamine and detomidine alone following intranasal administration in ring-necked parakeets. J Am Vet Med Assoc 2006;228(3):383–8.

142. Weiland LC, Kluge K, Kutter APN, et al. Clinical evaluation of intranasal medetomidine–ketamine and medetomidine–S(+)-ketamine for induction of anaesthesia in rabbits in two centres with two different administration techniques. Vet Anaesth Analg 2017;44(1):98–105.

143. Johnson DH. Intranasal midazolam for procedural sedation in miniature pigs (*Sus scrofa domesticus*). In: Proceedings ExoticsCon. Portland (OR): 2016. p. 611.

144. Schumacher J, Mans C. Anesthesia. In: Divers S, Mader D, editors. Current therapy in reptile medicine and surgery. 1st edition. St Louis (MO): Saunders Elsevier; 2014. p. 134–53.

145. Schnellbacher RW, Hernandez SM, Tuberville TD, et al. The efficacy of intranasal administration of dexmedetomidine and ketamine to yellow-bellied sliders (*Trachemys scripta scripta*). J Herp Med Surg 2012;22(3):91–8.

146. Emery L, Parsons G, Gerhardt L, et al. Sedative effects of intranasal midazolam and dexmedetomidine in 2 species of tortoises (*Chelonoidis carbonaria* and *Geochelone platynota*). J Exotic Pet Med 2014;23(4):380–3.

147. Chen KS, Bharaj SS, King EC. Induction and relief of nasal congestion in ferrets infected with influenza virus. Int J Exp Pathol 1995;76(1):55.

148. Yoshimoto J, Yagi S, Ono J, et al. Development of anti-influenza drugs: II. Improvement of oral and intranasal absorption and the anti-influenza activity of stachyflin derivatives. J Pharm Pharmacol 2000;52(10):1247–55.

149. Zhao Y, Tao T, Wu J, et al. Pharmacokinetics of tramadol in rat plasma and cerebrospinal fluid after intranasal administration. J Pharm Pharmacol 2008;60(9):1149–54.

150. Heard M. Anesthesia. In: Speer B, editor. Current therapy in avian medicine and surgery. 1st edition. St Louis (MO): Elsevier; 2016. p. 601–15.

151. Sadar M, Drazenovich KH, Paul-Murphy JR. Pharmacokinetics of buprenorphine in guinea pigs (*Cavia porcellus*): intravenous, intramuscular and oral transmucosal administration. In: Proceedings of the American Association of Zoo Veterinarians (AEMV). Orlando (FL): 2014.

152. Phillips BE, Harms CA, Messenger KM. Oral transmucosal detomidine gel for the sedation of the domestic ferret (*Mustela putorius furo*). J Exot Pet Med 2015;24(4):446–54.

153. Morici M, Interlandi C, Costa GL, et al. Sedation with intracloacal administration of dexmedetomidine and ketamine in yellow-bellied sliders (*Trachemys scripta scripta*). J Exotic Pet Med 2017;26(3):188–91.

154. Harrison GJ, Lightfoot TL, Flinchum GB. Emergency and critical care. In: Harrison GJ, Harrison LR, editors. Clinical avian medicine. 1st edition. Palm Beach (FL): Spix Publishing; 2006. p. 213–32.

155. Stout JD. Common emergencies in pet birds. Vet Clin North Am Exot Anim Pract 2016;19(2):513–41.

156. Lennox AM. Rhinotomy and rhinostomy for surgical treatment of chronic rhinitis in two rabbits. J Exotic Pet Med 2013;22(4):383–92.

157. Sousa J, Alves G, Oliveira P, et al. Intranasal delivery of ciprofloxacin to rats: a topical approach using a thermoreversible in situ gel. Eur J Pharm Sci 2017;97: 30–7.

158. Hasegawa-Baba Y, Kubota H, Takata A, et al. Intratracheal instillation methods and the distribution of administered material in the lung of the rat. J Toxicol Pathol 2014;27(3+ 4):197–204.

159. Krautwald-Junghanns M-E, Vorbrüggen S, Böhme J. Aspergillosis in birds: an overview of treatment options and regimens. J Exotic Pet Med 2015;24(3): 296–307.

160. Phillips A, Fiorello CV, Baden RM, et al. Amphotericin B concentrations in healthy mallard ducks (*Anas platyrhynchos*) following a single intratracheal dose of liposomal amphotericin B using an atomizer. Med Mycol 2017. [Epub ahead of print].

161. Hernandez-Divers SJ. Pulmonary candidiasis caused by *Candida albicans* in a Greek tortoise (*Testudo graeca*) and treatment with intrapulmonary amphotericin B. J Zoo Wildl Med 2001;32(3):352–9.

162. McArthur S. Feeding techniques and fluids. In: Meyer J, McArthur S, Wilkinson R, editors. Medicine and surgery of tortoises and turtles. 1st edition. Oxford (UK): Blackwell Publishing; 2004. p. 257–71.

163. Hernandez-Divers SJ. Endosurgical debridement and diode laser ablation of lung and air sac granulomas in psittacine birds. J Avian Med Surg 2002; 16(2):138–45.

164. Dyer DC, Alstine WGV. Antibiotic aerosolization: tissue and plasma oxytetracycline concentrations in parakeets. Avian Dis 1987;31(3):677.

165. Alstine WGV, Dyer DC. Antibiotic aerosolization: tissue and plasma oxytetracycline concentrations in turkey poults. Avian Dis 1985;29(2):430.

166. Junge RE, Naeger LL, LeBeau MA, et al. Pharmacokinetics of intramuscular and nebulized ceftriaxone in chickens. J Zoo Wildl Med 1994;25(2):224–8.

167. Emery LC, Cox SK, Souza MJ. Pharmacokinetics of nebulized terbinafine in Hispaniolan amazon parrots (*Amazona ventralis*). J Avian Med Surg 2012;26(3): 161–6.

168. Beernaert LA, Baert K, Marin P, et al. Designing voriconazole treatment for racing pigeons: balancing between hepatic enzyme auto induction and toxicity. Med Mycol 2009;47(3):276–85.

169. Carpenter JW, Hawkins MG, Barron H. Appendix 1 table of common drugs and approximate doses. In: Speer B, editor. Current therapy in avian medicine and surgery. 1st edition. St Louis (MO): Elsevier; 2016. p. 795–824.

170. Beaufrère H. Respiratory system. In: Tully TN, Mitchell ML, editors. Current therapy in exotic pet practice, vol. 1, 1st edition. St Louis (MO): Saunders; 2016. p. 76–150.

171. O'Callaghan C, Hardy J, Stammers J, et al. Evaluation of techniques for delivery of steroids to lungs of neonates using a rabbit model. Arch Dis Child 1992;67(1 Spec No):20–4.

172. Dijk PH, Heikamp A, Oetomo SB. Surfactant nebulisation: lung function, surfactant distribution and pulmonary blood flow distribution in lung lavaged rabbits. Intensive Care Med 1997;23(10):1070–6.

173. Corbanie EA, Matthijs MGR, van Eck JHH, et al. Deposition of differently sized airborne microspheres in the respiratory tract of chickens. Avian Pathol 2006; 35(6):475–85.

174. Schoemaker N, Westerhof I, van Zeeland Y. Distribution of nebulized fluorescein-labeled propylene glycol or saline in pigeons. In: Proceedings of the ExoticsCon. San Antonio (TX): 2015.

175. Tell LA, Stephens K, Teague SV, et al. Study of nebulization delivery of aerosolized fluorescent microspheres to the avian respiratory tract. Avian Dis 2012; 56(2):381–6.

176. Chow KE, Tyrrell D, Yang M, et al. Scintigraphic assessment of deposition of radiolabeled Fluticasone delivered from a nebulizer and metered dose inhaler in 10 healthy dogs. J Vet Intern Med 2017;31(6):1849–57.

177. Wenzel U, Heine J, Mengel H, et al. Efficacy of imidacloprid 10%/moxidectin 1% (Advocate®/Advantage Multi™) against fleas (Ctenocephalides felis felis) on ferrets (Mustela putorius furo). Parasitol Res 2008;103(1):231–4.

178. Dorrestein GM, Van der Horst HHA, Cremers HJWM, et al. Quill mite (Dermoglyphus passerinus) infestation of canaries (Serinus canaria): Diagnosis and treatment. Avian Pathol 1997;26(1):195–9.

179. Hahn A, D'Agostino J, Cole G, et al. Pharmacokinetics of selamectin in helmeted guineafowl (Numida meleagris) after topical administration. J Zoo Wildl Med 2014;45(1):176–8.

180. Schilliger L, Betremieux O, Rochet J, et al. Absorption and efficacy of a spot-on combination containing emodepside plus praziquantel in reptiles. Revue Med Vet 2009;160(12):557–61.

181. Mehlhorn H, Schmahl G, Mevissen I. Efficacy of a combination of imidacloprid and moxidectin against parasites of reptiles and rodents: case reports. Parasitol Res 2005;97(S01):S97–101.

182. Foley PL, Henderson AL, Bissonette EA, et al. Evaluation of fentanyl transdermal patches in rabbits: blood concentrations and physiologic response. Comp Med 2001;51(3):239–44.

183. Darrow BG, Myers GE, KuKanich B, et al. Fentanyl transdermal therapeutic system provides rapid systemic fentanyl absorption in two ball pythons (Python regius). J Herp Med Surg 2016;26(3–4):94–9.

184. Delaski KM, Gehring R, Heffron BT, et al. Plasma concentrations of fentanyl achieved with transdermal application in chickens. J Avian Med Surg 2017; 31(1):6–15.

185. Wack CL, Lovern MB, Woodley SK. Transdermal delivery of corticosterone in terrestrial amphibians. Gen Comp Endocrinol 2010;169(3):269–75.

186. Stone SM, Clark-Price SC, Boesch JM, et al. Evaluation of righting reflex in cane toads (Bufo marinus) after topical application of sevoflurane jelly. Am J Vet Res 2013;74(6):823–7.

187. Mombarg M, Claessen H, Lambrechts L, et al. Quantification of percutaneous absorption of metronidazole and levamisole in the fire-bellied toad (Bombina orientalis). J Vet Pharmacol Ther 1992;15(4):433–6.

188. Riviere JE, Shapiro DP, Coppoc GL. Percutaneous absorption of gentamicin by the leopard frog, Rana pipiens. J Vet Pharmacol Ther 1979;2:235–9.

189. Doss GA, Nevarez JG, Fowlkes N, et al. Evaluation of metomidate hydrochloride as an anesthetic in leopard frogs (Rana pipiens). J Zoo Wildl Med 2014;45(1): 53–9.

190. McMillan MW, Leece EA. Immersion and branchial/transcutaneous irrigation anaesthesia with alfaxalone in a Mexican axolotl. Vet Anaesth Analg 2011; 38(6):619–23.

191. Jenkins JR. Skin disorders of the rabbit. Vet Clin North Am Exot Anim Pract 2001;4(5):543–63.

192. Hernandez-Divers SM. Principles of wound management of small mammals: hedgehogs, prairie dogs, and sugar gliders. Vet Clin North Am Exot Anim Pract 2004;7(1):1–18.
193. Smith DA, Barker IK, Allen OB. The effect of certain topical medications on healing of cutaneous wounds in the common garter snake (*Thamnophis sirtalis*). Can J Vet Res 1988;52(1):129.
194. Negrini J, Mozos E, Escamilla A, et al. Effects of topical insulin on second-intention wound healing in the red-eared slider turtle (*Trachemys scripta elegans*) – a controlled study. BMC Vet Res 2017;13(1):160.
195. Sypniewski LA, Hahn A, Murray JK, et al. Novel shell wound care in the aquatic turtle. J Exotic Pet Med 2016;25(2):110–4.
196. Spadola F, Morici M. Treatment of turtle shell ulcerations using photopolymerizable nano-hybrid dental composite. J Exot Pet Med 2016;25(4):288–94.
197. Chow EP, Bennett RA, Dustin L. Ventral bulla osteotomy for treatment of otitis media in a rabbit. J Exotic Pet Med 2009;18(4):299–305.
198. Taylor WM, Beaufrère H, Mans C, et al. Long-term outcome of treatment of dental abscesses with a wound-packing technique in pet rabbits: 13 cases (1998–2007). J Am Vet Med Assoc 2010;237(12):1444–9.

Low-Stress Medication Techniques in Birds and Small Mammals

Brian L. Speer, DVM, DABVP (Avian Practice), DECZM (Avian)[a,*],
Melody Hennigh, RVT, KPA CTP[a], Bernice Muntz[b],
Yvonne R.A. van Zeeland, DVM, MVR, PhD, DECZM (Avian, Small Mammal)[c]

KEYWORDS

- Low stress • Treatment • Medication • Training • Learning • Welfare

KEY POINTS

- Forceful, coercive, and fear-evoking treatment methods can be behavioral harmful to the patient as well as result in lower prognosis and impaired clinical outcome.
- Many medical behaviors can be trained using science-based methods, often quickly and effectively, in a veterinary practice setting.
- Keys to implementation of low-stress medication techniques in practice require the ability to recognize fear and to use desensitization and counterconditioning and the use of versatility, adjusting methods to best fit the behavioral and medical needs of the patient at hand.
- Medication can be optimally delivered through the use of food vehicles and via operantly trained medication/treatment behaviors.
- Selective and appropriate use of conscious sedation and even general anesthesia may be appropriate in select cases at key times, but these pharmacologic interventions rarely should become the sole methods for maintaining long-term treatment or execution of medical procedures.

 Video content accompanies this article at http://www.vetexotic.theclinics. com/.

INTRODUCTION

Low-stress medication techniques are an important component of ethical and effective treatment. Paired with the medical details of patient management, by balancing medication techniques, success can be greatly enhanced. Low-stress medication

The authors have nothing to disclose.
[a] Medical Center for Birds, 3805 Main Street, Oakley, CA 94561, USA; [b] Dierentrainer, Mauvelaan 13, Leidschendam 2264 AJ, The Netherlands; [c] Division of Zoological Medicine, Department of Clinical Sciences of Companion Animals, Faculty of Veterinary Medicine, Utrecht University, Yalelaan 108, Utrecht 3584 CM, The Netherlands
* Corresponding author.
E-mail address: avnvet@aol.com

Vet Clin Exot Anim 21 (2018) 261–285
https://doi.org/10.1016/j.cvex.2018.01.016
1094-9194/18/© 2018 Elsevier Inc. All rights reserved.

techniques require careful assessment of body language, at times may use strategic and appropriate use of anxiolytics to facilitate some medical procedures, and often use the regular implementation of target training as a gateway to other trained medical behaviors as well as enrichment. The neurobiological aspects of the stages of memory formation, and how these stages may be influenced by stress and some therapeutics, are explored.

CAPTURE AND RESTRAINT

Many case reports, veterinary textbook references, conference proceedings, and discussions describe techniques and treatments used to provide medical care for birds using the term "capture and restraint," or fail to describe the methods used and assess their behavioral outcome on the patient. Loosely, "capture and restraint" often includes combinations of techniques that include physically overpowering the bird, sneaking up on or surprising the bird, or other means to quickly get the bird restrained and get the task at hand done. In addition, videos of these methods and techniques, good and bad, live in perpetuity on YouTube and other sources, are repeated, and are even referenced in current presentations. Conversely, medication techniques may also not even be described at all in scientific studies, case reports, or other descriptions of procedures requiring therapeutic administrations. These realities, in turn, can result in further confusion and misunderstanding about the "controversial" views on the topic.

Similar issues are encountered in small mammals because veterinarians are often trained to handle and restrain these animals using "traditional methods," such as applied in laboratory animals. Moreover, animals are often chased in their cage before being grabbed quickly and forcefully and held in the air with their feet off the ground. This activity in itself is likely innately aversive to the animal because it mimics the chase-and-capture action of a predator. However, additional stress and anxiety may result because of the aversive nature of the treatment that is being administered, especially if the procedure is recurring on a daily or twice-daily basis. As a result, it is not surprising that a large number of animals will show fear behaviors or resistance when being handled. For example, surveys among rabbit owners have shown that around 60% of rabbits will struggle if lifted or demonstrate fear-related aggression upon being approached.[1–4]

> By restraining pets in a forceful, crude or unskilled manner, you could be breaking your promise to do no harm. Such handling can make pets behaviorally worse and even lead to aggression and, ultimately, euthanasia.
>
> —Dr Sophia Yin

This quote really applies to how veterinary professionals interact with pets in all aspects of veterinary medicine, not only restraint.

Outdated methods or techniques that are not evaluated for effectiveness on all aspects, above and beyond outcome alone, typically overlook some of the more important ethical considerations and best practices for pet birds and small mammals. When veterinarians and health care personnel did not look back and critically evaluate the outcomes of restraint and medication methods, most people were quick but incorrect to pronounce those methods effective. This is especially true in parrots as an example, as their intelligence and learning capacity was often discounted. In reality, these "successes" were in fact often quite far from their ideal or intended mark. The adverse effects of our own failure to appreciate learned fear in the development of and shaping of behaviors during in-patient treatment and clinical procedures are immense. Inadvertent, unrecognized, or unaltered use of stressful or fear-evoking treatments can lead to significant adverse consequences. These perceived acute and chronic stressful situations can adversely affect the immediate and longer-term outcomes of an examination, a specific procedure or surgical event, patient-healing capacity, and the long-term quality of life of the animal. In addition, the observed changes to the pet's behavior can easily adversely affect a client's desire to return for further care or even annual wellness evaluations. Misconceptions about the use of training methods in birds and small mammals have to some degree become included as part of routine veterinary aspects of patient care.[5] Because welfare and the nature of learned experiences are considered more a part of veterinary health care, balanced behavioral science and these modern myths have become combined in in-patient management plans and have become included as part of outcome assessments. Fragments of popular pseudoscience, mixed and blended with more current scientific information in the same discussion, presentation, or publication, can become challenging for even the most critical veterinary minds struggling to separate fact from fiction pertinent to their patient's care decisions. Conflict, confusion, and variable levels of understanding and assessments of outcomes of treatment effectiveness abound. There is enough scientific evidence that the use of force-, coercion-, and "capture"-oriented methods and positive punishment or negative reinforcement as the primary means with which to guide behavior, more than ever before, are increasingly less appropriate for most of the animals in our stewardship and care.[6,7]

Low-stress techniques also do not have the same problems associated with forceful treatment, such as increased learned fear-eliciting stimuli, increased learned aggression, increased risks to the bird and handlers, increased risk of problems during medical procedures, and increased difficulty interpreting some laboratory diagnostics due to iatrogenic and stress-influenced changes. Low-stress handling techniques are time-effective and can directly enhance the comfort of the avian and small mammal patient in daily clinical practice. These basic skills and techniques are essential not only to avoid the old "capture and restraint" methods and their adverse consequences but also to enable veterinarians and technicians to be more ethical and effective in their health care delivery for companion birds and small mammals and to enable training of medical behaviors in the present and the future. In the practice setting, encouraging staff to take low-stress medicating into their own hands helps empower staff and share what they learn with other coworkers and ultimately clients. In the examination room and with hospitalized patients, it is easy to adjust timing, scheduling, and service prices to benefit the patient and the veterinary practice.

The training of medical behaviors is becoming increasingly more common in zoologic institutions.[7] Nevertheless, training birds and small mammals to cooperate in their own medical care unfortunately still is a comparatively new, but key aspect of treatment (**Box 1**). Methods should be focused on positive reinforcement and should be a component of most treatment plans, almost regardless of the nature of the problem or problems being addressed. Trainable medical behaviors for birds include standing on scales, allowing restraint in a towel, being comfortable with a tactile examination, voluntarily presenting feet for nail trims, voluntary participation in venipuncture, medical treatment plans, and more.[8] Trainable behaviors for small mammals include, for example, crating, being picked up and handled (or stepping voluntarily onto the hand), toweling, standing still and allowing an examination to be performed, targeting (eg, to direct the animal to get onto and off of a scale, coming out of a cage), administering medication (topical, oral, parenteral), and voluntarily undergoing grooming procedures (eg, nail trimming, brushing) (Videos 1–4).[9]

Box 1
Benefits of training health care behaviors in birds and exotic small mammals

- Creates a patient that willingly participates in health care procedures, significantly reducing stress on the patient, the veterinary staff, and the caregiver.
- Reduces patient aggressive behavior toward the veterinary staff or caregiver.
- Preempts the need for heavy-handed or chemical restraint.
- Increases behavioral resiliency when it is necessary to expose the animal to an aversive experience. Animals will "bounce back" more easily.
- Builds a relationship of trust between caregiver and animal, reducing the animal's anxiety and fear in its daily life.
- Creates empowering problem-solving opportunities for the animal, resulting in behavioral enrichment and an increase in the animal's behavioral repertoire.

Adapted from Brown S. Small mammal training in the veterinary practice. Vet Clin North Am Exot Anim Pract 2012;15:471; with permission.

THE ABCs OF DESCRIBING BEHAVIOR

The simplest manner of describing an initial evaluation of a behavior is through the use of the ABC's of behavior.[10,11]

The letters stand for the 3 elements of a simplified behavioral "equation," which includes the *Antecedents*, *Behavior*, and *Consequences*. With this simple descriptive and analytical strategy, we seek to identify through careful observation the events and conditions that occur before a specific behavior: *Antecedents*, as well as identifying the results that follow the *Behavior*: its *Consequences*. When paired with keen observation skills and creative problem-solving abilities, the ABCs help clarify the way in which the basic components of behavior are interrelated. It is this clarity that leads to important insights and more effective teaching or training strategies. The ABCs can also be used to help identify problem situations and consequences that also have a formative role in some behaviors. By describing a behavior in the context that it is occurring, one is more optimally positioned to describe problem behavioral situations and therefore has more opportunity to alter them. There are 6 steps to analyzing and using the ABCs in a behavior-change strategy: (1) describe the target behavior in clear and observable terms; (2) describe the antecedent events that occur and conditions that exist immediately before the behavior happens; (3) describe the consequences that immediately follow the behavior; (4) examine the antecedents, the behavior, and the consequence in sequence; (5) devise new antecedents and/or consequences to teach new behaviors or change existing ones; (6) evaluate the outcome.

The ABCs are used to enable critical employment of operant behavior changes with the learner and can be put in better context with the use of paradigms of reinforcement and punishment (**Table 1**).

Table 1
Basic paradigms of reinforcement and punishment

	Operant Response Increases	Operant Response Decreases
Stimulus presentation	Positive reinforcement (R+)	Positive punishment (P+)
Stimulus removal	Negative reinforcement (R−)	Negative punishment (P−)

Reading from the left, if a stimulus is being presented to the learner, this is represented as a positive. Then, evaluating the frequency or probable frequency of the behavioral consequence of this presented stimulus, one can assess if the stimulus is functioning as a positive reinforcer (R+), or a positive punisher (P+). If the behavior increases, the introduced stimulus is functioning as a reinforcer, and if the behavior decreases, the introduced stimulus is a punisher. If a stimulus is being removed from the learner as a result of its behavior, it is represented as a negative. Based on the observed frequency or probable frequency of the behavioral consequence of this removed stimulus, we can also assess whether the stimulus is functioning as a negative reinforcer (R−), or a negative punisher (P−).

In a review article of 17 different studies on the effects of training dogs, it was concluded that using aversive training methods (positive punishment and negative reinforcement) can jeopardize both the physical and the mental health of dogs. Although positive punishment could be effective, there was no evidence that it was more effective than positive reinforcement, and more potential that it could be less effective.[12]

BODY LANGUAGE: WHAT IT IS AND WHAT IT IS NOT

In order to effectively train and guide behaviors, clear descriptions of what is seen are important. When describing any behavior, it is important to describe observable actions (ie, what we see and can be seen easily by others). What body language and observed behavior are not are labels. These types of labeled descriptors often have different meanings to different people. For example, an "aggressive" bird may look like a bird slamming its toys around the cage to one person, but to another person "aggressive" may look like a lunging, biting bird. The same applies to a "territorial" rabbit, which can be used as a label to describe a rabbit scent-marking and spraying while roaming freely through the house, a rabbit grunting, lunging, or biting upon being approached by a human handler while in its enclosure, or a rabbit that will fight with other rabbits with which it is housed. Another common label that is used in popular practice is the "hormonal" label, which may be used to justify treatment without a clear description of what behavior or behaviors are being observed. Similarly, people may refer to a "depressed" animal, which needs to be petted constantly to be "happy." "Happy" and "depressed" can have many different meanings to different people, yet they are very commonly used as explanations for why an animal behaves the way that it does. One seeks to describe the animal's personality (the veterinary staff might say, "That's just how the animal is!") or its state of mind, but these labels rarely, if ever, can be objectively and accurately assessed. As a result, these can easily predispose veterinarians to incomplete, imbalanced, and sometimes less comprehensive treatment strategies, rather than to help design a concrete behavior-modification plan that would be considered the best treatment practice for the patient before them. Without taking time to paint a clear picture of an animal's behavior, veterinarians can sometimes be a greater hindrance than help for the patients and clients. As such, veterinarians are encouraged to describe the actual behavior, something the animal is doing, that can be measured, observed, and repeated, as well as the conditions under which it occurs, because these descriptors provide the best indicators for what is going on and why, thereby rendering it more likely to design a concrete behavior-modification plan that will result in the desired behavioral changes.

IDENTIFY FEAR AND EMPLOY DESENSITIZATION AND COUNTERCONDITIONING

Desensitization and counterconditioning are both techniques that can be used to address elicited fear responses in patients. Desensitization is the process of incrementally exposing the animal to the aversive stimulus without crossing the threshold, causing the animal to show any fear response. Desensitization and counterconditioning are focused on altering respondent behavior and are very effective especially when used together. Careful observation of the animal's body language is crucial, because it is the animal's "comfort" level that decides whether to decrease proximity to the aversive stimulus. For example, a bird may show an elicited fear response (eg, increased respiratory rate when observed from a distance, screaming, flattening of the feathers against the body; **Table 2**) upon being presented with a towel at close proximity, for example, when the towel is brought within 8 feet of the bird. However, the same bird may be preening when the towel is presented at a far enough distance, for example, within 10 feet of it. Based on these observations, we know that 10 feet would be an appropriate distance to start, because the bird is displaying "calm" body language by preening. Small approximations are subsequently used to bring the towel closer to the bird without it demonstrating fear or escape behavior, the size of the approximation being dependent on the bird and its response. Aside from objects, desensitization can also be applied to potentially aversive sounds (eg, clipping of nails or noise of a nebulizer), for which the animal may be gradually desensitized by keeping the animal at a distance and slowly increasing proximity to the noise-producing object, and/or starting with the sound at a low frequency or short duration (eg, one clip, turning on the nebulizer for 1 second) and gradually increasing the frequency or duration. Alternatively, the sound can be recorded and initially played at a soft intensity followed by a slow increase of the intensity, while ensuring that the animal is displaying calm behavior before continuing to the next approximation (and taking a step back when a fear response is elicited; see **Table 2**). Once the animal is desensitized to the sound or object and displays calm behavior in proximity of the object, the next step would be to gradually desensitize to the touch of the towel, nail clippers, or the face mask, and so forth.

Counterconditioning focuses on pairing a desired or appetitive stimulus with the aversive stimulus (the undesirable stimulus that the animal avoids and causes a fear response) to change the stimulus from aversive to valued. The appetitive stimulus should elicit a stronger response from the animal than the aversive stimulus. In the previous example, if a bird shows elicited fear of the towel, and if we know that this individual bird enjoys peanuts and scrambled eggs, we can pair the appetitive response from eating the food with the towel, thereby overriding the fear response. The same pairing would be possible for an aversive sound, for example, if a rabbit shows a fear response (eg, ears flattened against the body) upon hearing the nail clippers, and we know that this rabbit highly favors banana, we can present this food item to the rabbit while simultaneously exposing the rabbit to the sound of the nail clippers. Many birds and small mammals have several food items that may be used as a reward during counterconditioning (**Figs. 1** and **2**, **Table 3** also supplies examples). Reserve the animal's favorite, that is, a very highly valued food item, for this exercise. In the aforementioned example, if when the towel is presented, the bird will not eat the peanut, then it may be wise to try a different food. If the bird readily eats scrambled eggs when the towel is presented, we know we have a food item that is high enough value to outweigh the aversiveness of the towel in the manner it is being presented. It is fair to assume that an animal that is stressed or does no' feel "safe" will not eat treats. Slowly, the end result is an animal that does not show a fear response when it is confronted with the aversive stimulus (ie, the towel or sound of the nail clippers in the aforementioned examples) because it was successfully paired with the appetitive response of eating its favored treats (ie, the scrambled eggs in the case of the bird or the strawberries and bananas in the case of the rabbit).

Table 2
Common behavioral indicators of fear in birds and small mammals

	Freeze Response (Fright)	Flight Response: Escape and Avoidance Behaviors	Fight-Response: Defensive of Fear-Related Aggression (Usually Last Resort for Prey Species When Cornered)	Other Remarks
Birds	Flattening of feathers Muscle tensing Body still and tensed Hunched/crouched posture Vision oriented toward the threat, following its every movement	Leaning backwards Flying or running away from the perceived threat Shelter-seeking behaviors, for example, hiding in a corner or underneath an object Wing flapping Falling from perch Struggling and wing flapping while being caught or restrained Screaming (high-pitched vocalizations)	Eye pinning Feathers either fluffed or flattened against the body Lying on back, kicking with feet Tail fanning Lunging forward with beak Biting (often short, quick bite) Screaming (high-pitched vocalizations)	Sounds produced can vary per species
Rabbits	Eyes wide open and unblinking, into the eye socket Ears initially pointed forward, then laid back flat against body	Running away from the perceived threat Shelter-seeking behaviors, for example, by hiding in a corner or underneath furniture Guinea pigs, rats, and hamsters: repeated nudging of and digging in cage bedding, trying to bury itself in it Struggling and scratching or kicking while caught or being restrained Running away from perceived threat, shelter-seeking behaviors	Body leaning backwards, with the weight placed on in back legs Lunging forward with head and front feet toward the perceived threat Growling, grunting Biting	Eyes can either bulge slightly or be retracted in the eye socket Position of the ears can be more difficult to observe in lop-eared rabbits
Lip-licking	Body still and tensed (freeze response), body flattened to the ground, oriented toward the threat; foot thumping, but no other movements			
Guinea pigs	Eyes wide open (white of the eye may be visible), lowered head and ears, head stretched forward Shivering		Growling, teeth chattering Lunging and biting (rarely)	

(continued on next page)

Table 2
(continued)

	Freeze Response (Fright)	Flight Response: Escape and Avoidance Behaviors	Fight-Response: Defensive of Fear-Related Aggression (Usually Last Resort for Prey Species When Cornered)	Other Remarks
	Muscle tensing, stiffening of front legs Standing tall or sitting still, frozen, feigning death Body often oriented toward the perceived threat Growling, shrieking, whining			
Chinchillas	Stiff body with weight in hind legs, or standing upright Ears forward or flattened on the back Sitting still, with body Directed toward perceived threat		Teeth chattering, barking, screaming, grunting, whistling Urine spraying Lunging, biting	
Rats	Piloerection Standing on hind legs, slapping tail Body tensed and still, lowered to the ground and oriented toward the threat Defecating and urinating		Flip onto back with mouth open, ears flattened against head High-pitched squeal, low-pitched squeak, hissing, teeth chattering Revealing lower teeth Lunging and biting	
Hamsters	Body stiffness, standing upright, flattened to the ground, washing face continuously Defecating and urinating		Flip onto back with mouth open, ears flattened against head Screaming, tooth clicking Revealing teeth Lunging and biting	
Ferrets	Piloerection on tail and sometimes body Standing still, with arched back; body tensed and oriented toward the perceived threat Anal gland expression		Hissing, huffing, screaming Backing up with mouth open Flip onto back with mouth open Lunging and biting	Note that backing up with mouth open can also be observed during play

Note: In all species, these behavioral responses are often accompanied by sympathetic responses (eg, increase in heart rate, respiratory rate, blood pressure).
Data from Refs. [13–17]

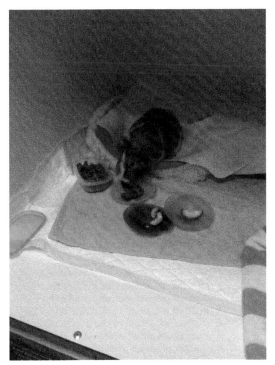

Fig. 1. To identify which food items are favorites, preference tests can be performed. Here, a Guinea pig is allowed to select which food items (carrot, banana, cucumber, pellets) it prefers to eat. The most favored item can subsequently be used in training sessions.

Desensitization and counterconditioning work very well together by combining the pairing of stimuli from counterconditioning at each approximation used with desensitization. In the aforementioned examples, the towel would be brought close to the bird or a single sound of the nail clippers would be produced in proximity of the rabbit, and if no fear response or escape behavior were shown, small pieces of food (scrambled egg or banana, respectively) would be offered. Each successful approximation of decreased distance between the towel and bird (or increased frequency of the nail clipper sound produced in proximity of the rabbit) is reinforced with a positive stimulus, which makes the appetitive stimulus dependent (contingent) on the behavior.[11,14–20]

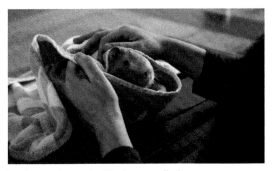

Fig. 2. Towel training in a guinea pig (*Cavia porcellus*).

Table 3	
Food items that can be used as reinforcers during training for birds and small mammals[a]	
Birds	• Dried or fresh fruit, cut into smaller pieces (grapes, apple, banana) • Nuts: shelled, unsalted, and cut into smaller pieces (for example, almonds, pine nuts, palm nuts, macadamia nuts) • Sunflower or safflower seeds, cereals and grains, dried peppers • Treat foods • Other highly favored food items often include foods for human consumption (eg, cheese, cooked pasta, peanut butter, bread, popcorn)
Herbivorous small mammals (eg, rabbits, guinea pigs, chinchillas)	• High-fiber pellets • Fresh greens and vegetables (eg, [dried] parsnip, [dried] cucumber carrot) • Canned unsweetened pumpkin or squash, unsweetened fruit juice, unsweetened vegetable juice • Grains (whole oats, barley, plain popcorn) • Dried fruit with no added sugar (dried mango and papaya) or fresh fruit (eg, apple, banana) • Treat foods • Fruit or vegetable baby food puree
Small rodents (hamsters, mice, gerbils, rats)	• Pelleted rodent food broken into tiny pieces • Unsalted raw seeds or nuts and grains (as listed for rabbits) • Unsweetened fresh or dried fruit, herbs, or vegetables (eg, coconut flakes, dried white man's foot or dandelion leaves) • Liquid foods, such as those described for rabbits, yoghurt (eg, coconut flavored) • Fresh or dried mealworms of appropriate size • Treat foods and other highly favored food items, such as mentioned for birds (eg, cooked pasta) • Fruit or vegetable baby food puree
Ferrets and other carnivorous species	• Dried ferret food that is slightly moistened to facilitate chewing • Cooked meat (eg, chicken, turkey, organ meat) or eggs • Fatty acid supplement in small squeeze bottle or syringe or presented on a spoon (maximum ½ teaspoon a day per ferret) • All-meat baby food on a spoon or tongue depressor or in a syringe (diluted with water or meat broth) • Liquid recovery diets (eg, Convalescence support [Royal Canin], Emeraid Carnivore [Lafeber Company], Critical Care for Carnivores [Oxbow])

[a] Up to the daily limit.

Adapted from Brown S. Small mammal training in the veterinary practice. Vet Clin North Am Exot Anim Pract 2012;15:478; with permission.

A video example of desensitization and counterconditioning can be found at https://youtu.be/wm3tWFmWa0c.

THE APPROPRIATE USE OF CONSCIOUS SEDATION

Where indicated, conscious sedation or even general anesthesia should be considered in particularly stressed or fearful patients. Although these maneuvers can be very effective, they should not be uniformly used in all patients and should not be viewed as a means with which to avoid the need for low-stress handling methods. The choice to use conscious sedation or general anesthesia may also depend on the frequency with which the procedure needs to be repeated. For treatments that are common and frequently recurring, it might be beneficial to train; for those that only occur incidentally, training may be less important, and low-stress methods possibly aided with the use of sedation or anesthesia may be more appropriate.

Midazolam 0.5 to 1 mg/kg intramuscularly (IM), paired with butorphanol 1 to 2 mg/kg IM, can produce effective conscious sedation for many, but not all, companion bird species, and midazolam 2 mg/kg intranasally can also be used where appropriate.[21–24] Similarly, benzodiazepines (eg, midazolam 0.2–0.5 mg/kg) can be used, with or without butorphanol (dose 0.1–1 mg/kg), in small mammals. When injecting these medicaments, the subcutaneous route is preferred over the IM route because it produces equivalent effects, but is far less likely to cause discomfort (and thereby fear or resistance) to the animal.[25,26]

The advantages that conscious sedation offers include minimal cardiopulmonary effects and the potential for an amnesia effect as is described in humans.[27] If training of medical behaviors is a goal of the treatment plan, however, these same sedatives may be less appropriate. However, benzodiazepines, including midazolam, are not analgesics. Although sometimes referred to as "sedated" with isoflurane, volatile anesthetics are not sedatives and render the patient entirely unconscious. Even though volatile anesthetics offer a relatively wide margin of safety, they are not benign and can produce apnea and hypotension, especially at the higher concentrations required when used as sole agents. In addition, the process of mask induction can be quite stressful and fear-evoking for both birds and small mammals, and undesired learned fear responses still may be generated.[28] Although the task at hand may be able to be accomplished, the greater goal of minimizing fear and stress and facilitating learned cooperative interaction between the animal and staff is reduced.

MEDICATION TRAINING

Birds and small mammals can be taught numerous medical behaviors using target training. By this method, the animal can be taught that if it "targets" (touches with a body part, eg, its beak or nose) an object (such as a chopstick, or closed hand), it will receive a favorable outcome, that is, positive reinforcement. Target training is used very commonly to train a large number of animal species, particularly in zoos. Target training can be used to train birds to do anything from play basketball, allow IM injections, to enter and exit the carrier. Similarly, target training can be used in small mammals to teach them to get onto and off of a scale voluntarily, stand still while being treated/examined, or enter or exit a carrier or its enclosure. Using small approximations and the individual strength of different reinforcers, new behaviors can be created. A reinforcer is any consequence that increases the strength or frequency of the behavior. A very simple example of target training is when teaching a bird, rabbit, ferret, or rodent to take medication directly from a syringe. Initially, the animal is reinforced just for touching the tip of the syringe: the owner holds the syringe up to the animal's beak or mouth (antecedent); the animal touches the tip of the syringe with its beak or mouth (behavior); owner gives the animal a treat (consequence). Assuming that treat provided (eg, millet, fruit, piece of meat; see **Table 3**) is a reinforcer for this individual animal, it can be predicted that the animal will continue to touch the target to get a nibble of millet or a piece of fruit or meat. Approximations are small steps taken to get to an end behavior. Each approximation should be repeated a few times or until the animal is comfortable before progressing to the next step. One can guess that the animal understands what is being asked when it can perform the desired behavior readily/without hesitation.

It may be helpful to list out the desired approximations before starting medication training with an animal so that you have a reminder of how you would like the training to progress. Although writing out a shaping plan may help with organization, keep open to the idea that there are several different ways to teach a behavior and the plan may need to be changed as it progresses. The learner, the bird, rabbit, ferret, or rodent, should control how quickly you progress to the next approximation, how small or large you break up the approximations, and whether you need to go back to the drawing board to make a new shaping plan.[29] Ideally, training sessions are kept short, giving the teacher time to review progress and adjust the shaping plan, and to make any needed changes to the environment, type of reinforcer, and so forth. For the purpose of training and shaping medical behaviors, many times these initial steps can be trialed while the patient is hospitalized. Short training sessions, 1 to 3 minutes for example, are recommended. Short sessions are easier to keep the animal engaged. If the animal loses interest before this time frame, end the session and try again later. Alternatively, some animals may prefer to train for hours. Keeping the sessions brief builds excitement for the next training session.

There are many reasons an animal may choose not to engage in a training session. For example, motivation may be low because the animal is already satiated or becoming satiated during the session. In birds, the following signs may indicate a satiated animal: rubbing or cleaning the beak on the perch, tucking the head back to preen, beak grinding. Satiated ferrets will often start licking their lips and rub their face against the floor or a cloth or other item, whereas resting and grooming behavior (eg, washing of the face and body) can be seen in all small mammal species. Animals might also fail to interact in a training session when it is unsure what you are asking of it (ie, does not understand how to get reinforcement). In this situation, try asking for a previously completed approximation to maintain interest while you assess the need to change the shaping plan (Are smaller steps needed? What might be unclear to the animal?). Check the environment for fear-evoking stimuli or other potential barriers to the learning experience. Check the patient's body language for clues to what signals may be missed. An animal that does no't feel safe is not likely to accept reinforcement of any kind, eat, or engage in a training session. Similarly, the animal may be distracted because of training sessions taking to long. It is therefore recommended to keep training sessions short to ensure an optimal attention span. Dependent on the species and engagement of the individual, durations of training sessions may vary from 1-3 minutes to periods of 10 to 20 minutes. Inclusion of short breaks, in which the animal is allowed to do something else (eg, play with a toy or other type of enrichment) can also help to keep it engaged longer.

As stated previously, there are numerous possible paths to get the desired behavior. Dependent in part on the already learned behaviors of the patient and its level of fearfulness, there may be different starting points for planned approximations. A few examples for medication training in birds and small mammals are provided, including different approximation paths that can be used to achieve the desired target behavior.

Shaping plan: learning a bird to accept medication from a syringe

Shaping Plan A

1. Bird drinks medication from syringe without restraint
2. Bird touches syringe to receive reinforcement
3. Bird touches syringe filled with water to receive reinforcement
4. Bird touch syringe with drop of water at the end to receive reinforcement
5. Bird drinks small amount of water from syringe to receive reinforcement
6. Bird touches syringe filled with medication to receive reinforcement
7. Bird drinks small amount of medication from syringe to receive reinforcement

Shaping Plan B

1. Bird drinks medication from syringe without restraint
2. Bird looks at syringe to receive reinforcement
3. Bird touches syringe to receive reinforcement
4. Bird bites syringe to receive reinforcement
5. Bird bites syringe filled with water to receive reinforcement
6. Bird bites syringe with drop of water at the end to receive reinforcement
7. Bird bites syringe filled with juice to receive reinforcement
8. Bird bites syringe with drop of juice at the end to receive reinforcement
9. Bird drinks small amount of water from the syringe to receive reinforcement
10. Bird drinks small amount of juice from the syringe to receive reinforcement
11. Bird drinks small amount of juice mixed with medicine to receive reinforcement

Shaping plan: toweling and using a face mask to anesthetize a guinea pig that routinely needs gas anesthesia for a dental examination and correction

*Behavior 1: accept toweling (see **Fig. 1**)*

Start with towel at the distance of approximately 1 m; guinea pig looks at the towel and displays calm behavior to receive reinforcement

Slight (eg, 10 cm) decrease of distance between towel and guinea pig, calm behavior displayed to receive reinforcement

Gradual decrease in distance; calm behavior displayed to receive reinforcement; repeat step until distance between towel and guinea pig has minimized

Place towel on the table near the guinea pig; look at towel to receive reinforcement (while maintaining calm behavior)

Guinea pig touches the towel with its nose to receive reinforcement

Guinea pig touches towel for longer periods to receive reinforcement

Guinea pig steps on towel to receive reinforcement

Guinea pig stands on towel for longer time to receive reinforcement

Guinea pig stands still while towel is lifted slightly to receive reinforcement

Guinea pig stands still while towel is gradually lifted higher to receive reinforcement

Guinea pig stands still while towel is gradually held above its head to receive reinforcement

Guinea pig stands still while towel is held above its head and lowered slightly so that a piece of towel touches its back shortly to receive reinforcement

Guinea pig stands still while towel is held above its head and lowered slightly so that a piece of towel touches its back for longer periods of time to receive reinforcement

Guinea pig stands still while towel is gently dropped over it for short period to receive reinforcement

Guinea pig stands still while towel is placed over it for longer periods to receive reinforcement

Guinea pig held in towel by hand while remaining calm to receive reinforcement (initially only for a short second, then gradually increase the duration)

> Behavior 2: accepting facemask
>
> Present the facemask at a large enough distance to not elicit a fear response and gradually decrease the distance while reinforcing calm behavior (as described for the towel) until the distance between the facemask and guinea pig has minimized
>
> Guinea pig looks at the facemask to receive reinforcement
>
> Guinea pig moves toward facemask to receive reinforcement
>
> Guinea pig touches the facemask with its nose to receive reinforcement
>
> Guinea pig touches the facemask with its nose while the facemask is held in correct position to receive reinforcement
>
> Guinea pig touches the facemask with its nose while facemask is held in position for longer duration to receive reinforcement

Once a reinforcer and a delivery method have been established, begin targeting to the syringe. Reinforcement may be given for any interaction with the syringe to start, including biting. There are a few ways to address "attacking" (biting/lunging) at the syringe. Biting the syringe is interacting with the syringe and close to the goal behavior of drinking medication from the syringe, so one way to address this is to reinforce it! By capturing a behavior, we reinforce a behavior the animal is already offering. Think of taking a photograph of the behavior. This photograph is what you choose to reinforce. Any behavior reinforced is a behavior that is likely to be repeated, giving you more opportunities to reinforce biting the syringe and build your shaping plan from that point. Another option is to mark and reinforce when the animal is reaching to bite the syringe, so it may help to hold the syringe slightly out of reach. After reinforcing the behavior of reaching for the syringe, shape touching the syringe by offering the syringe closer (**Fig. 3**). Aside from medication training, target training is an important exercise in communication and strengthening the bond that can be started with clients during new pet/client examinations and wellness checks. Target training has multiple other practical applications in teaching animals to go into their carriers, for towel training, and for several medical uses, and is very useful when working with "aggressive" animals. Essentially, target training is the perfect way to start integrating training into the examination rooms, by making veterinarian visits fun for your patients and clients.

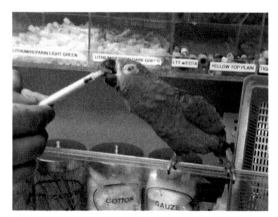

Fig. 3. Dusky-headed conure (*Aratinga wedellii*) demonstrating willingness to participate in drinking medication by leaning toward the syringe with open beak.

Links to step-by-step videos to help clarify the in-house use of approximations for medication training are available for viewing at https://youtu.be/3RufY4U_bnM.

FOOD VEHICLES

We all wish on occasion that medication administration could be as simple as stuffing a pill in a piece of cheese for a dog, but even that may not be as straightforward as we hope. After considering the health status of the animal and other factors, the decision to give medication in food is up to you and the pet owner. If the patient is a suitable candidate for receiving medication in food, this may be a minimally stressful method of delivery. The best food vehicle is small enough to encourage rapid consumption, but large enough to hide the taste of the medication, and most importantly, is a food item that is very high value for the animal. Food that mixes easily or acts as an absorbent, like bread, scrambled eggs, oatmeal, peanut butter, or pastries, generally works well with liquid medication (**Fig. 4**). For ferrets, you may consider including pate as a food vehicle. If the animal likes a juice, applesauce, or yogurt, you can mix these easily with the medication and offer in a spoon or bowl, whichever the animal prefers. With the help of a compounding pharmacy, medication can be made at a higher concentration, resulting in a smaller volume to put in food. However, medication at a higher concentration may have a stronger flavor, which might be harder to disguise in food. It may also be possible to hide medication by injecting it or hiding it in a small piece of fruit (eg, grape, banana) or a prey animal that is being fed to predators (birds of

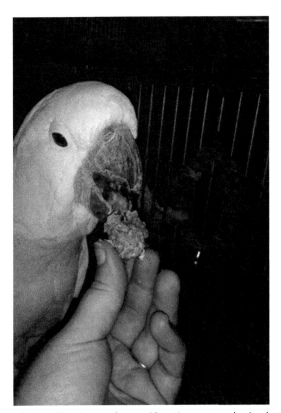

Fig. 4. Moluccan cockatoo (*Cacatua moluccensis*) eating oatmeal mixed with medication.

prey, ferrets). Similarly, for medicating poultry or waterfowl, a pill can be hidden in their favorite treat, like what is often done for medicating dogs. Grapes, cheese, tomatoes, and bread seem to work well for this, depending on what the bird prefers. If trying a new food, offer it first without medication to see if the animal will eat it. Ideally, the food has a very high value for the animal, which can take some trial and error to discover. When offering new foods, try several to see what the animal likes. Many tame birds and some small mammals like rats are highly interested in food that comes off our plate, which we can use to our advantage. Birds especially that are over threshold outside of the cage are not likely to eat or try new foods. For these birds, offer a variety of food to sample in the cage and come back in a few hours to see what the favorites were. The purpose of delivering medication in food is as a less stressful method, not to trick our animals into taking medication. If the flavor of the medication is too strong or apparent and/or the food vehicle not appealing enough to the animal, it might refuse to eat the food. Withholding the animal's normal diet until the medication is eaten rarely works in the authors' experience. Occasionally, an animal will taste medication in its favorite foods, resulting in it refusing to eat not only the food vehicle but also other treats/food offered outside of the normal diet. In this situation, even for animals that do not tolerate handling well, it is best to move to a different technique, like target training for medication.

TEACHING ANIMALS TO TAKE MEDICATION FROM A SYRINGE

Teaching an animal to drink medication from the syringe is an option that should be strongly considered for aggressive or fearful individuals because there is no restraint necessary. Although we can help our animals acclimate to a towel or handling, in many situations it is much more reinforcing to provide the opportunity for the animal to take part in its training, giving it control over the outcome, and then to restrain them or wrap them in the towel for medication.

Mixing medication with juice or another (semi)liquid substance (eg, recovery or critical care formula) may help your patient's willingness to drink a foul-tasting medication. Offer the juice or liquid substance to the animal first in a bowl or spoon to see if it likes the taste. For an animal that does not like the taste of the liquid, you may be making more work for yourself by teaching it to drink 2 foul-tasting liquids AND increasing the total volume you are asking it to drink from the syringe. Teaching an animal to drink from a syringe works well for any animal, regardless of whether it is "tame" or not by teaching the animal how to target to the syringe through cage bars while it is inside the cage (**Fig. 5**). First ensure that you have a reinforcer and a way to deliver the

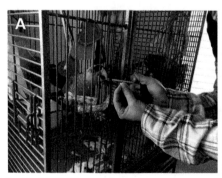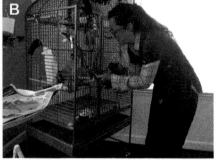

Fig. 5. (*A, B*) Lilac-crowned Amazon parrot (*Amazona finschi*) learning to target to the syringe through the cage bars.

reinforcer. Depending on the animal's response (is it showing escape/avoidance behaviors, is it lunging/trying to bite), you may need to be creative with how you deliver reinforcement. For example, a bird that flees to the opposite side of the cage when you hold up your hand might not be willing to take a treat from the hand. Offing a treat from a spoon may add distance between the bird and your hand and lessen anxiety should proximity to your hand be fear evoking. For smaller birds, offer a bite from an entire millet sprig, rather than a bite from a tiny piece in your hands. Another option is to fasten a "treat bowl" in the cage, which is a bowl that only holds treats. With some practice, using a treat bowl should feel safe for both human and bird. Remember that both teacher and student have a reinforcement history, and although one may have learned to avoid hands, the other may have learned to avoid beaks. It is important to take both into consideration for a successful shaping plan. By using a specific bowl and location in the cage, we teach the bird that there is a preferred place to perch, essentially teaching them to station for training (**Fig. 6**). Similar methods can be applied to small mammal species as well to teach them to accept medication from a syringe.

IN-PATIENT MANAGEMENT

Patients who are hospitalized or boarding are in an excellent position to begin medication training. Owners of animals that may require long-term medication often can recognize the merits of the ability to treat the animal without restraint, as a happy alternative to, for example, wrangling their bird, rabbit, or ferret in the towel. Compliance with treatment plans can be greatly enhanced. Also, it seems that a surprising number of clients are interested in beginning medication training *before* their pet even needs it! This framework can be facilitated with young animals while still in the appropriate socialization window or with adult animals just the same.

Particularly in birds, boarding patients for the purpose of training can enlist help with "problem" behaviors like lunging, training step-up behaviors, and especially medication training, just to name a few. There does not always have to be a behavior problem to go the extra mile with training. Medication training can easily be incorporated into daily treatments and documented on the patient's chart to note progress. Adjustments can be made to fees and treatment sheets to ensure time with technicians, according to what works best for your hospital. Hospitalized and boarding patients are also a

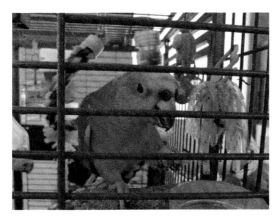

Fig. 6. Birds that cannot easily or safely come out of the cage, like this yellow-naped Amazon parrot (*Amazona auropalliata*), can be taught to station at a designated perch where training sessions occur. This helps set the stage for training lessons: When you come to this perch, we have a training session, that is, there are multiple opportunities for reinforcement.

great learning opportunity for the rest of the hospital staff. Including staff with the training and behavioral plan for patients opens the stage for them to ask questions and practice, which will ultimately allow them to help educate clients.

FINDING TIME

Perhaps the most challenging part of integrating training and low-stress methods into daily practice is competing with a busy schedule and time constraints. Training sessions should be short, 1 to 3 minutes ideally, which can make planning time during the work day a bit easier to manage. Longer training sessions may overwhelm, frustrate, and cause the patient to lose interest. For hospitals that have very busy treatment areas, use an empty examination room and place on the appointment schedule. Time will need to be set aside for client communication, which can be scheduled during the patient discharge. Visual aids, such as handouts and videos, may make this process easier for the clients to adjust to and help with time management.

EXAMINATION ROOM AND OUTPATIENT MANAGEMENT

Examination room setup can be easily tailored to meet the needs of the patients. Items like appropriate-sized perches for birds, or boxes, towels, or blankets for small mammals to hide in, and a room with minimal (visual, olfactory, and auditory) distractions will help patients feel comfortable. Any supplies you may need for the examination, training, or test sample collection should be stored in the examination room to minimize the amount of time the animal needs to be restrained. A variety of treats and training supplies like target sticks and a clicker can easily be stored in the examination room. Although it can be tricky storing properly sized items for various sizes and species of animals (perches, scales, towels/blankets/mats, hiding boxes, toys, treats), having these items readily available cuts down on restraint time and stress, which is important for both birds and small mammals. While handling, ensure that the animal is restrained as loosely as possible, and, especially in rabbits and rodents, allow the hind feet to have contact with a solid, nonslippery surface (bathmats usually work well for this purpose). Flooding, where an animal is restrained too long or excessively, which then causes the animal to not struggle anymore, should be avoided if at all possible for ethical and humane reasons.

In the examination room, it is not difficult to find a client who wants to make giving oral medication easier. It is also not difficult to find a client who wants to put their animal back in the cage without the animal attempting to bite, struggle, or escape. Who wouldn't want that? For most veterinary practices, *time* is the biggest obstacle to helping clients with their behavior questions and dilemmas. After addressing the primary reason for the examination, there may be hardly any time to delve into low-stress medicating let alone questions about the pet's behavior. Another complicating factor is that there are so many variations of behavior problems and questions, a short question may have a mile-long answer! Or even worse, several answers! For example, questions about how to give medication from a syringe may entail several different techniques, explanations of positive reinforcement, and successive approximations. It may also include less forceful handling and toweling methods. Delegate these tasks to your staff. Just like many tasks in the veterinary practice setting, educating clients about behavior and low-stress medicating is not a one-person job! By using regular, staff-wide continuing education, a more uniform practice team can be developed. The more advanced training opportunities that a veterinary practice staff has had the ability to pursue and put to work, the better the collaborative power the practice has to effect favorable change for their clients and patients. **Box 2** provides training opportunities and other great resources about behavior and training.

Box 2
Behavior and training resources

Veterinary Specialty Groups

- American College of Veterinary Behaviorists http://www.dacvb.org/
- American College of Animal Welfare http://www.acaw.org/
- European College of Animal Welfare and Behavioural Medicine www.ecawbm.com
- International Society for Applied Ethology www.isae.org

Behavior Associations

- Animal Behavior Management Alliance (ABMA) www.theabma.org
- Animal Behavior Society www.animalbehaviorsociety.org
- American Veterinary Society of Animal Behavior (AVSAB) www.avsabonline.org
- International Association of Animal Behavior Consultants (IAABC) www.iaabc.org

Exotic Animal Behavior/Training texts and videos

- Bunny Training 101 (Video). Heidenreich B. 2011. www.bunnytraining.com
- Exotic Pet Behavior: Birds, Reptiles, and Small Mammals. Bradley Bays T, Lightfoot T, Mayer J. Saunders Elsevier; 2006.
- Behavior of Exotic Pets. Tynes V, editor. Wiley Blackwell; 2010.
- Manual of Parrot Behavior. Luescher AU. Blackwell Publishing; 2006.
- Parrot training. Heidenreich B. http://www.goodbirdinc.com/

Web sites

- www.behaviorworks.org
- www.bunnytraining.com
- www.clickertraining.com
- www.drsophiayin.com
- www.kenramireztraining.com
- www.medicalcenterforbirds.com/training.pml

Adapted from Brown S. Small mammal training in the veterinary practice. Vet Clin North Am Exot Anim Pract 2012;15:472; with permission.

Although there are several different approaches and changes that can be made to accommodate necessary time for behavior talk with clients, it is important to find what works best for *your* hospital. Behavior questionnaires for clients are easily available and can be adapted to fit your client needs. Handouts can be a great way to provide clients with information and give "homework" between visits. Follow-up is important and can be accomplished via recheck examinations, technician appointments, telephone calls, or e-mail. Most importantly, however, is that follow-up is not dismissed, and that the behavioral health and welfare of the patient remain the focus, above and beyond the mere medical model of the current problem of concern.

FORAGING AND ENRICHMENT

Foraging is a necessary form of enrichment, especially for animals in captivity. Applied optimally, foraging can be used as a means of enrichment to redirect an animal's attention and behavior, as a part of a DS/CC (desensitization/counterconditioning) plan, to avoid the need for use of restraint collars and to avoid the need for some medical treatments to suppress undesired behaviors (particularly in birds). Foraging functions as a means with which to enrich the welfare of the animals themselves. Working for food by means of searching through boxes, toys, or puzzles, and shredding or chewing through paper or cardboard are great ways to keep your bird, rodent, and rabbit patients busy (**Figs. 7** and **8**). For ferrets, provision of a "foraging mat" or puzzle feeders and toys similar to those used in cats and dogs will work great too. Many animals will need to be taught these very natural behaviors, because they are not innate and are oftentimes very limited in the lifestyles of many companion animals. The need for training natural behaviors may be particularly the case when some natural chewing behaviors are considered a nuisance by the pet owner and discouraged. Beginning

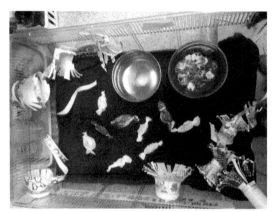

Fig. 7. Example of foraging for food in a hospital isolette for a small bird, which includes paper cups for shredding and food wrapped in paper for foraging.

foraging behaviors and shredding can be taught by demonstration in the examination room and continued at home (**Fig. 9**). These food acquisition activities can range from very simple hidden treats in half-covered bowls, wrapping food in pieces of paper, or hanging it at a more difficult to reach location (particularly for rabbits and rodents) to very complex puzzles and time-consuming boxes to untie or open for parrots. By increasing foraging in daily activities, oftentimes undesired behaviors can be eliminated or lessened, and quality of life can be enhanced. Enrichment and foraging are skills that can easily be developed in many settings while a patient is hospitalized and then transferred as a value-added skill set directed toward longer-term lifestyle changes at home. These enrichments are best viewed as lifelong lesson plans, and veterinarians can deliver their best impact by following through with patients and their stewards, coaching both from the side and tailoring recommendations to best fit patient needs.

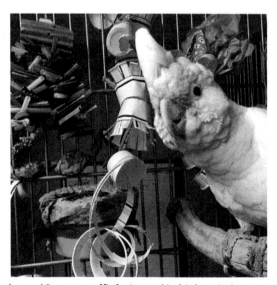

Fig. 8. Goffin's cockatoo (*Cacatua goffini*) pictured in his hospital cage with food hidden in paper cups, packaging paper, and a paper-covered food dish.

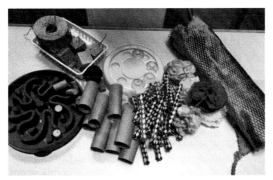

Fig. 9. Example of some different foraging supplies kept at the veterinary hospital.

THE POTENTIAL FOR INFLUENCE OF DRUG THERAPIES ON MEMORY AND LEARNING

Some treatments that patients receive as well as treatment methods can also influence memory and learning. There are some endocrine and drug-related influences on learning and memory retention, outside of a reinforcing consequence alone. For example, several studies have shown that psychological stress (eg, predator exposure) impairs spatial memory in rats.[30–32] Gonadal sex hormones can also affect memory and learning, as demonstrated in rats, in which acquisition, consolidation, and retrieval of inhibitory avoidance learning and memory were found to be impaired following intrahippocampal injections of testosterone.[33] Similarly, domestic chicks pretreated with testosterone, or treated within 30 minutes after exposure, were less able to retain aversion-trained stimuli. Without evidence from juvenile and adult birds to the same effect, it is not yet possible to conclude that such effects exist as a result of manipulation of gonadal steroids within physiologic ranges.[34] Estradiol plays a necessary role in auditory processing and memory of zebra finches (*Poephila guttata*). Estradiol depletion negatively affected the neuronal memory for vocalizations in that species, lending additional support that sex steroids have a role in memory and memory processing.[35] There are other endocrine influences on the development of long-term memory. Day-old chicks trained on a single-trial passive discrimination-avoidance task showed improved long-term memory with weakly reinforced tasks, when treated with noradrenaline, corticotropin, and vasopressin in close proximity to the training trial. The net effect mimicked the outcome of strongly reinforced learning and of retaining the weakly reinforced tasks.[36] There is a phase of memory in the day-old chick that is susceptible to interference by drugs affecting noradrenergic processes. The intermediate phase of memory processing of day-old chicks, to passive discrimination-avoidance tasks, was inhibited by the subcutaneous administration of propranolol. This effect was seen in chicks with strongly reinforced training, and with weakly reinforced training presented twice or coupled with a selected dose of the stress-related hormone corticotropin.[37]

Although the concept of a stress-free learning environment seems good, stress to a certain degree can facilitate memory and learning. In mice, corticotropin-releasing factor and acute stress were found to facilitate long-term potentiation of the hippocampus and enhance context-dependent fear conditioning.[38] Long-term memory for a passive avoidance task in day-old chicks has been shown to depend upon an action of the adrenal steroid corticosterone through specific receptors in a brain region, and corticosteroid synthesis inhibitors can inhibit long-term memory formation for passive avoidance tasks in day-old chicks.[39] Corticosteroid synthesis inhibitors were shown to impair long-term memory for a passive avoidance task in day-old chicks.[40]

Passive avoidance training results in increased cell proliferation in day-old chicks in areas of the brain known to be loci of memory formation.[41] Of course, not all levels of stress are necessarily a good thing. Stress functions to facilitate the consolidation of contextual fear memory. In rats, midazolam attenuated the stress-induced promotion of fear memory formation.[42] What this may mean, in practical applications, is that the appropriate and timely use of benzodiazepines may be important but not necessarily a requisite, along the long-term course and goal of not requiring continual use in patient treatment and management, in order to help avoid the development of learned fear in patients. Behavioral assessment and enrichment, combined with the physiologic and neurobiological aspects of learning, remain key. Short-term enrichment of housing conditions in chickens has been shown to have favorable, immediate effects on chickens by reducing behaviors that are likely to reflect fearfulness and by favorably affecting learning performance. This effect did not translate to long-term retention, however. In essence, a low-stress hospital environment, with strategic enrichment used, can help reduce perceived stress and can function to enhance operant conditioning of therapeutic procedures and treatments.[43]

Three memory developmental stages are known in birds and mammals: 2 short term and 1 long term. There is a long-term, antibiotic-sensitive, and likely protein synthesis–dependent stage of memory development.[44] Passive avoidance training memory was shown to be inhibited by the use of intracranial chloramphenicol.[45] Similarly, amnestic effects have been observed from antibiotic use in mammals.[46] Cyclooxygenases are induced during training, and cyclooxygenase products are of importance in memory formation of the chick.[47] Intracerebral injections of the cyclooxygenase inhibitors indomethacin, naproxen, and ibuprofen caused amnestic effects at all concentrations tested when injected either before (in chicks) or after training (in rats).[48,49]

Dopamine modulation of late-memory formation may be attenuated by haloperidol.[50] This attenuation of late memory does not necessarily imply that learning is critically impaired in patients being treated with haloperidol. In cases where feather-plucking sulfur-crested cockatoos (*Cacatua galerita*) were being treated medically (haloperidol), and with socialization, training, and feeding enrichment, the most successful treatments included the training sessions. These sessions provided much needed social attention as well as mental stimulation.[51] Desensitization, counterconditioning, enrichment, and pharmacologic intervention can be combined in case management. In a case report of a cockatiel with a history of repetitive chewing of the third digit of the right foot, the hypothesized causes of the behavior were presumed to be multifactorial, involving neurochemical changes, learning or owner reinforcement, and anxiety-induced displacement activity. Case management components that led to resolution of the problem included antecedent arrangement strategies (removal of stimuli that were associated with an increase in the problem behavior), enrichment (altered and enhanced social interactions with the stewards of the bird in the home), removal of hypothesized reinforcements for the problem behavior (successful attention acquisition), and reinforcement of alternative behaviors (counterconditioning) paired with desensitization. Fluoxetine was prescribed at 1 mg/kg orally every 24 hours as a pharmacologic intervention intended to aid in downsizing impulse control concerns. Enrichment of alternative behaviors and cessation of the problem behavior were accomplished over 1 month, and fluoxetine was reduced in dose and ultimately discontinued by 5 months.[52] Although some drugs can certainly have influence on the perception of stress and learning, there is even stronger support that with a balance of appropriate medication choices, training, enrichment, and socialization, there is an excellent opportunity for most effective and least intrusive treatment strategies to be formulated and implemented.

SUPPLEMENTARY DATA

Supplementary data related to this article can be found online at https://doi.org/10.1016/j.cvex.2018.01.016.

REFERENCES

1. Schepers F, Koene P, Beerda B. Welfare assessment in pet rabbits. Anim Welf 2009;18:477–85.
2. Normando S, Gelli D. Behavioral complaints and owners' satisfaction in rabbits, mustelids, and rodents kept as pets. J Vet Behav 2011;6:337–42.
3. Rooney NJ, Blackwell EJ, Mullan SM, et al. The current state of welfare, housing and husbandry of the English pet rabbit population. BMC Res Notes 2014;7:942.
4. Bradbury AG, Dickens GJE. Appropriate handling of pet rabbits: a literature review. J Small Anim Pract 2016;57:503–9.
5. Heidenreich B. Myths and misconceptions about parrot behavior and training. Proceedings of AAV, held at Savannah (GA), August 9–14, 2008. p. 375–9.
6. O'Heare J. The least intrusive effective behavior intervention (LIEBI) algorithm and levels of intrusiveness table: a proposed best-practices model. Journal of Applied Companion Animal Behavior 2009;3(1):7–25.
7. Heidenreich B. Using science-based training technology to train avian, exotics, and zoo animals to cooperate in medical care. Proceedings of Vet Behav Symposium held at San Antonio (TX), Aug 5, 2016.
8. Heidenreich B. A formalized program for in-house parrot training classes. Proceedings of AAV held at Savannah (GA), August 9–14, 2008. p. 169–72.
9. Brown SA. Small mammal training in the veterinary practice. Vet Clin North Am Exot Anim Pract 2012;15:468–87.
10. vanZeeland YRA, Friedman SG, Bergman L. Behavior. In: Speer BL, editor. Current vet therapy in avian med and surg. St Louis (MO): Elsevier; 2016. p. 177–251.
11. Friedman SG, Edling TM, Cheney CD. Concepts in behavior: section I, the natural science of behavior. In: Harrison G, Lightfoot T, editors. Clinical avian medicine. Palm Beach (FL): Spix Publishing Inc; 2006. p. 46–59.
12. Ziv G. The effects of using aversive training methods in dogs – a review. J Vet Behav 2017;19:50–60.
13. Bradley Bays TB. Rabbit behavior. In: Bradley Bays T, Lightfoot T, Mayer J, editors. Exotic pet behavior: birds, reptiles, and small mammals. St Louis (MO): Saunders Elsevier; 2006. p. 1–49.
14. Lightfoot T. Psittacine behavior. In: Bradley Bays T, Lightfoot T, Mayer J, editors. Exotic pet behavior: birds, reptiles, and small mammals. St Louis (MO): Saunders Elsevier; 2006. p. 51–101.
15. Fisher PG. Ferret behavior. In: Bradley Bays T, Lightfoot T, Mayer J, editors. Exotic pet behavior: birds, reptiles, and small mammals. St Louis (MO): Saunders Elsevier; 2006. p. 163–205.
16. Bradley Bays TB. Guinea pig behavior. In: Bradley Bays T, Lightfoot T, Mayer J, editors. Exotic pet behavior: birds, reptiles, and small mammals. St Louis (MO): Saunders Elsevier; 2006. p. 207–38.
17. Evans E. Small rodent behavior: mice, rats, gerbils and hamsters. In: Bradley Bays T, Lightfoot T, Mayer J, editors. Exotic pet behavior: birds, reptiles, and small mammals. St Louis (MO): Saunders Elsevier; 2006. p. 239–61.

18. Friedman SG, Haug L. From parrots to pigs to pythons: universal principles and procedures of learning. In: Tynes VV, editor. The behavior of exotic pets. Blackwell Publishing; 2010.

19. Friedman SG, Haug LI. From parrots to pigs to pythons: universal principles and procedures of learning. Behavior of Exotic Pets. Ames (IA): Wiley-Blackwell; 2010. p. 190–205.

20. Friedman SG, Martin S, Brinker B. Behavior analysis and parrot learning. In: Luescher AU, editor. Manual of parrot behavior. Ames (IA): Blackwell Publishing; 2006. p. 147–64.

21. Vesal N, Eskandari MH. Sedative effects of midazolam and xylazine with or without ketamine and detomidine alone following intranasal administration in Ring-necked Parakeets. J Am Vet Med Assoc 2006;228(3):383–8.

22. Vesal N, Zare P. Clinical evaluation of intranasal benzodiazepines, α2-agonists and their antagonists in canaries. Vet Anaesth Analg 2006;33:143–8.

23. Moghadam AZ, Sadegh AB, Sharifi S, et al. Comparison of intranasal administration of diazepam: clinical evaluation. Iranian Journal of Veterinary Science and Technology 2009;1(1):19–26.

24. Mans C, Guzman DSM, Lahner LL, et al. Sedation and physiologic response to manual restraint after intranasal administration of midazolam in Hispaniolan Amazon parrots (Amazona ventralis). J Avian Med Surg 2009;26:130–9.

25. Hedenqvist P, Orr HE, Roughan JV, et al. Anaesthesia with ketamine/medetomidine in the rabbit: influence of route of administration and the effect of combination with butorphanol. Vet Anaesth Analg 2002;29:14–9.

26. Lennox AM. Sedation of exotic companion mammals. In Proceedings of the 31st AAV Conference and Expo. San Diego (CA), August 2–5, 2010. p. 117–20.

27. Thiébot MH. Some evidence for amnesic-like effects of benzodiazepines in animals. Neurosci Biobehav Rev 1985;9:95–100.

28. Flecknell PA, Roughan JV, Hedenqvist P. Induction of anaesthesia with sevoflurane and isoflurane in the rabbit. Lab Anim 1999;33:41–6.

29. Heidenreich B. An introduction to the application of science-based training technology. Vet Clin North Am Exot Anim Pract 2012;15:371–85.

30. Diamond DM, Park CR, Heman KL, et al. Exposing rats to a predator impairs spatial working memory in the radial arm water maze. Hippocampus 1999;9(5):542–52.

31. Mesches MH, Fleshner M, Heman KL, et al. Exposing rats to a predator blocks primed burst potentiation in the hippocampus in vitro. J Neurosci 1999;19(14):RC18.

32. Woodson JC, Macintosh D, Fleshner M, et al. Emotion-induced amnesia in rats: working memory-specific impairment, corticosterone-memory correlation, and fear versus arousal effects on memory. Learn Mem 2003;10(5):326–36.

33. Harooni HE, Naghdi N, Rohani AH. Intra hippocampal injection of testosterone impaired acquisition, consolidation and retrieval of inhibitory avoidance learning and memory in adult male rats. Behav Brain Res 2008;188:71–7.

34. Clifton PG, Andrew RJ, Gibbs ME. Limited period of action of testosterone on memory formation in the chick. J Comp Physiol Psychol 1982;96(2):212–22.

35. Yoder KM, Lu K, Vicario DS. Blocking estradiol synthesis affects memory for songs in auditory forebrain of male zebra finches. Neuroreport 2012;23:922–6.

36. Crowe SF, Ng KT, Gibbs ME. Memory consolidation of weak training experiences by hormonal treatments. Pharmacol Biochem Behav 1990;37:729–34.

37. Crowe SF, Ng KT, Gibbs ME. Possible noradrenergic involvement in training stimulus intensity. Pharmacol Biochem Behav 1991;39:717–22.

38. Blank T, Nijholt I, Eckart K, et al. Priming of long-term potentiation in mouse hippocampus by corticotropin-releasing factor and acute stress: implications for hippocampus-dependent learning. J Neurosci 2002;22(9):3788–94.
39. Sandi C, Rose SP, Mileusnic R, et al. Corticosterone facilitates long-term memory formation via enhanced glycoprotein synthesis. Neuroscience 1995;69:1087–93.
40. Loscertales M, Rose SP, Sandi C. The corticosteroid synthesis inhibitors metyrapone and aminoglutethimide impair long-term memory for a passive avoidance task in day-old chicks. Brain Res 1997;769:357–61.
41. Dermon CR, Zikopoulos B, Panagis L, et al. Passive avoidance training enhances cell proliferation in 1-day old chicks. Eur J Neurosci 2002;16:1267–74.
42. Maldonado NM, Martijena ID, Molina VA. Facilitating influence of stress on the consolidation of fear memory induced by a weak training: reversal by midazolam pretreatment. Behav Brain Res 2011;225:77–84.
43. Krause T, Naguib M, Trillmich F, et al. The effects of short term enrichment on learning in chickens from a laying strain (Gallus gallus domesticus). Appl Anim Behav Sci 2006;101:318–27.
44. Ng KT, Gibbs ME, Crowe SF, et al. Molecular mechanisms of memory formation. Mol Neurobiol 1991;6:333–50.
45. Freeman FM, Young G. Chloramphenicol-induced amnesia for passive avoidance training in the day-old chick. Neurobiol Learn Mem 1999;71:80–93.
46. Barraco RA, Stettner LJ. Antibiotics and memory. Psychol Bull 1976;83:242.
47. Clifton PG, Andrew RJ, Gibbs ME. Prostaglandins play a role in memory consolidation in the chick. J Comp Physiol Psychol 1982;96:212–22.
48. Hölscher C. Inhibitors of cyclooxygenases produce amnesia for a passive avoidance task in the chick. Eur J Neurosci 1995;7:1360–5.
49. Sharifzadeh M, Naghdi N, Khosrovani S, et al. Post-training intrahippocampal infusion of the COX-2 inhibitor celecoxib impaired spatial memory retention in rats. Eur J Pharmacol 2005;511:159–66.
50. Hale MW, Crowe SF. The effects of apomorphine and haloperidol on memory consolidation in the day-old chick. Behav Neurosci 2001;115:376–83.
51. Jen-Lung Peng S, Hessey J, Tsay T, et al. Assessment and treatment of feather plucking in sulphur-crested cockatoos (Cacatua galerita). J Anim Vet Adv 2014;13:51–61.
52. Seibert LM. Animal behavior case of the month. J Am Vet Med Assoc 2004;224: 1433–5.

Techniques for Monitoring Drug Efficacy

Marike Visser, DVM*

KEYWORDS

- Therapeutic drug monitoring • Compounded drug • Dose-response curve
- Therapeutic index • Effective dose • Lethal dose

KEY POINTS

- Drug efficacy is based on a dose-response curve, requiring a combination of pharmacokinetic and pharmacodynamic data.
- Monitoring drug efficacy includes monitoring for adverse events and should be tailored based on the drug and any reported toxicities within the species.
- Monitoring includes therapeutic drug monitoring, monitoring clinical response, imaging, and diagnostics such as complete blood count, biochemistry, and urinalysis.
- Therapeutic drug monitoring can offer an effective method to determine plasma drug concentration in the individual patient and tailor the dose based on clinical signs or adverse drug events.

INTRODUCTION

Assessing drug efficacy can be a challenge in exotic medicine due to the limited pharmacokinetic (PK) data and even fewer pharmacodynamic (PD) studies. PK reports what the body does to the drug, from absorption to metabolism, distribution, and excretion. In contrast, PD describes what the drug does to the body in a dose-dependent manner, including anticipated and unanticipated (adverse) responses. The definition of what is considered efficacious varies based on the treatment protocol, the purpose of the selected drug, the dose selection, and the dosing interval. Drug efficacy is furthermore influenced by the pharmaceutical formulation, with clinically relevant differences reported in some compounded medications compared with the approved formulations. The clinician must, therefore, critically weigh the use of compounded drugs, especially if there is a concern of therapeutic failure or an adverse event (AE). Before discussing the methods of monitoring drug efficacy, an overview of how drug efficacy is established is required.

Disclosure Statement: The author does not have any conflict of interest to declare.
Department of Anatomy, Physiology and Pharmacology, Auburn University, 1500 Wire Road, Auburn, AL 36849, USA
* 137 North Park Street, Kalamazoo, MI 49007.
E-mail address: visserm0512@gmail.com

DRUG EFFICACY
Dose-Response Relationship

One of the fathers of toxicology, Paracelsus, is credited with the well-known saying, "All things are poison and nothing is without poison, only the dose makes that a thing is no poison."[1] Drug efficacy and toxicity is based on the dose-response relationship **(Fig. 1)** of a given drug, which illustrates the effect (response) associated with a given dose. The maximum effect a drug can have (ie, $e = 1$ or 100%) is defined as a full response and encompasses both therapeutic effects and AE. For example, at a dose corresponding to $e = 1$, the analgesic effects of fentanyl are accompanied by significant respiratory depression. Two drugs in the same class are compared and contrasted by potency and efficacy. Potency describes the dose needed for 2 drugs to provide the same magnitude of effect, whereas efficacy compares the effect that the drug has at the site of action (eg, morphine vs buprenorphine). Drugs are considered to be equal in efficacy if both induce the same magnitude of clinical response, but the drug causing the clinical response at a lower dose is considered more potent. For example, fentanyl and hydromorphone are equally effective, but a lower dose of fentanyl is required to elicit the desired response; therefore, fentanyl is more potent.[2]

Establishment of the Therapeutic Window

Once the dose-response relationship has been described, a therapeutic window can be designed for a given drug. The window reports a plasma drug maximum concentration (C_{max}) above which there is an increased risk of AE and a plasma drug minimum concentration (C_{min}) below which concentrations are ineffective **(Fig. 2)**.[2] The therapeutic window is based on population statistics of the median effective dose (ED_{50}) at which at least 50% of the population has the desired response. In contrast, the median lethal dose (LD_{50}) is defined as the dose at which 50% of the population has a lethal response **(Fig. 3)**. Dividing the LD_{50} by the ED_{50} establishes a therapeutic index (TI) and the larger the TI, the safer the drug.[1] This TI can vary between species

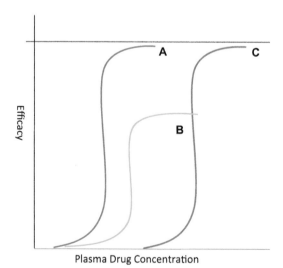

Plasma Drug Concentration

Fig. 1. Drug A and C are similarly effective; however, drug A is more potent because less of the drug is necessary. Drug A is more effective than drug B because it is 100% effective compared with the 50% effectiveness of drug B.

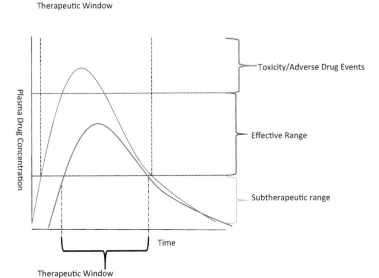

Fig. 2. Comparison between the area under the curve for the same drug given at 2 different doses. At higher concentrations, the C_{max} is within the adverse drug event or a toxicity range. At the lower dose, the C_{max} is within the effective range but will be within the subtherapeutic range faster, requiring more frequent dosing.

based on physiologic differences; hence caution should always be used when applying a TI to a species with an unknown dose-response curve. An example of suspected differences in TI between species is the use of fenbendazole,[3] which is reported to have a wide TI. It is so wide that a toxic dose could not be established in

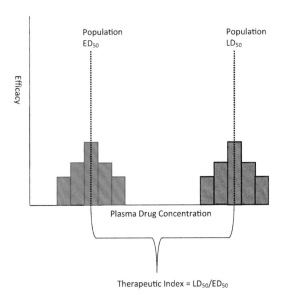

Fig. 3. Development of a therapeutic index, based on the effective dose (ED_{50}) in 50% of the population and the lethal dose (LD_{50}) in 50% of the population.

dogs, cats, and a variety of ruminants.[4] However, bone marrow necrosis has been reported in pelicans and storks receiving doses that are safe in dogs and cats.[5,6] Whereas the TI reports the fold difference between efficacious and toxic dose, the therapeutic window is the plasma drug concentration (PDC) at which most animals have the desired effect with the least risk of toxicity.[7,8]

WHAT CONSTITUTES DRUG EFFICACY MONITORING?

Therapeutic windows for exotic species are rarely known owing to the lack of species-specific PK and PD data, preventing the description of a dose-response relationship. Therefore, the clinician must use indirect methods to monitor drug efficacy, tailored by drug class, species, and the risk of AE, which may range from mild signs, such as anorexia, vomiting, and diarrhea, to severe clinical signs of renal or hepatic failure, or even death. Information regarding used dosages and AE are reported in case reports or series; larger, controlled toxicity studies or clinical trials; and derived from clinical experience. All published cases and information regarding a specific drug should always be critically evaluated by the clinician to develop a better understanding of the drug and to develop a dose and dosing interval that is effective while minimizing risk of AE to the individual patient. After initiation of a treatment regimen, a combination of monitoring techniques can be used to indirectly evaluate the drug's efficacy and presence of AE. Common methods that are used for this purpose include[9]

- Clinical examination (including history) to evaluate clinical response (improvement or deterioration)
- Complete blood count; for example, myelosuppression, hemolysis, resolution of leukocytosis, and resolution of hemoparasite infection
- Biochemistry; for example, liver and renal toxicity, blood glucose, and protein electrophoresis
- Hormone analysis; for example, total thyroxine to evaluate development of hypothyroidism due to sulfonamides and to monitor efficacy of hyperthyroidism treatment
- Urinalysis; for example, renal toxicity, resolution of glucosuria in diabetes mellitus, proteinuria, and resolution of urinary tract or kidney infection.
- Fecal examination; for example, presence or resolution of endoparasite infestation, and occult blood
- Culture and sensitivity to identify presence or absence of a pathogen and select the appropriate antimicrobial drug and dose
- Imaging (eg, radiography, ultrasonography, advanced imaging, endoscopy) and resolution or progression of disease
- Electrocardiogram for development or resolution of arrhythmia
- Blood pressure monitoring for development or resolution of hypovolemia, hypotension, hypervolemia, or hypertension
- Tonometry for changes in intraocular pressure (eg, uveitis, glaucoma)
- Therapeutic drug monitoring (TDM); tailor the dose to the patient to minimize AE.

Based on the disease present and the drugs used, a selection can be made using the previously mentioned list to ensure that the monitoring is tailored to fit the individual patient's needs (**Table 1**). Species differences are important to take into account because some drugs or drug classes have known reported risks across most species, whereas others are only reported to be toxic in certain species (eg, diclofenac in vultures[10] and fenbendazole in pelicans, storks, and porcupines[5,6,11]). In addition, species-specific dose sensitivity and clinical signs can vary, even within each drug

Table 1
Modalities to monitor drug efficacy for commonly used drug classes in exotic species

Drug Class	Monitoring for Drug Efficacy
Nonsteroidal antiinflammatory drugs	CBC, biochemistry (renal function), UA
Cardiac drugs	CBC, biochemistry (renal and liver function, protein, electrolytes, cardiac troponin[a]), UA, imaging, ECG, BPM, TDM
Anticonvulsants	Clinical monitoring of seizure frequency, CBC, biochemistry (particularly liver function), TDM, T4[b]
Immunosuppressant	CBC, biochemistry (liver, renal function), UA, TDM
Antimicrobials	Culture and sensitivity, CBC, UA, biochemistry (protein electrophoresis), imaging
Antifungals	Culture and sensitivity, CBC, biochemistry (protein electrophoresis), Imaging, TDM
Parasiticides	Fecal examination, CBC, biochemistry (eg, liver, renal function)

Note that these are general recommendations that should be tailored to the individual based on the drug used and the reported AEs within each species.

Abbreviations: BPM, blood pressure measurement; CBC, complete blood count; ECG, electrocardiography; T4, thyroxine; TDM, therapeutic drug monitoring; UA, urinalysis.

[a] Available in ferrets.

[b] In case of zonisamide because long-term administration of this drug can result in hypothyroidism.

class. For example, vultures have been found to be extremely sensitive to ketoprofen and diclofenac, whereas meloxicam is reported to be safe.[10,12,13]

THERAPEUTIC DRUG MONITORING

One of the most direct methods of correlating dose, PDC, and effect is through the use of TDM. TDM is the use of serum or PDCs combined with clinical observation to aid in therapeutic decision-making.[14,15] TDM can range from establishing or maintaining a patient within a therapeutic window, decreasing the risk of AE, or calculating a dosing interval. In veterinary medicine, TDM ranges from monitoring for drug residues in food animals and unapproved drugs in performance animals to determining dosing intervals for the individual patient. There are no reports in veterinary medicine concerning the beneficial impact of TDM; however, in humans, a meta-analysis reports a significant increase in clinical efficacy and a decrease in nephrotoxicity with TDM implementation (**Table 2**).[16]

Several diagnostic laboratories offer TDM for a variety of drugs, including anticonvulsants (phenobarbital, potassium bromide, levetiracetam, zonisamide, and diazepam), cardiac drugs (digoxin, lidocaine, and quinidine), antifungals (itraconazole), antimicrobials (amikacin and gentamicin), immunosuppressants (cyclosporine and leflunomide), psychoactive drugs (paroxetine and amitriptyline), and bronchodilators (theophylline).

Before submitting samples, be sure to contact the laboratory to inquire

1. How the sample should be collected (eg, what type of container to use), handled (eg, centrifuging, freezing), and shipped (eg, cooled or on dry ice)
2. What additional demographic (age, sex, species) and/or clinical information (current disease, treatments, perceived efficacy) needs to be included with the sample[2]
3. If the assay been validated with the target species.

Table 2
Potential applications of therapeutic drug monitoring in exotic animal medicine

Aim	Which Parameter to Target	When to Collect Sample
Decrease the risk of AE	C_{max}	Collect 2–4 h after dose administration
Identify subtherapeutic level	C_{min}	Collect right before next dose
Determine a dosing interval	C_{max}, C_{min}	Collect 1 sample 2–4 h after dose and 1 sample right before next dose
Determine if there has been a change in the PDC if patient suddenly starts to show clinical signs or AE	C_{max} or C_{min}	Collect at time previous sample had been collected to allow for comparison

A variety of TDM methods have been developed for the drugs, each requiring a very specific assay. Species differences in plasma proteins and viscosity can alter the ability of the assay to accurately quantify PDC and the clinician should enquire about validation techniques with the laboratory.[9,17]

Despite TDM offering several benefits for patient monitoring, there are also some drawbacks and limitations that should be taken into consideration (**Table 3**). A discussion with the laboratory is usually warranted to determine whether TDM will answer the clinical question.

Interpretation of Therapeutic Drug Monitoring Results

A clinical pharmacologist can help in interpretation of a result, and will usually ask for additional demographic and clinical information.

Information to include on a submission includes

- Species, age, and gender
- Reason for submission: therapeutic failure versus maintenance versus new formulation versus toxicity
- Perceived drug efficacy
- Any additional medications that the patient is receiving, including all herbal or nutritional supplements
- Dosing formulation, dose, and dosing interval
- Collection times relative to the time since dosing, especially if 2 samples are submitted.

Table 3
Advantages and disadvantages of therapeutic drug monitoring in exotic patients

Advantages	Disadvantages
Ability to determine an individualized dosing interval	Lack of assay validation in exotic species
Ability to monitor changes in PDC with changes in disease state	Lack of species-specific therapeutic window
Ability to correlate PDC with additional diagnostics such as C&S, CBC, biochemistry	Amount of serum or plasma that may need to be submitted

Abbreviation: C&S, culture and susceptibility.
Data from Lainesse C. Quick and easy therapeutic drug monitoring from the comfort of your own desk. Paper presented at: Western Veterinary Conference. Las Vegas, Febuary 19–23, 2012.

In addition to interpretation of the results based on the supplied data, dosing adjustments can be made using a few selected equations. Using the measured PDC along with the time, simple PK equations (**Box 1**) can be used to adjust the patient's dose. Causes for dose adjustment include the presence of hepatic or renal disease that could alter elimination, therapeutic failure, or suspect drug interactions.

Example Problem

One of the most common reasons for dose adjustment is determining a dosing interval for efficacy or safety, particularly if a therapeutic dose has not been established. For example, it is recommended that amikacin PDC is less than 5 μg/dL in dogs to prevent acute renal toxicosis, but it is recommended that the PDC is less than 1 μg/dL before dosing again. In an exotic patient with unknown PK parameters, the half time ($t_{1/2}$) can be calculated and then used to determine when the PDC would be less than 1 μg/dL.

If the C_{max} PDC is 20 μg/dL at 2 hours after administration and the C_{min} PDC is 5 μg/dL at 8 hours (k_{el} is the elimination constant, In is the natural log, and $t_{1/2}$ is the half-life):

$$k_{el} = \ln\frac{\frac{20}{5}}{8-2} = 0.23$$

$$t_{1/2} = \frac{0.693}{0.23} = 3\ h$$

This exotic species seems to have a prolonged half-life compared with the 1 hour reported in dogs.[2] Now calculate the least amount of time the clinician should wait before dosing again (e is the constant and t is time):

$$1\ \mu g/dL = (20\ \mu g/dL)e^{-0.23t}$$

$$t = 13\ h$$

The clinician should wait at least 13 hours before dosing again. In the case of amikacin, it is recommended that animals are dosed once a day. This exotic animal will be safe with dosing once a day.

DETERMINING THE EFFICACY OF COMPOUNDED MEDICATIONS

Compounded medications are frequently used in veterinary medicine and are absolutely essential in exotic veterinary practice. Two important concepts are used when

---

Box 1
Calculations for dosing adjustment

- Dose adjustment: Dose = Current dose × $\frac{Target\ PDC}{Measured\ PDC}$
- Dosing interval adjustment: Interval = Current interval × $\frac{Measured\ PDC}{Target\ PDC}$
- Drug elimination constant: $k_{el} = \frac{\ln\frac{peak\ PDC}{trough\ PDC}}{t_{trough}-t_{peak}}$
- Half-life: $t_{1/2} = \frac{0.693}{k_{el}}$
- $C = C_{max}e^{-k_{el}t}$

Abbreviations: C, PDC at a given time; C_{max}, maximum concentration; k_{el}, elimination constant; PDC, plasma drug concentration; t, time.
Data from Lainesse C. Quick and easy therapeutic drug monitoring from the comfort of your own desk. Paper presented at: Western Veterinary Conference. Las Vegas, 2012.

comparing an approved (pilot) pharmaceutical to its compounded counterpart. The first is bioequivalence, which compares the active pharmaceutical ingredient administered via the same route and but in different formulations. Two drugs are considered bioequivalent if the PK parameters, bioavailability, and area under the curve are within 90% to 110% of each other.[18,19] Bioavailability is the second important concept and refers to the percentage of a drug that reaches systemic distribution, with absolute bioavailability comparing intravenous administration to an extravenous route and relative bioavailability comparing 2 extravenous routes.[2] Ideally, a compounded product is bioequivalent to an approved drug; however, this information is frequently unavailable and the clinician must assess the product's stability and efficacy via TDM and use of the US Pharmacopeia guidelines.[20] (See Lauren V. Powers and Gigi Davidson's article, "Compounding and Extralabel Use of Drugs in Exotic Animal Medicine," in this issue.)

SUMMARY

There is no single correct method to assess drug efficacy in the absence of a species-specific TI and therapeutic window. The clinician should use a combination of clinical observation; any reported PK, PD, AE, and data; and tailored drug monitoring to determine drug efficacy. The monitoring should be based on the purpose for a selected drug and the potential for AE, as well as the formulation selected. If a compounded drug is used, both product stability and bioequivalence can influence drug efficacy and needs to be evaluated. Using multiple techniques, drug efficacy can be critically assessed and changed if there is no improvement.

REFERENCES

1. Brunton L, Chabner BA, Knollman B. 12 edition. Goodman and Gilman's the pharmacological basis of therapeutics, vol. 1549. New York: McGraw-Hill New York; 2010.
2. Boothe DM. Principles of drug therapy. St. Louis (MO): Saunders; 2012.
3. Schwartz RD, Donoghue AR, Baggs RB, et al. Evaluation of the safety of fenbendazole in cats. Am J Vet Res 2000;61(3):330–2.
4. McKellar Q, Scott E. The benzimidazole anthelmintic agents-a review. J Vet Pharmacol Ther 1990;13(3):223–47.
5. Lindemann DM, Eshar D, Nietfeld JC, et al. Suspected fenbendazole toxicity in an American white pelican (Pelecanus erythrorhynchos). J Zoo Wildl Med 2016; 47(2):681–5.
6. Weber MA, Miller MA, Neiffer DL, et al. Presumptive fenbendazole toxicosis in North American porcupines. J Am Vet Med Assoc 2006;228(8):1240–2.
7. Trepanier LA. Applying pharmacokinetics to veterinary clinical practice. Vet Clin North Am Small Anim Pract 2013;43(5):1013–26.
8. Riviere JE. Comparative pharmacokinetics: principles, techniques and applications. Ames (IO): John Wiley & Sons; 2011.
9. Flanagan R, Brown N, Whelpton R. Therapeutic drug monitoring (TDM). CPD Clin Biochem 2008;9(1):3–21.
10. Swan G, Naidoo V, Cuthbert R, et al. Removing the threat of diclofenac to critically endangered Asian vultures. PLoS Biol 2006;4(3):e66.
11. Weber MA, Terrell SP, Neiffer DL, et al. Bone marrow hypoplasia and intestinal crypt cell necrosis associated with fenbendazole administration in five painted storks. J Am Vet Med Assoc 2002;221(3):417–9, 369.

12. Naidoo V, Wolter K, Cromarty D, et al. Toxicity of non-steroidal anti-inflammatory drugs to Gyps vultures: a new threat from ketoprofen. Biol Lett 2010;6(3):339–41.
13. Naidoo V, Wolter K, Cromarty AD, et al. The pharmacokinetics of meloxicam in vultures. J Vet Pharmacol Ther 2008;31(2):128–34.
14. Shaw LM, Figurski M, Milone MC, et al. Therapeutic drug monitoring of mycophenolic acid. Clin J Am Soc Nephrol 2007;2(5):1062–72.
15. Jorga A, Holt DW, Johnston A. Therapeutic drug monitoring of cyclosporine. Transplant Proc 2004;36(2 Suppl):396S–403S.
16. Ye ZK, Tang HL, Zhai SD. Benefits of therapeutic drug monitoring of vancomycin: a systematic review and meta-analysis. PLoS One 2013;8(10):e77169.
17. Schumacher GE, Barr JT. Therapeutic drug monitoring. Clin Pharmacokinet 2001; 40(6):405–9.
18. Tett SE, Saint-Marcoux F, Staatz CE, et al. Mycophenolate, clinical pharmacokinetics, formulations, and methods for assessing drug exposure. Transplant Rev (Orlando) 2011;25(2):47–57.
19. Johnson JR, Stell AL, Delavari P. Canine feces as a reservoir of extraintestinal pathogenic Escherichia coli. Infect Immun 2001;69(3):1306–14.
20. Pharmaceutical compounding-nonsterial preparataions (general chapter 795). The United States Pharmacopenia 38th rev., and the National Formulary, 33rd edition. Rockville (MD): The United States Pharmacopeial Convention; 2015. p. 559–67.

Group Treatment Strategies for Animals in a Zoologic Setting

Katie W. Delk, DVM, Dipl ACZM[a],
Christine M. Molter, DVM, Dipl ACZM[b],*

KEYWORDS

- Group treatment • Zoo • Multispecies • Amphibian • Avian • Hoofstock
- Herd health • Aviary health

KEY POINTS

- Group treatments vary between taxa, but all have benefits and risks that should be considered before therapy administration.
- Treatments administered topically on or milled into food, solubilized in drinking water, and mixed into a bath are common routes of administration for groups of animals.
- Sick animals should be treated individually to ensure compliance, because group treatments are often only effective against highly susceptible pathogens.

INTRODUCTION

Providing care for groups of animals is a major part of practicing zoologic medicine. Herd health is key to the mindset of a zoo clinician no matter the species encountered, be it avian or artiodactylid. In addition to the classic examples of group treatment involving chemotherapeutics (discussed in detail later), zoo clinicians also practice herd health by preventing disease from entering the collection. Before traveling to a new institution, most animals undergo a preshipment examination, which serves as a screening tool for common infectious diseases specific to that taxa, and provides a snapshot of that individual's health. Diagnostics commonly included in a preshipment examination are a complete blood count, serum or plasma biochemistry, imaging, and fecal examination. On arrival to a new institution, most animals undergo a quarantine period, often 30 to 90 days, in addition to another thorough examination. All of these precautionary measures are vital to ensure that infectious disease does not enter an institution, and also provide the opportunity for targeted therapy if

Disclosure Statement: The authors have nothing to disclose.
[a] Veterinary Services, The North Carolina Zoo, 4401 Zoo Parkway, Asheboro, NC 27205, USA;
[b] Houston Zoo, Inc., 1513 Cambridge Street, Houston, TX 77030, USA
* Corresponding author.
E-mail address: cmolter@houstonzoo.org

needed, before the animal is placed within its new social group. It is highly recommended that all animals that die within a zoologic setting receive a thorough gross necropsy with histopathology to try and determine the cause of death. Then, if an infectious cause is diagnosed, therapy for the remaining group of animals is based on the pathology findings.

Another way that zoo clinicians can try to limit the need for group treatment is to have a working knowledge of which taxa can be safely housed together. In addition to such factors as size and potential for trauma, knowledge of how certain infectious diseases interact with various species can prevent future outbreaks. For example, *Entamoeba invadens* is transmitted from clinically healthy herbivorous tortoises to snakes when they are housed together, causing the snakes to develop severe ulcerative colitis and hepatitis.[1] If a disease outbreak does occur, practicing vigilant biosecurity to try and limit transmission is key to decreasing the number of animals affected and needing treatment. Depending on the etiologic agent footbaths, isolation, and appropriate personal protective equipment may be used.[2]

When treatment is needed in a zoologic setting it presents unique challenges. One obstacle commonly encountered is that few pharmacokinetic studies have been performed in the species commonly found in zoos, so doses are often extrapolated from their closest domestic relative. Although extrapolation from domestics is done easily for some taxa, such as exotic canids, felids, or equids, there are species with no domestic counterpart, such as marsupials or invertebrates. Several different types of interspecies scaling have been described in the literature, with allometric scaling considered the most accurate.[3] However, there are limiting factors to consider when using allometric scaling, such as the route of elimination and the extent of metabolism of the selected therapeutic agent.[3] An additional challenge is that often accurate body weights cannot be obtained, so estimated weights are used, which can increase the risk of underdosing or overdosing an animal.[4] Group treatment is not common for some taxa, such as large carnivores, and individual treatment is advised when possible. Once a dosage has been selected and a weight obtained or estimated, the next question is how to administer the drug to the animal. Treatment options are heavily dependent on the species, and are covered in detail in the following sections. Group treatment is not standard for all taxa, so only the most common species are discussed.

AMPHIBIANS

Terrestrial and aquatic amphibians may be housed in single-species or mixed species exhibits, and individually. Regardless of species, morbidity and mortality is best prevented with appropriate environments, husbandry, nutrition, and biosecurity.[5–8] Separating ill or injured individuals from a group for individualized treatment is advised. Aquatic amphibians including premetamorphic larvae, neotenic salamanders, and aquatic newts and frogs inherently have a greater potential need for group treatments because of their aquatic existence; however, the potential exists for the need to treat a variety of amphibians as a group.

Terrestrial and aquatic amphibians living in a group may be separated for individualized treatments and this is generally well-tolerated. Individual animals may be temporarily moved out from the group enclosure to a separate enclosure for treatments and may remain separated for the duration of the treatment or be moved for short periods of time on a routine basis (**Fig. 1**). Individualized housing for medical care may be simplistic, but is acceptable as long as husbandry needs are adequately met.[5] Benefits of individualized treatments are assurance of medication compliance, ability to closely monitor clinical condition, reduced risk of infectious disease spread,

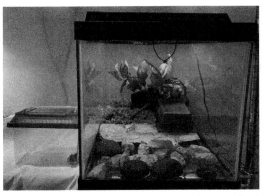

Fig. 1. A Panamanian golden frog (*Atelopus zeteki*) is moved into a plastic covered container for daily medicated bath treatments. After treatments, the animal is moved back into a more elaborate enclosure.

and elimination of extraneous treatments for healthy animals or nontarget species as compared with group treatments. Risks of individualized treatments include potential social and behavioral stress, and epithelial trauma from handling.[9]

Skin of amphibians is vascular and highly permeable, allowing for gas, water, and electrolyte exchange, and should absorb medications effectively transcutaneously.[10,11] In terrestrial and semiaquatic systems, topical medications may be administered to individuals living within the group as spot-on treatments without handling and may be a useful strategy when handling or removal from the group is not desired. Alternatively, animals may be restrained on a routine basis for medicating and be replaced back into the group. If spot-on topical medications are desired for aquatic animals, some duration of dry docking out of water is needed for the drug to absorb before being returned to water. This should not be done if the animal is unable to tolerate a period out of water because of lack of respiration or dehydration. Topical medications are particularly useful for very small animals.[12] Care should be taken to accurately calculate the intended dose. Dilute compounded drug formulations and calibrated micropipettes for delivery help facilitate small animal treatments and prevent overdosing.[13] Evidence for spot-on topical treatments in amphibians is primarily anecdotal, but common in practice and suggested dosages are available.[14]

Bath treatments are a common therapeutic modality for amphibians, terrestrial and aquatic. For terrestrial species, bath treatments are achieved by placing the individual to be treated in a container, such as a vented plastic carrier, filled with the solution just to the point where it covers the ventral drink patch to allow for adequate absorption (**Fig. 2**). Multiple animals may be treated in the same bath simultaneously, as space and temperament allows (**Figs. 3** and **4**). For aquatic species, the medicated bath should ideally be separate from the animal's home enclosure to prevent treatment of nontarget species, adverse effects on the biofilter, or damage to living plants. Additionally, using an animal's home enclosure water may be necessary for aquatic species to prevent sudden changes in water quality leading to electrolyte imbalance and stress. An air stone to provide oxygenation may be considered for lengthy treatments. However, if treatment in the primary enclosure's water system is desired, medications may be added directly into the water system. After the desired length of treatment, the medicated water should be cleared by a water change or high flow rate filtration to prevent an unnecessarily long exposure.[15] Typical bath treatments include electrolyte, antibiotic, and

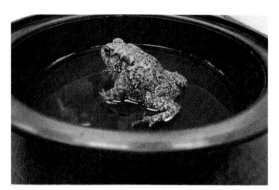

Fig. 2. A single Houston toad (*Anaxyrus houstonensis*) soaks in an electrolyte solution with the ventral drink patch completely submerged. Ideally, the container should have a cover to prevent the animal from exiting the space and to ensure adequate contact or compliance throughout the entire treatment period.

antifungal solutions that are calculated to be a certain dosage per volume of water over a specified period of time at set intervals. For example, chytrid fungus (*Batrachochytrium dendrobatidis*) treatment may include a bath of 0.01% itraconazole (100 ppm or 1 mg/L) in an electrolyte solution for 5 minutes daily for up to 14 days.[16] The total volume to be administered depends on the size container for medication and the size of animal, so that the drink patch is covered. The benefits of group bath treatments are that it is time and resource efficient and reduces handling. For topical spot-on and bath treatments, the pH of the desired medication should be checked and ensured to be neutral. This may be done with in-house pH strips to prevent caustic dermal from either acidic or alkaline products.

Injectable medications may also be administered with intramuscular or intralymphatic injections being common.[12] These routes of administration are more invasive and require additional handling compared with topical treatments, thus making these

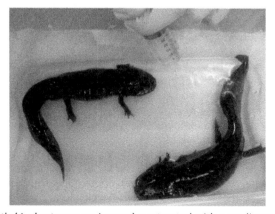

Fig. 3. Two axolotls (*Ambystoma mexicanum*) are treated with a medicated electrolyte solution bath in tandem. These animals were moved from their primary enclosure into a clean plastic container containing the medicated solution. A 60-mL syringe is being used to apply the solution topically to the dorsum because these animals are not completely submerged for the duration of treatment.

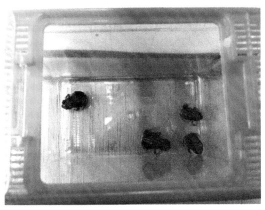

Fig. 4. Four Houston toadlets (*Anaxyrus houstonensis*) share a medicated bath solution that is deep enough to cover the ventral drink patch within a vented plastic carrier.

less common for group treatments. Long-acting medications in depo-formulations, such as ceftiofur crystalline-free acid antibiotics, may allow for less frequent handling and minimize disruption to the amphibian group, but have not been well-studied in amphibians, so any potential use should be done with caution.

Oral medications may be given to terrestrial and aquatic individuals into the oral cavity with a syringe or pipette or gavaged deeper into the esophagus or stomach with a metal ball–tipped feeding tube, a pliable red-rubber catheter, or similar device. Individuals require handling for this route of administration, which may prove challenging in vigorous aquatic species. Handling trauma, regurgitation with aspiration into the glottis or contamination of the gills, are risks. In debilitated animals, oral medications may be given with nutritional support.

Oral group treatments may be administered prophylactically, such as part of a preventative medicine program, or may be in response to disease. These treatments are generally administered as topical applications onto insects or fed to insects before feeding out to amphibians. This method allows for a completely hands-off approach to treatment and is rapid for large groups. However, the method is also problematic because the medication may easily dissolve or dislodge off the insect and relies on all amphibians consuming medicated prey items immediately and equally, so dosage received by an individual may be over or under the target. Animals that consume more than the anticipated number of medicated insects should be monitored for adverse reactions or toxicities.[17] For example, a study in Houston toads (*Anaxyrus houstonensis*) demonstrated that fenbendazole reduced the number of nematode eggs, larvae, and adults observed on fecal examination. This was achieved by dusting crickets with finely ground fenbendazole granules and feeding them once daily for 3 consecutive days. The dosage for this treatment was higher than most other published doses and was estimated based on how much fenbendazole dust adhered to the cricket.[18] Considerations should also be made for the welfare of insects being treated before being fed out to prevent undue distress.

Environmental changes, such as temperature adjustments, are reported as effective therapies and may be applied readily to groups of terrestrial and aquatic amphibians.[19,20] For example, caecilians (*Typhlonectes natans*) with subclinical chytridiomycosis have been successfully treated by gradually elevating their tank water temperature by 2°C to 3°C per day until a temperature of to 32.2°C (90°F) was reached and this was sustained for 72 hours. After treatment, the tank water was gradually returned to normal over 3 to 4 days.[19] Not all species tolerate therapeutic temperature changes and it may be most useful in combination with other therapies.[8]

Preventative medicine in terrestrial amphibians varies by species and institution, but may include routine deworming. Groups of amphibians may be treated topically with anthelmintics, by injections, oral medications either directly gavaged to the animal or on prey items, or via bath solution. Fecal parasite screenings are recommended to determine which treatments to administer and efficacy of medications.

When treating larval amphibians, dosages may be lower than that used for adults and are likely species specific. Therefore, caution and conservative dosing may be prudent when treating groups of larval amphibians. For example, midwife toad (*Alytes muletensis*) tadpoles cleared *B dendrobatidis* infections at less concentrated intraconazole bath solutions than adults, but developed epidermal depigmentation, thought to be caused by hepatotoxicity.[21]

BIRDS

Aviary populations are highly variable and may consist of single or multiple species. Avian group medicine focuses on prevention of and rapid response to disease in flocks of birds.[22] Birds housed in groups may have drugs administered individually via injectable, topical, oral, or inhalational routes or as group treatments via oral routes in water or food based on several factors, including, but not limited to clinical condition, population of birds within the group, drug availability, frequency of administration, and risks of treatment.[23]

For birds requiring medical treatments, separating the individual from the group is advantageous to ensure compliance and provide close monitoring, but may also come with social and behavioral stress, along with risks of repeated manual restraint. In ill birds, if compliance cannot be achieved by a particular route of administration, an alternative route, hospitalization, or isolation from the group may be needed.[24] Intramuscular and subcutaneous injections ensure compliance, but are invasive and may traumatize or irritate tissues. Long-acting depo-formulations of drugs are available, such as ceftiofur crystalline-free acid, which may be given less frequently than other antibiotics and may reduce handling for a bird still living within a group.[25–27] Intravenous and intraosseous injections have similar risks and benefits as other injections, but these are most commonly performed in sedated or critically ill patients.[23] Nebulization, intratracheal, and topical routes of administration are also possible for individuals.[23] Oral medications may be administered to the individual directly in the oral cavity or via gavage tube passed into the crop or esophagus. Advantages include ensured accurate compliance and an opportunity to provide nutritional supplementation for sick individuals. Disadvantages include frequent restraint, stress, aspiration, or regurgitation.[23]

Oral medications may also be provided topically on food items, to individually or group housed bird (**Fig. 5**). Powders, crushed tablets, and oral suspensions may be added to favored or high value food items. This administration strategy is simple; depends on the bird self-medicating through food consumption; and does not require handling, which may be a significant advantage in large, potentially challenging flocks, such as with ratites.[28] Chicks may be medicated via the parents by adding medications to the adult diet. Disadvantages include that food items may reduce drug absorption, sick birds in most need of medication may consume less food, and food may be unpalatable or refused or conversely overconsumed resulting in toxicoses.[23,29,30] In general, it is difficult to achieve therapeutic concentrations of drugs with this strategy and only very susceptible pathogens are likely treated.[23] However,

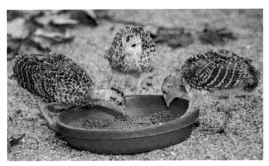

Fig. 5. A group of Attwater's prairie chicken chicks (*Tympanuchus cupido attwateri*) may be treated as a group topically on pelleted food to avoid catching individuals housed in large communal enclosures.

there are some situations where this strategy may be useful, such as when treating flocks of cockatiels (*Nymphicus hollandicus*) for *Chlamydia psittaci* with doxycycline-medicated pelleted diets.[30] Dosing is often based on the mass of food to be treated or on the average body weight of birds in the flock multiplied by population size. Specific references are available.[31]

Formulated diets that contain medications milled directly into the food item are also commercially available.[23] Compliance with this type of food item may be increased by gradually introducing the medicated food in replacement of or in addition to the regular diet.[32]

Oral medications may be provided in water-sources and are most successful in treating mild infections where local effect in the gastrointestinal tract is desirable or when widespread zoonoses treatment is imperative, such as adding antifungals or doxycycline to drinking water for pigeons with candidiasis or chlamydiosis, respectively.[33,34] Like medications applied on food; administering medications in water is simple; depends on the bird self-medicating through drinking, and does not require handling. Medicated water may decrease disease transmission via medicated drinking water.[23] Disadvantages include that water consumption is more erratic than food consumption for birds in general and may not be appropriate for every species. For example, frugivorous birds stay hydrated through fruit consumption and raptors do not consistently drink water.[32,35] Environmental temperatures may affect water consumption, whereas in hot weather, birds may consume large volumes of medicated water resulting in toxicoses.[36] Moreover, medicated water may be unpalatable and reduced water consumption may decrease the achieved drug concentration and may result in dehydration. Furthermore, not all drugs are stable or soluble in water, so drug choice may be limited and potency may degrade over time.[32] In most cases, medicated water does not reach therapeutic concentrations in the animal to adequately treat most diseases, because birds usually fail to drink enough, especially if ill. If water is consumed, low drug concentrations are sustained, which will likely be effective only to a highly susceptible pathogen. Remaining pathogens could develop resistance and become established within a flock, which would be detrimental to flock health if treated nonspecifically or at subtherapeutic levels.[23] Because of these factors, water-based treatments are not appropriate for sick birds alone, but may be used as an ancillary treatment to direct drug administration or in situations where individual treatment is impossible. For example, in Attwater's prairie chickens (*Tympanuchus cupido attwateri*) with *Clostridium coli* infections, tylosin powder was provided in the only source of drinking water in addition to the birds receiving parenteral antibiotics. Dosing is often based on the volume of water to be treated and references are available.[31]

In mixed-species aviaries, birds occupying the same ecologic niche may compete for space, food, water, and other resources resulting in antagonism.[2] Birds occupying different niches may allow for the targeted species to be adequately medicated, they would not contact the same feeders or occupy the same space[37]; however, this does not prevent nontarget species from accessing medicated food items. For example, in a mixed species exhibit, arboreal birds may be medicated on food in elevated feeders, but if food is spilled from the feeder, terrestrial species may have access to this and consume it.

Preventative medicine for the flock typically consists of, but is not limited to, anthelmintic treatments. Fecal parasite screenings are recommended to determine which treatments to administer and efficacy of medications. Preventative treatments may also include probiotics. Probiotics may improve gastrointestinal microbiota and health by providing balance and inhibiting pathogenic bacteria. This type of medication may be added prophylactically or responsively to food or water sources for flocks (**Fig. 6**).[38]

MAMMALS

Group treatment of mammals is challenging and not practiced as widely as group treatment of other taxa. Most mammals are treated individually, or are not housed in cohorts as large as those commonly found in other species. However, exotic hoofstock are commonly housed in large herds, and therefore are the focus of this section. Two of the most common reasons for mass treatment of hoofstock are contraception and gastrointestinal parasites. Contraception can be administered to a group of animals by milling a chemotherapeutic agent into the feed, such as melengestrol acetate,

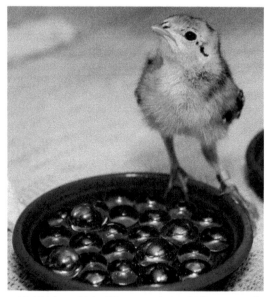

Fig. 6. Attwater's prairie chicken chicks (*Tympanuchus cupido attwateri*) may be treated as a group by adding medication, such as probiotics into the water source within the enclosure. When chicks are less than 2 weeks old, glass marbles are added to shallow plastic dishes to prevent chicks from turning over the dish or from soaking feathers.

which is a synthetic progestin.[39] This method has been used to reduce fertility in herds of barasingha (*Cervus duvauceli*), axis (*Cervus axis*), sambar (*Cervus unicolor*), and sika (*Cervus nippon taiwanaus*) deer, and blackbuck antelope (*Antilopa cervicapra*) under human care.[40] These species were fed melengestrol acetate at a concentration of 0.000154% in pelleted feed, which significantly decreased birth rates. However, posttreatment reproductive rates were lower than pretreatment rates, an effect that has also been seen in cattle.[41] A clinician should be aware of the potential risks of lowered fertility in a herd before mass treatment, and may elect for individual treatment instead.

Gastrointestinal parasitism is the most common reason for mass therapy for exotic hoofstock, and there are two main strategies. The first strategy is administering a large amount of medication to a group of mammals, for an average dose, and hoping that each animal consumes the correct amount. For example, this is done with deworming agents mixed into pelleted feeds.[42] Risks include overdosing and underdosing animals, which in addition to having potential toxic effects, can select for anthelmintic resistance in the parasites.[42,43] Social dynamics can have an impact on this medication strategy, because often the low-ranking individuals are denied access to the feeding stations, but they are usually the animals with the heaviest parasite burden.[42] Dose range via group feeding can only be roughly estimated, and the drug used should have a wide margin of safety, so that if animals do not eat the same amount every day, they are to be sufficiently treated after a period of time. If the group is treated, then often group fecals are to be used to track anthelmintic efficacy. Group sampling involves taking several samples from the herd and recording the median and range number of parasites observed, or pooling samples from many different fecal piles and mixing the sample before examination.[42] Although this route may be easier for the practitioner, it does not provide the most accurate representation of the effectiveness of the chosen drug therapy. Certain classes of animals tend to carry the highest parasite load (eg, calves), and if group samples are examined then the parasite load per animal is diluted and therefore not accurately represented.[42,44]

The second strategy for administering deworming agents to a large herd of hoofstock is targeted therapy. Administration may be done via physical restraint if a facility has the proper equipment, such as drop chutes or hydraulic squeeze chutes. If physical restraint is not possible because of either facilities limitations or the animal's size or temperament, then chemical immobilization must be used. The risks and benefits of chemical immobilization of an individual animal must be weighed against the benefit of the deworming procedure. If the animal is heavily parasitized, then a thorough physical examination with ancillary testing, such as a complete blood count, serum biochemistry analysis, and mineral panel, may help elucidate the underlying reason an animal has a high parasite load. While the animal is anesthetized a fecal sample can be collected from the rectum for individual sample analysis.

If neither medicated feed nor chemical and physical restraint are possible, then anthelmintics may be darted to individual animals. The benefit of this technique is targeted therapy and limited stress to the animal. However, most injectable anthelmintics are not labeled to be administered intramuscularly, but subcutaneously, so the efficacy may be reduced. Additionally, darting an animal carries inherent risk of trauma if there is poor dart placement, and if follow-up treatment is needed, or multiple animals in a herd need to be darted, the subsequent darting attempts may be difficult because of the suspicious nature of the animals.

Because of the many difficulties of administering anthelmintics to large groups of hoofstock, nonchemotherapeutic methods should be judiciously used. For example, pasture management is a key strategy, because increased stocking density of animals on a habitat leads to increased fecal contamination and infective larval load.[2,4,42,45,46] Pasture rotation and combining animals of different taxa, such as bovids and equids, are highly effective strategies to reduce the fecal load in a habitat. Mixing browsing and grazing species can reduce grass length, which reduces worm burden on the pasture, and also increases refugia.[43,47] Refugia are species that are not clinically susceptible to the parasites of interest, and therefore dilute the resistant alleles of the parasites.[43] There are tools, such as paddock vacuum cleaners, that can facilitate fecal pick up in large habitats; however, such equipment is expensive, and the benefit may be offset by the stress imposed on the animals living in that habitat.[42]

Other nonchemotherapeutic options for managing gastrointestinal parasites in hoofstock include copper oxide wire pellets, condensed tannins, and nematophagous fungus. Copper wire oxide pellets are administered orally, most often in gelatin capsules, and when dissolved in the forestomachs, interact with parasites to cause expulsion or parasite death.[48] Copper oxide wire particles have been demonstrated to reduce trichostrongyle fecal egg count in several exotic hoofstock species including schmitar horned oryx (Oryx dammah), blackbuck (Antilopa cervicapra), roan antelope (Hippotragus equinus), and blesbok (Damaliscus pygargus).[49] Condensed tannins, such as Sericea lespedeza, can be fed to hoofstock either as hay or in pelleted form.[50,51] Once ingested, the tannins bind and disrupt the cuticle of the parasite causing reduced worm burden and reduced fecal egg count.[48] One last nonchemotherapeutic option for parasite control is nematophagous fungus. This fungus is ingested by the target animal, but actually does not work inside the animal that has consumed it. Instead, the fungal spores are passed in the animal's feces, where they germinate and then trap the developing nematode within the feces. Thus, because of the different mechanism of action of this agent, it does not impact the fecal load of the animal, and instead reduces the possibility of reinfection.[4] One nematophagous fungus, Arthrobotrys flagrans, has been used to lengthen the time until egg reappearance in a herd of equids within a zoo. When a mixed herd of plains zebra (Equus quagga), Falabella miniature horse (Equus caballus), European donkey (Equus asinus), and African wild ass (Equus africanus asinus) were treated with antiparasitic agents combined with the fungus, the egg reappearance was delayed by several months, compared with just deworming agents alone.[52] This and other studies have shown that combining chemotherapeutic and nontraditional deworming agents provides the zoo clinician with a variety of tools to try and facilitate group treatment of mammals.[42,45,46,49,52]

SUMMARY

Group treatments are most common in amphibian, avian, and certain mammalian species that may live in a zoologic setting. All taxa have various group treatment strategies that exist with advantages and limitations that should be considered before therapy administration. Preventative measures, such as infectious agent screening and biosecurity, are advantageous to reduce the need for group treatments in response to disease. Medications administered topically on or milled into food, solubilized in drinking water, and mixed into a bath are common routes of administration for groups of animals. Sick or debilitated animals should be treated individually, because group treatments are often only effective against highly susceptible pathogens. Group therapies may be a beneficial strategy when treating animals in a zoologic setting and may be used, provided the risks and benefits are considered, in a variety of species.

REFERENCES

1. Lock BA, Wellehan J. Ophidia (snakes). In: Fowler ME, Miller RE, editors. Fowler's zoo and wild animal medicine. 8th edition. St Louis (MO): Saunders Elsevier; 2015. p. 60–74.

2. Kaandrop J. Veterinary challenges of mixed species exhibits. In: Fowler ME, Miller RE, editors. Zoo and wild animal medicine current therapy. 7th edition. St Louis (MO): Saunders Elsevier; 2012. p. 24–31.

3. Hunter RP, Isaza R. Concepts and issues with interspecies scaling in zoological pharmacology. J Zoo Wildl Med 2008;39(4):517–26.

4. Fontenot DK, Miller JE. Alternatives for gastrointestinal parasite control in exotic ruminants. In: Fowler ME, Miller RE, editors. Zoo and wild animal medicine current therapy. 7th edition. St Louis (MO): Saunders Elsevier; 2012. p. 581–8.

5. Barnett SL, Cover JF, Wright KM. Amphibian husbandry and housing. In: Wright KM, Whitaker BR, editors. Amphibian medicine and captive husbandry. Malabar (FL): Krieger Publishing Company; 2001. p. 35–61.

6. Baitchman EJ, Herman TA. Caudata (Urodela): tailed amphibians. In: Fowler ME, Miller RE, editors. Fowler's zoo and wild animal medicine. 8th edition. St Louis (MO): Saunders Elsevier; 2015. p. 13–20.

7. Clayton LA, Mylniczenko ND. Caecilians. In: Fowler ME, Miller RE, editors. Fowler's zoo and wild animal medicine. 8th edition. St Louis (MO): Saunders Elsevier; 2015. p. 20–6.

8. Pessier AP, Mendelson JR. A manual for control of infectious diseases in amphibian survival assurance colonies and reintroduction programs. Apple Valley (MN): IUCN/SSP Conservation Breeding Specialist Group; 2010. Available at: www.cbsg.org.

9. Helmer PJ, Whiteside DP. Amphibian anatomy and physiology. In: O'Malley B, editor. Clinical anatomy and physiology of exotic species. 1st edition. Philadelphia, PA: Elsevier; 2005. p. 3–14.

10. Baitchman E, Stetter M. Amphibians. In: West G, Heard D, Caulkett N, editors. Zoo animal and wildlife immobilization and anesthesia. 2nd edition. Hoboken (NJ): John Wiley & Sons, Inc; 2014. p. 303–11.

11. Valitutto MT, Raphael BL, Calle PP, et al. Tissue concentrations of enrofloxacin and its metabolite ciprofloxacin after a single topical dose in the coqui frog (*Eleutherodactylus coqui*). J Herp Med Surg 2013;23(3–4):69–73.

12. Chai N. Anurans. In: Fowler ME, Miller RE, editors. Fowler's zoo and wild animal medicine. 8th edition. St Louis (MO): Saunders Elsevier; 2015. p. 1–13.

13. Clayton LA, Nelson J, Payton ME, et al. Clinical signs, management and outcome of presumptive ivermectin overdose in a group of dendrobatid frogs. J Herp Med Surg 2012;22(1–2):5–11.

14. Wright K, DeVoe RS. Amphibians. In: Carpenter JW, editor. Exotic animal formulary. 4th edition. St Louis (MO): Saunders Elsevier; 2013. p. 54–84.

15. Wright KM, Whitaker BR. Clinical techniques. In: Wright KM, Whitaker BR, editors. Amphibian medicine and captive husbandry. Malabar (FL): Krieger Publishing Company; 2001. p. 89–110.

16. Georoff TA, Moore RP, Rodriguez C, et al. Efficacy of treatment and long-term follow-up of *Batrachochytrium dendrobatidis* PCR-positive anurans following itraconazole bath treatment. J Zoo Wildl Med 2003;44(2):395–403.

17. Wright KM, Whitaker BR. Pharmacotherapeutics. In: Wright KM, Whitaker BR, editors. Amphibian medicine and captive husbandry. Malabar (FL): Krieger Publishing Company; 2001. p. 309–30.

18. Bianchi CM, Johnson CB, Howard LL, et al. Efficacy of fenbendazole and levamisole treatments in captive Houston toads (*Bufo [Anaxyrus] houstonensis*). J Zoo Wildl Med 2014;45(3):564–8.

19. Churgin SM, Raphael BL, Pramuk JB, et al. *Batrachochytridum dendrobatidis* in aquatic caecilians (*Typhlonectes natans*): a series of cases from two institutions. J Zoo Wildl Med 2013;44(4):1002–9.

20. Geiger CC, Küpfer E, Schär S, et al. Elevated temperature clears chytrid fungus infections from tadpoles of the midwife toad, *Alytes obstetricans*. Amphib-Reptil 2011;32:276–80.

21. Garner TWJ, Garcia G, Carroll B, et al. Using itraconazole to clear *Batrachochytrium dendrobatidis* infection, and subsequent depigmentation of *Alytes muletensis* tadpoles. Dis Aquat Org 2009;83:257–60.

22. Clubb SL, Flammer K. The avian flock. In: Ritchie BW, Harrison GJ, Harrison L, editors. Avian medicine: principles and application. Lake Worth (FL): Wingers Publishing, Inc; 1994. p. 45–62.

23. Flammer K. Antimicrobial therapy. In: Ritchie BW, Harrison GJ, Harrison L, editors. Avian medicine: principles and application. Lake Worth (FL): Wingers Publishing, Inc; 1994. p. 432–56.

24. Tully TN. An avian formulary. In: Coles BH, editor. Essentials of avian medicine and surgery. 3rd edition. Ames (IA): Blackwell Publishing; 2007. p. 219–65.

25. Kilburn JJ, Cox SK, Backues KA. Pharmacokinetics of ceftiofur crystalline free acid, a long-acting cephalosporin, in American flamingos (*Phoenicopterus ruber*). J Zoo Wildl Med 2016;47(2):457–62.

26. Wojick KB, Langan JN, Adkesson MJ, et al. Pharmacokinetics of long-acting ceftiofur crystalline-free acid in helmeted guineafowl (*Numida meleagris*) after a single intramuscular injection. Am J Vet Res 2011;72(11):1514–8.

27. Hope KL, Tell LA, Byrne BA, et al. Pharmacokinetics of a single intramuscular injection of ceftiofur crystalline-free acid in American black ducks (*Anas rubripes*). Am J Vet Res 2012;73(5):620–7.

28. Doneley B. Management of captive ratites. In: Harrison GJ, Lightfoot TL, editors. Clinical avian medicine. Palm Beach (FL): Spix Publishing, Inc; 2006. p. 957–90.

29. Powers LV, Flammer K, Papich M. Preliminary investigation of doxycycline plasma concentrations in cockatiels (*Nyphicus hollandicus*) after administration by injection or in water or feed. J Avian Med Surg 2000;14(1):23–30.

30. Flammer K, Massey JG, Roudybush T, et al. Assessment of plasma concentrations and potential adverse effects of doxycycline in cockatiels (*Nymphicus hollandicus*) fed a medicated pelleted diet. J Avian Med Surg 2013;27(3):187–93.

31. Hawkins MG, Barron HW, Speer BL, et al. Birds. In: Carpenter JW, editor. Exotic animal formulary. 4th edition. St Louis (MO): Elsevier Saunders; 2013. p. 183–437.

32. Coles BH. Medication and administration of drugs. In: Coles BH, editor. Essentials of avian medicine and surgery. 3rd edition. Ames (IA): Blackwell Publishing; 2007. p. 115–23.

33. Dahlhausen RD. Implications of mycoses in clinical disorders. In: Harrison GJ, Lightfoot TL, editors. Clinical avian medicine. Palm Beach (FL): Spix Publishing, Inc; 2006. p. 691–704.

34. Padilla LR, Flammer K, Miller RE. Doxycycline-medicated drinking water for treatment of *Chlamydophila psittaci* in exotic doves. J Avian Med Surg 2005;19(2): 88–91.

35. Samour J. Management of raptors. In: Harrison GJ, Lightfoot TL, editors. Clinical avian medicine. Palm Beach (FL): Spix Publishing, Inc; 2006. p. 915–56.

36. Sandmeier P, Coutteel P. Management of canaries, finches and mynahs. In: Harrison GJ, Lightfoot TL, editors. Clinical avian medicine. Palm Beach (FL): Spix Publishing, Inc; 2006. p. 879–914.

37. Crosta L, Timossi L, Burkle M. Management of zoo and park birds. In: Harrison GJ, Lightfoot TL, editors. Clinical avian medicine. Palm Beach (FL): Spix Publishing, Inc; 2006. p. 991–1003.
38. Seeley KE, Baitchman E, Bartlett S, et al. Investigation and control of an attaching and effacing *Escherichia coli* outbreak in a colony of captive budgerigars (*Melopsittacus undulatus*). J Zoo Wildl Med 2014;45(4):875–82.
39. Perry GA, Welshons WV, Bott RC, et al. Basis of melengestrol acetate action as a progestin. Domest Anim Endocrinol 2005;28(2):147–61.
40. Raphael BL, Kalk P, Thomas P, et al. Use of melengestrol acetate in feed for contraception in herds of captive ungulates. Zoo Biol 2003;22:455–63.
41. Patterson DJ, Kiracofe GH, Stevenson JS, et al. Control of the bovine estrous cycle with melengestrol acetate (MGA): a review. J Anim Sci 1989;67(8): 1895–906.
42. Flach E. Gastrointestinal nematodiasis in hoofstock. In: Fowler ME, Miller RE, editors. Zoo and wild animal medicine current therapy. 6th edition. St Louis (MO): Saunders Elsevier; 2008. p. 416–22.
43. Garretson PD, Hammond EE, Craig TM, et al. Anthelmintic resistant *Haemonchus contortus* in a Giraffe (*Giraffa camelopardalis*) in Florida. J Zoo Wildl Med 2009; 40(1):131–9.
44. Ramsay EC. Management of cryptosporidiosis in a hoofstock contact area. In: Fowler ME, Miller RE, editors. Zoo and wild animal medicine current therapy. 7th edition. St Louis (MO): Saunders Elsevier; 2012. p. 570–2.
45. Epe C, Kings M, Stoye M, et al. The prevalence and transmission to exotic equids (*Equus quagga antiquorum, Equus przewalskii, Equus africanus*) of intestinal nematodes in contaminated pasture in two wild animal parks. J Zoo Wildl Med 2001;32(2):209–16.
46. Lih-Chiann Wang L, Ho H, Yu J. A 20-year disease survey of captive Formosan serows (*Capricornis swinhoei*) at the Taipei zoo (1991-2011). J Zoo Wildl Med 2014;45(3):487–91.
47. Stringer AP, Linklater W. Everything in moderation: principles of parasite control for wildlife conservation. Bio Science 2014;64:932–7.
48. Williamson LH. Anti-parasitic use of *Sericea lespedeza* and copper oxide wire particles in small ruminants. Conf Proc Ann Conf Amer Assoc Bovine Pract 2016;49:105–9.
49. Fontenot DK, Kinney-Moscona A, Kaplan RM, et al. Effects of copper oxide wire particle bolus therapy on trichostrongyle fecal egg counts in exotic artiodactylids. J Zoo Wildl Med 2008;39(4):642–5.
50. Terrill TH, Mosjidis JA, Moore DA, et al. Effect of pelleting on efficacy of *Sericea lespedeza* hay as a natural dewormer in goats. Vet Parasitol 2007;146:117–22.
51. Shaik SA, Terrill TH, Miller JE, et al. *Sericea lespedeza* hay as a natural deworming agent against gastrointestinal nematode infection in goats. Vet Parasitol 2006; 139:150–7.
52. Arias M, Cazapal-Monteiro C, Valderrabano E, et al. A preliminary study of the biological control of strongyles affecting equids in a zoological park. J Equine Vet Sci 2013;33:1115–20.

Considerations for Treatment of Large Zoologic Collections: Fish

Claire D. Erlacher-Reid, DVM, DACZM

KEYWORDS

- Fish • Immersion • Nutrition • Parasites • Quarantine • Salinity • Vaccines
- Water quality

KEY POINTS

- The health of the environment is intimately connected to the health and medical care of aquatic species.
- Fish health should be maintained by ensuring appropriate husbandry and nutrition for the housed aquarium species. Medications may be delivered orally, by immersion, topically, or by injection.
- Prevention and early diagnosis of infectious diseases are recommended by establishing a thorough quarantine and preventative medicine protocol.
- Treatments for fish are generally multimodal involving environmental and/or nutritional management first, followed by targeted pharmacologic treatment to control a specific pathogen if needed.
- The relationship between and among water quality parameters, targeted pathogens, aquarium species, and medications should be investigated thoroughly before selecting a treatment regimen.

INTRODUCTION

Aquatic species live most or all their lives in water; therefore, the health of the environment is intimately connected to the health and medical care of these species. Understanding and maintaining appropriate nutrition, temperature, water quality, filtration, substrate, and stocking density are necessary to sustain health. Most diseases of fish are secondary opportunistic infections; therefore, it is recommended to establish a thorough quarantine and biosecurity protocol (**Box 1**) to reduce the risks of introducing infectious diseases to an established aquarium system.[1–4] Implementing a thorough routine preventive medicine protocol (**Box 2**) will also facilitate diagnosis and guide treatment and/or management decisions for when health concerns of established aquarium collections do present.

Disclosure Statement: The author has nothing to disclose.
Zoological Operations, Department of Veterinary Services, SeaWorld Orlando, 7007 Sea World Drive, Orlando, FL 32821, USA
E-mail address: Claire.Erlacher-Reid@SeaWorld.com

Vet Clin Exot Anim 21 (2018) 311–325
https://doi.org/10.1016/j.cvex.2018.01.008
1094-9194/18/© 2018 Elsevier Inc. All rights reserved.

Box 1
Quarantine considerations for fish maintained in public display aquaria

All new incoming fish species should be placed in quarantine for a minimum of 30 days (45–60 days usually recommended for cold water species).

Entrance and exit examinations

Entrance and exit examinations on a subset of the population (approximately 2%-5%) should occur within 1 week of quarantine arrival and 1 week before quarantine departure. The following criteria should be met when possible during both of those examinations:
- Visual inspection;
- Body weight;
- Skin scrape (with or without fin clip) wet mount examination;
- Gill clip wet mount examination when feasible;
- Blood sampling for hematology and plasma biochemistry, especially in moray eel and elasmobranch species (not recommended in fish <8 cm total length); and
- Thorough necropsy of all deceased fish when possible, including postmortem wet mount samples of skin scrapes, fin clips, gill biopsies, and all internal organs.

Treatments

Treatment protocols should be designated by veterinary staff. This may include prophylactic treatment of quarantine fish to prevent parasite introduction to established systems (eg, praziquantel, formalin, fenbendazole, copper, etc) and/or specific treatment based on diagnostic examinations.

Medical records

Written or computerized records should be maintained for each system documenting the following criteria daily to monitor trends during the quarantine period:
- Water quality parameters;
- Number of mortalities;
- Treatments administered (eg, dose, duration/frequency, and route); and
- Estimated percentage of food intake for the population.

Biosecurity

- Fish should ideally be quarantined in an isolated facility located away from collection animals.
- Teleost fish, elasmobranchs, and invertebrate species should be quarantined in separate systems by taxa when possible.
- There should be designated staff members assigned to work only in the quarantine facility. Alternatively, if that is not possible, collection fish should be handled first prior to employees entering the quarantine facility for the day.
- Foot baths should be maintained at all quarantine entryways and exits, and if possible, between systems.
- Designated nets and equipment should be assigned to each system. Alternatively, if that is not possible, gloves, hand washing stations, and net disinfection stations should be readily available and easy to access.

Data from Hadfield CA, Clayton LA. Fish quarantine: current practices in public zoos and aquaria. J Zoo Wildl Med 2011;42:641–50; and Hadfield CA. Quarantine of fish and aquatic invertebrates in public display aquaria. In: Miller RE, Fowler ME, editors. Zoo and wild animal medicine: current therapy, 7th edition. St Louis (MO): Elsevier; 2012. p. 202–9.

PATIENT EVALUATION AND DIAGNOSTICS

Diagnostics should first consist of evaluation of the environment, water quality, nutrition, and visual observation of the species. **Table 1** provides general guidelines for what may be considered acceptable water quality ranges in many species of fish,

---

Box 2
Routine preventative medicine considerations for fish maintained in public display aquaria

Elasmobranchs
Routine health evaluations: At a minimum, all elasmobranchs should be visually examined by a staff veterinarian annually. When feasible, handling an elasmobranch for a brief physical examination once a year is advised and should be discussed among staff veterinarians and aquarium leadership. The decision to handle should be based on species, human and animal safety, enclosure and ability to catch, available equipment, and available space. If handled for a physical examination, the following sampling criteria should be met when possible:
- Appropriate restraint for select species to ensure both animal and human safety (eg, tonic clonic immobilization, oxygen narcosis, behavioral or manual restraint in a net or sling, or chemical);
- Body weight and morphometric measurements;
- Blood sampling for hematology, plasma chemistries, and point-of-care analyzer (eg, blood gasses and lactate);
- Skin scrape and gill biopsy wet mount examination when possible;
- Ultrasound examination, especially females;
- Coelomic wash for species considered susceptible to *E southwelli* (eg, cownose rays); and
- Radiographs for select species (eg, sand tiger sharks with suspected spinal deformity).

Teleost fish
Routine health evaluations: At minimum all teleost fish should be visually examined by a staff veterinarian annually. If a fish is handled for any cause, the following minimal physical examination criteria should be performed when feasible:
- Appropriate restraint for select species to ensure both animal and human safety (eg, manual restraint in a net/sling or chemical);
- Weight and appropriate morphometric measurements;
- Skin scrape (with or without fin clip) wet mount examination;
- Gill clip wet mount examination when feasible; and
- Blood sampling for hematology and plasma biochemistry when possible (not recommended in fish <8 cm total length).

---

but it is important to be aware of species-specific differences.[5,6] African cichlids prefer hard alkaline water, for example, whereas piranhas tend to prefer slightly acidic conditions.[2] Fish are extremely diverse; therefore, it is important to research the species of concern to become familiar with what may be considered normal or abnormal behavior and appearance. Clinical signs in fish are typically nonspecific and may include abnormal or erratic swimming, abnormal buoyancy, flashing (ie, rubbing body across surfaces), clamped fins (ie, holding fins close to body), changes in respiratory rate or character, color changes to skin and/or gills, excessive mucous on skin and/or gills, raised nodules, ulcerative and/or erosive lesions on the skin, loss of scales and/or fins, exophthalmia, enophthalmia, cloudy eyes, coelomic distension, emaciation, or visual observation of large external parasites. The majority of diseases in fish can be diagnosed by evaluation of water quality and wet mount examination of tissues with light microscopy.[7] Therefore, skin scrapes, fin clips, and gill biopsy wet mount examination with light microscopy should be considered the minimum diagnostic database for most species of fish when presented for a physical examination. These diagnostics may help to identify external parasites or granulomas, gas emboli, fungal organisms, some bacteria (eg, *Flavobacterium columnarae*), and provide a presumptive diagnosis for some viral diseases (eg, lymphocystis). To avoid potential parasitic detachment, which could decrease the sensitivity of the skin scrape or gill clip, it is best to acquire these samples before sedation while ensuring human and animal safety are still prioritized.[7] Other diagnostics that may be pursued to evaluate the health of fish include hematology (when fish are ≥8 cm in total length), fecal examination, tissue biopsies,

Table 1
Acceptable water quality parameters for many species of fish[a]

Parameter	Freshwater Fish	Saltwater Fish
Dissolved oxygen	Saturation (typically ≥5 mg/L)	Saturation (typically ≥5 mg/L)
Carbon dioxide	<12–20 mg/L	<12–20 mg/L
pH	6.0–9.0	7.8–8.4
Total ammonia nitrogen	Can usually tolerate <1 mg/L	Can usually tolerate <0.5 mg/L
Ammonia (toxic unionized)	0.00–0.05 mg/L	0.00–0.05 mg/L
Nitrite	0.00–0.10 mg/L	0.00–0.10 mg/L
Nitrate	20–100 mg/L	70–100 mg/L
Total alkalinity	>100 mg/L $CaCO_3$	>175–250 mg/L $CaCO_3$
Total hardness	>20 mg/L $CaCO_3$	>250 mg/L $CaCO_3$
Total chlorine	0 mg/L	0 mg/L
Free chlorine	0 mg/L	0 mg/L

[a] This table is a general representation of acceptable water quality parameters for many species of fish, but it is important to exercise caution and be aware of species-specific differences.

Data from Francis-Floyd R. Aquatic systems. In: Aiello SE, Moses MA, editors. The Merck veterinary manual. 11th edition. New Jersey: Merck & Co, Inc; 2016; and Petty BD. Basic water quality for fish. In: Proceedings of the North American veterinary conference: small animal edition, vol. 20. 2006. Available at: http://www.ivis.org/proceedings/navc/2006/SAE/549.pdf?LA=1. Accessed November 20, 2017.

coelomic saline flush when applicable, or diagnostic imaging (eg, radiographs, ultrasound imaging, endoscopy, computed tomography scans, or MRI). When there is high morbidity and mortality in a collection of fish and antemortem diagnostics have not revealed a definitive diagnosis, humane euthanasia and necropsy on a subset of fish including wet mount examination of internal organs, cultures, and histopathology may be considered a reasonable and valuable diagnostic tool.

TREATMENT

Treatments for fish may include both nonpharmacologic and pharmacologic methods, including environmental manipulation (eg, temperature or salinity changes), the addition of biological control for parasites (eg, blue-lined cleaner wrasse, cleaner shrimp), manual removal of large parasites, nutritional supplementation, and/or various chemical medications delivered orally, by immersion, topically, or by injection (eg, intracoelomic, intramuscular, or intravenous). In most cases, therapy is multimodal, involving environmental management first followed by targeted therapy to control specific pathogens if needed.[8]

NONPHARMACOLOGIC TREATMENT OPTIONS: ENVIRONMENTAL AND NUTRITIONAL MANAGEMENT

Most disease conditions of fish are secondary and stem from improper water quality and husbandry. Therefore, animal health should be maintained by ensuring that appropriate filtration, substrate, lighting, stocking density, water quality, and nutrition are provided for the housed aquarium species. If errors in water quality are identified, they should be corrected immediately (**Table 2**). Illnesses derived directly from abnormal water quality include but are not limited to supersaturation, hypoxia, old tank syndrome, and toxicities to ammonia, nitrite, nitrate, and chlorine.[5–7]

Table 2
Common water quality–related illnesses and treatment in fish

Problem	Common Findings	Treatment and Prevention
Supersaturation or gas bubble disease Often owing to excess nitrogen gas	Lethargy, buoyancy problems, exophthalmos, gas emboli in tissues, mortality	A saturometer is the best tool for direct detection of the condition Vigorous aeration to volatilize excess gas, degasser, and correction of underlying mechanical problems and faulty equipment
Hypoxia Low dissolved oxygen	Piping from surface, gathering around inflow, lethargy, flared gills, mortality Large fish usually more affected than small fish	Increase aeration and evaluate husbandry for potential causes Increases in temperature, salinity, altitude, stocking density, feeding frequency, and reduced aeration can favor hypoxic conditions
Old tank syndrome	Markedly reduced or absent total alkalinity, decreased pH (<5–6), and high total ammonia nitrogen (>20 mg/L) may result in lethargy, poor appetite, and chronic mortality	Perform daily small water changes to avoid a marked increase in pH and toxic unionized ammonia levels A large water change could be catastrophic Caused by exhaustion of buffering capacity within a system, often owing to chronic small and infrequent water changes Once corrected, the system should receive regular, large water changes to prevent recurrence
Ammonia toxicity or new tank syndrome Unionized ammonia most toxic and of greatest concern	Can result in acute mortality when unionized ammonia >1 mg/L, but chronic measurements of 0.05 mg/L can lead to gill damage and reduced growth	Addition of nitrifying bacteria, allowing biological filtration to mature, water changes as needed, decrease feeding, decrease stocking density, and evaluate husbandry practices for potential causes Elevated pH, increased temperatures, decreased salinity, increased stocking density, and high frequency of feeding can favor the presence of toxic unionized ammonia New tank syndrome occurs when biological filtration has not had time to establish and mature in a new aquarium system
Nitrite toxicity	Nitrite >0.1 mg/L, dyspnea, piping at surface, dark brown gills and blood, species variability (eg, centrarchids are more tolerant of high levels)	Addition of chloride (NaCl or CaCl), water change, addition of nitrifying bacteria/biological filtration, and evaluate husbandry for potential causes (eg, feeding frequency, stocking density)

(continued on next page)

Problem	Common Findings	Treatment and Prevention
Table 2 **(continued)**		
Nitrate toxicity	Nitrate >70 mg/L, lethargy, evidence of goiter	Water changes, anaerobic denitrification, and evaluate husbandry for potential causes (eg, increased stocking density)
Chlorine toxicity	Adverse effects may be seen when levels reach 0.003–0.02 mg/L Mortality may occur when levels reach 0.04–0.05 mg/L Sublethal exposure may result in dyspnea, gill necrosis, clouding of corneas, and increased mucus production	Addition of sodium thiosulfate to neutralize chlorine, activated carbon also will remove chlorine

Data from Refs.[5–7]

Adjusting environmental salinity has many uses in fish medicine, including managing or minimizing parasitic load, inhibiting fungal and bacterial growth, minimizing osmoregulatory stress, improving penetration of medicated immersions, and reducing uptake of nitrites.[7,8] This may be in the form of a short-term dip (5–15 minutes) where salinity is temporarily reduced to 0 g/L for saltwater fish and increased to 27 to 30 g/L for freshwater fish or in the form of a prolonged immersion, where salinity is reduced to 15 to 25 g/L for saltwater fish and increased to 1 to 3 g/L for freshwater fish. Most species of fish tolerate short-term dips well if executed appropriately and closely monitored; however, there are reports of sensitive species in which this technique should be avoided (eg, many catfish species).[3,7] Similarly, most freshwater species of fish seem to tolerate 1 to 3 g/L of salt indefinitely, but potential species sensitivities should be researched before using this method.[7,9] Salinity adjustments are especially a valuable tool for large, mixed species exhibits where chemical treatments are troublesome owing to cost, volume, differences in species sensitivities, difficulty in maintaining therapeutic levels, and bacterial degradation of the medication. There has been anecdotal evidence to suggest that the short-term use of hyposalinity (15–18 g/L) along with temperature increases may aid in resolution of *Cryptocaryon irritans* infections in large tropical marine mixed-species exhibits (Heym K, personal communication, March 16, 2017). Indefinite hyposalinity (20–24 g/L) has also proven successful at preventing recurrent outbreaks of external monogenean (*Neobenedenia spp*) parasites in a large marine mixed species exhibit housing teleosts, elasmobranchs, and sea turtles (Heym K, personal communication, March 16, 2017). It is important to reduce the salinity slowly by 5 to 10 g/L each day when commencing chronic hyposalinity treatment.[7] Biological control with various species of cleaner fish (eg, blue-lined cleaner wrasse, neon gobies, juvenile butterflyfish and angelfish, cleaner shrimp) may also be a viable nonpharmacologic solution for reducing parasitic load in large aquarium exhibits.[7]

Temperature seems to be an important factor in the development and/or treatment of many infectious diseases in fish. It is important to become familiar with the temperature range at which common fish diseases will proliferate. Koi herpesvirus is a warm water disease in koi that seems to develop when water temperatures range between 64°F and 81°F (between 18°C and 27°C), whereas spring viremia of carp seems to develop in koi at cooler water temperatures ranging between 41°F and 64°F (between

5°C and 18°C).[5] *Fusarium solani* infections seem to respond to adjustments in temperature when attempts at chemotherapy have been ineffective.[5,9] Clinical disease has been reported in bonnethead sharks (*Sphyrna tiburo*) and scalloped hammerhead sharks (*Sphyrna lewini*), causing ulceration and granulomatous dermatitis of the head, lateral line canal system, and fins.[10,11] Several species of marine fish also seem to be particularly susceptible including parrotfish, angelfish, triggerfish, and filefish.[9] This fungal pathogen seems to proliferate at temperatures of less than 80°F (26°C); therefore, successful resolution requires warming the water to greater than 80°F (26°C).[8,9] Similarly, *Saprolegnia spp* have been associated with suboptimal environmental temperatures, and increasing water temperatures are thought to improve response to pharmacologic treatment.[5]

When selecting a diet for managed fish populations, it is important to consider any known species-specific dietary requirements, anatomic differences, feeding habits or strategies of the species, health status, and age class of the animals. It is also important to avoid nutritional diseases by storing the food appropriately and ensuring that all fish are eating adequate amounts of food for their body weight and expected growth rate. Mixed species exhibits typically require several types of feed items to meet the nutritional needs of all occupants. Overall, providing appropriate nutrition to fish is challenging, because the nutritional requirements for most species of fish remain unknown. Nutritional deficiencies may result in reduced survival, anorexia, poor growth, scoliosis and/or deformed gill cartilage (eg, deficiencies in vitamin C), anemia (eg, oxidation of unsaturated fatty acids or deficiencies in vitamins C, B_{12}, E, K, folic acid, niacin, pantothenic acid, pyridoxine, and/or iron), cataracts or other ocular abnormalities (eg, deficiencies in riboflavin, tryptophan, methionine, manganese, zinc, and/or vitamin A), thyroid hyperplasia (eg, deficiencies in iodine), and neurologic disorders (eg, deficiencies in thiamine and/or pyridoxine).[2,8]

Goiter and spinal deformity are 2 common health problems in aquarium-maintained elasmobranchs believed to involve both nutritional and environmental etiologies with potential species-specific sensitivities.[11-15] Goiter has been well-documented in white-spotted bamboo sharks (*Chiloscyllium plagiosum*), brown-banded bamboo sharks (*Chiloscyllium punctatum*), and swell sharks (*Cephaloscyllium ventriosum*).[11-13] Elasmobranchs with goiter may present with lethargy, decreased appetite, and subcutaneous swelling on the ventral midline immediately caudal to the mouth in the anatomic region of the thyorid.[12] Elevated nitrate levels (short-term exposure to levels >70 mg/L or chronic exposure to levels at 35 mg/L), exposure to ozone, and insufficient dietary or environmental iodine have all been associated with this disease.[12,13] Recommendations for the prevention and treatment of goiter in elasmobranchs include a reduction of nitrate concentrations with water changes or anaerobic denitrification, discontinuing ozone, and maintaining sufficient quantities of environmental iodide (minimum concentration of 0.10–0.15 μmol/L) in addition to routine dietary supplementation of iodine.[12,13] Providing dietary supplementation alone may not be adequate, because most of the iodine needed is absorbed from the environment.[12]

Spinal deformity has been well-documented in sandtiger sharks (*Carcharias taurus*) with deformities commonly occurring anterior to the cranial dorsal fin. Gingival hyperplasia, jaw protrusion, and curled pectoral fins are commonly seen associated clinical signs.[14] Multiple environmental and nutritional factors have been associated with disease, including capture by pound net at a small size; deficiencies in potassium, zinc, and vitamins C and E; increased swim to glide ratio; increased body condition; increase tail beat duration; and decreased horizontal distance of enclosure pool (<20 m).[14,15] Recommendations for the prevention of spinal deformities in this species include minimizing or eliminating trauma at time of capture; supplementing diets with additional potassium; zinc, and vitamins C and E, providing a complex pool design to discourage stereotypical behaviors (eg, circling); and providing behavioral and feeding enrichment.[14,15] Treatment is likely unsuccessful once the disease process has become chronic; however, there is some preliminary evidence that onabotulinumtoxin A (Botox) injections may be helpful for treating early onset disease or slowing the progression in chronic cases.[16]

PHARMACOLOGIC TREATMENT OVERVIEW

Numerous factors must be taken into consideration when deciding on a pharmacologic treatment plan, including routes of delivery for the medication, environment and water quality, species to be treated, and the targeted pathogen. It is important to remember to complete a thorough physical examination to determine if more than 1 pathogen may be ailing the fish, necessitating additional medications and supportive care.

Medications in fish may be delivered orally, by immersion, topically, or by injection. Deciding on the method of delivery for treatment may depend on the location of the infection, the number of fish requiring treatment (individual vs population), available formulations for the selected treatment, the appetite of the animal(s), the ability to handle the animal(s), type of system and volume of water involved, and potential consequences for filtration or mixed species within the exhibit. Immersion and topical treatments are usually advantageous when treating external infections (eg, superficial wounds, ocular lesions, or external parasites).[8] However, many environmental factors (eg, temperature, salinity, dissolved oxygen, alkalinity, filtration, and microbe community) may influence chemical treatment selection, monitoring, and efficacy when immersion formulations are used. Reduced alkalinity, for example, may enhance heavy metal toxicity. Therefore, copper immersion treatment is not advised when alkalinity is less than 50 mg/L.[17] Increasing aeration and closely monitoring dissolved oxygen are essential when treating with formalin immersion, because formalin will deplete 1 mg/L of oxygen for each 5 mg/L added to a system.[1] Calcium and magnesium will bind to oxytetracyline and tetracycline when used for immersion treatments; thus, as water hardness increases, the doses of these medications must also increase.[8,18] Removal of activated carbon from the filter system and maintaining a closed system during treatment is typically used to prevent the removal and dilution of immersion medications; however, recent research has also indicated that the microbial population within an aquarium system might degrade praziquantel and formalin immersion treatments below targeted therapeutic levels.[19,20] It is also important to know the consequences the selected treatment may have on the biological filtration, plants, or other animal species within the environment before treating. Copper, formalin, and organophosphates are toxic to invertebrates, harmful to most plants, and are not well-tolerated by most elasmobranchs; therefore, these species must be removed from the system before using these chemical immersions or an alternative treatment should be selected.[8]

When treating large populations of fish, broadcast feeding of oral medications and prolonged immersions are often used. However, oral treatments are typically more cost effective, efficient, and less detrimental to water quality and biological filtration when compared with immersion treatments.[18] Many drugs are also available in premixed medicated feeds for convenience. When oral medications are chosen, the animal's current appetite and the food preference of the species typically guides the formulation selected (eg, bioencapsulation in brine shrimp or medicated flakes, gel, pellet, or gruel). In general, medicated food and parenteral treatments are most appropriate for internal infections.[8] Although parenteral treatment is typically the most direct and effective way to control the amount of medication delivered, it can be labor intensive and is often reserved for treating individual or anorectic fish.[8,18] Similarly, medications and nutrition may also be gavaged orally to individuals when appetite is poor.

Therapeutic options in fish approved by the US Food and Drug Administration are available for parasitic, bacterial, and fungal infections but are limited; therefore, it is imperative to become familiar with these medications if treating fish that are intended for human consumption (**Box 3**).[8,18,21] Veterinarians are recommended to visit the following website for the most current information regarding medications approved for use in select aquaculture species: https://www.fda.gov/animalveterinary/developmentapprovalprocess/aquaculture/.

In a zoologic setting, therapeutic management of fish commonly requires extralabel use of drugs and available pharmacokinetic data are extremely limited. When selecting a medication for use in a fish species, veterinarians are encouraged to use caution, perform a thorough literature search, reference reliable veterinary formularies, and discuss treatment options with experienced colleagues. If species-specific sensitivities or toxicities are not known for a selected treatment, it is advised to treat a smaller number of fish or use surrogate species and monitor them closely before treating an entire system or population to avoid unexpected adverse results.[1]

In general, prophylactic medication in the absence of diagnostic testing may contribute to resistant infections and other complications, and is not typically

---

Box 3
Medications approved for use by the US Food and Drug Administration in the treatment or control of specific parasitic, bacterial, and fungal infections in select aquaculture species*

Florfenicol (Aquaflor)
- *Aeromonas salmonicida* (furunculosis)
- *Flavobacterium psychrophilum* (coldwater disease)
- *Flavobacterium columnare* (columnaris)
- *Edwardsiella ictaluri* (*enteric septicemia*)
- *Streptococcus iniae*

Formalin (Parasite-S, Formalin-F, and Formacide-B)
- *Saprolegnia* spp.
- External protozoa
- Monogenetic trematodes

Hydrogen peroxide (35% Perox-Aid)
- *Saprolegnia* spp.
- *Flavobacterium columnare* (columnaris)
- *Flavobacterium branchiophilum* (bacterial gill disease)

Oxytetracycline dihydrate (Terramycin 200)
- *Aeromona salmonicida* (furunculosis)
- *Haemophilus piscium* (ulcer disease)
- *Aeromonas liquefaciens* (bacterial hemorrhagic septicemia)
- *Pseudomonas* spp.
- *Flavobacterium psychrophilum* (coldwater disease)
- *Flavobacterium columnare* (columnaris)

Sulfadimethoxine plus ormetoprim (Romet 30 and Romet TC)
- *Aeromonas salmonicida* (furunculosis)
- *Edwardsiella ictaluri* (enteric septicemia)

*The information in this table was current as of December 2017.
Data from Refs.[8,18,21,28]

recommended.[8] With that being said, the sensitivity of skin, fin, and gill wet mount diagnostic examinations may be low in subclinical or minimally affected fish because the acquired sample represents only a small portion of the actual tissue. Therefore, a negative test result does not ensure that the population of fish examined is truly free of disease.[22] For this reason, prophylactic treatments may be considered at the veterinarian's discretion as part of a quarantine protocol to prevent the introduction of infectious organisms into an established system (see **Box 1**).[3,4] However, a definitive diagnosis should be obtained whenever possible, because knowledge of the pathogen, its pathogenesis, and its life cycle (if applicable) will guide treatment choices. For parasitic infections, identification of the parasite to species or genus is not always required to determine an initial therapeutic course of action (**Box 4**).[7] However, knowledge of the life cycle of the parasite and the temperature at which it optimally grows is imperative for deciding the duration and frequency of treatment. Oviparous parasitic species, for example, usually require multiple repeated treatments and a longer duration of treatment when compared with viviparous parasitic species. The life cycle of some parasites, including *C irritans* and *Ichthyophthirius multifiliis*, will slow with lower environmental temperatures, usually requiring a longer treatment duration at colder temperatures.[7]

The majority of bacteria that cause disease in fish are gram negative.[18] However, culture and sensitivity testing should be used when possible for selecting appropriate antibiotics and guiding treatment. Injectable antibiotics commonly used in public aquaria at various doses have included but are not limited to amikacin, ampicillin,

---

Box 4
Common antiparasitic medications and the category of parasites they primarily target

Chloroquine
- Protozoan ectoparasites (primarily *Cryptocaryon irritans* and *Amyloodinium ocellatum*)

Copper
- Protozoan ectoparasites
- Some monogeneans

Fenbendazole and levamisole
- Gastrointestinal nematodes (nonencysted)

Formalin (37% formaldehyde)
- Protozoan ectoparasites
- Some monogeneans
- Parasite-S, Formalin-F, and Formacide-B labeled for use to treat protozoan parasites and monogeneans in select aquaculture species

Metronidazole
- Internal flagellates (especially Spironucleus *spp.* in freshwater cichlids)
- May have activity against some external protozoa (eg, scuticociliatosis/*Uronemia spp.*)

Organophosphates and chitin inhibitors
- Crustaceans
- Leeches
- Some monogeneans

Potassium permanganate (freshwater use only)
- Protozoa

Praziquantel
- Monogeneans
- Cestodes
- Digeneans

ceftazidime, ceftiofur crystalline free acid (Excede), danofloxacin, enrofloxacin, erythromycin, florfenicol, and gentamicin. Antibiotics commonly used in the public aquaria industry in oral and/or immersion formulations at various doses have included but are not limited to ampicillin, amoxicillin, ciprofloxacin, enrofloxacin, erythromycin, florfenicol, kanamycin, nalidixic acid, neomycin, nitrofurazone, metronidazole, oxolinic acid, oxytetracycline, sulfadimethoxine/ormetoprim, tetracycline, and trimethoprim/sulfamethoxazole. Generally, the penicillins and erythromycin are effective against gram-positive bacteria and may not be a good first choice for empirical treatment of bacterial infections in fish unless indicated in culture and sensitivity results.[8,18,23]

Vaccines for protection against bacterial and viral diseases have been used successfully in some aquaculture industries for years, especially in the salmon industry, and have been delivered to fish orally, by immersion, and by injection. Licensed vaccines have been developed for numerous bacterial and viral diseases including *Aeromonas salmonicida* (furunulosis), *Yersinia ruckeri* (enteric redmouth disease), *Renibacterium salmoninarum* (bacterial kidney disease), *Edwardsiella ictaluri* (channel catfish septicemia), *Flavobacterium columnare* (columnaris), infectious salmon anemia virus, infectious hematopoietic necrosis virus, and cyprinid herpesvirus type 3 (koi herpesvirus). Autogenous vaccines have also been created for facilities with continual or cyclical disease outbreaks. These vaccines are derived from a pathogen that has been isolated from diseased fish at a specific facility when a licensed commercial vaccine was not available. The use of vaccines in warm water fish production and zoologic facilities is rare and limited, but research is ongoing.[24]

Fungal infections in fish are typically secondary to improper husbandry, poor nutrition, bacterial infections, parasitic infections, and/or trauma; therefore, early diagnosis and prevention with appropriate management are key. Once fungal infections are present, errors in husbandry and nutrition must first be corrected and adjusting temperature or salinity may help to control or resolve some infections. In many cases, pharmacologic treatments have demonstrated limited efficacy and seem to be largely ineffective, but medications that have been used in an attempt to treat or control fungal infections at various doses have included potassium permanganate, formalin, povidone iodine solutions, hydrogen peroxide, copper sulfate, miconazole, fluconazole, ketoconazole, itraconazole, voriconazole, and terbinafine.[8,9,23]

TREATMENT CHALLENGES
Parasite Management in Large Mixed Species Exhibits

When dealing with parasitic infections, it is usually recommended to treat the entire aquarium environment when possible and when applicable for the best chance of successful therapy.[1] However, once parasites are introduced to an established system, treatment may become problematic, especially when involving large mixed species aquariums with complex life support systems. When that does occur, efforts are usually focused on parasite management by maintaining animal health and adjusting temperature, water quality, filtration, substrate, or stocking density as needed for the housed aquarium species to prevent parasite flare-ups and subsequent morbidity and mortality. In cases of parasite flare-ups in which a specific species is markedly compromised and the entire system cannot be treated, it may become necessary to remove those fish from the environment and treat them individually.

Hyposalinity has been a valuable tool for managing capsalids in large mixed species exhibits. Capsaloidea or capsalids, including the genera *Neobenedenia* and *Benedenia*, are large oviparous monopisthocotylean flatworms (approximately 3–10 mm) commonly found in tropical saltwater aquariums.[7] They may infest the skin, gills, and eyes of teleost fish and elasmobranchs causing flashing, erratic swimming, scale loss, erosions of the skin, ulcerations of the skin and eyes, and subsequently may lead to death. Diagnosis may be made with gross observation of the parasites, wet mount examination of the skin and gills, or histopathology. The parasites may also easily be recovered from the bottom of a bucket or tank after a freshwater dip and this method is often used to reduce parasitic loads in heavily parasitized fish before further treatments. Capsalids produce many triangular-shaped eggs (>80 in a day in some species) that may take 4 to 21 or more days to hatch depending on environmental temperature.[7] These eggs also contain long sticky threads that are used for attachment to fish, substrate, nets, and other objects. For these reasons, they are extremely difficult to eliminate from a system once established and efforts are usually focused on management to reduce outbreaks. Chemical treatments are often difficult in large aquarium systems owing to cost, volume, differences in species sensitivities, difficulty maintaining therapeutic levels, and bacterial degradation of the medication. Thus, chronic exposure to reduced salinity is thought to reduce egg viability and may be a useful tool in the management of capsalids in large aquarium systems when chemical treatment is not a viable option. Indefinite hyposalinity (20–24 g/L) has proven successful at preventing recurrent outbreaks of external monogeneans (Neobenedenia spp) in a 500,000-gallon mixed species exhibit housing sea turtles, sand tiger sharks (C taurus), nurse sharks (Ginglymostoma cirratum), southern stingrays (Dasyatis americana), spiny lobsters (Panulirus argus), and teleost fish (Heym K, personal communication, March 16, 2017). Hyposalinity has been maintained in this exhibit since 2011 with no obvious adverse effects observed in the collection species. Only when attempts were made to increase the salinity did outbreaks and resultant morbidity and mortality reoccur.

Temporarily removing affected fish and treating them individually has aided in the management of Branchellion torpedinis leech infestations in large mixed species exhibits. These marine leeches exclusively parasitize elasmobranchs, resulting in ulcerations at attachment sites, lethargy, anorexia, anemia, and potential death in as few as 5 days (McDermott A, personal communication, January 26, 2017).[7,25] Leeches may also serve as vectors for infectious diseases. Affected species have included sawfish (Pristis pristis), guitarfish (Rhina ancylostoma), zebra sharks (Stegostoma fasciatum), spotted eagle rays (Aetobatus narinari), manta rays (Manta birostris), southern stingrays (D americana), and experimentally yellow stingrays (Urobatis jamaicensis; McDermott A, personal communication, January 26, 2017).[25] Leeches are most commonly recovered from the claspers, pectoral fins, eyes, oral cavity, and cephalic lobes, and seem to remain permanently attached to the host if not removed. Manual removal when leeches are easily accessible is a treatment option, but the process is time consuming. Trichlorfon (Dylox) at 0.25 to 0.4 mg/L for a 5- to 6-hour bath has been used with success; however, it is strongly recommended to premedicate with atropine at 0.04 to 0.08 mg/kg intramuscularly approximately 45 to 60 minutes before trichlorfon treatment (McDermott A, personal communication, January 26, 2017). It is also important to remember, when calculating the dose, that commercial preparations of organophosphates vary in percentage of active ingredients.[7] Spotted eagle rays may be more sensitive to this treatment; therefore, caution is advised and premedication with atropine is highly advised (McDermott A, personal communication, January 26, 2017). Leech cocoons will hatch in approximately 30 days; therefore, repeated treatment may become necessary at that time.[25] Topical or systemic antibiotic administration and blood transfusions have also been helpful in the supportive care and recovery of the affected host when deemed necessary by the veterinarian.

Future studies to establish pharmacokinetic effects and safety for trichlorfon in various species of elasmobranchs are warranted.

Degradation of Praziquantel and Formalin in Recirculating Systems

Recent research has discovered significant degradation of both praziquantel and formalin immersion treatments in saltwater aquariums when using standard published doses and frequencies.[19,20] Failure to maintain therapeutic concentrations in a system could lead to decreased efficacy, recurrence of the pathogen, and possibly the development of resistance.[26] The microbial population within the aquarium system is thought to be the primary contributing factor for the degradation of these treatments. Degradation rates seem to increase with subsequent dosing of these medications, possibly related to increased bacterial activity or bacterial growth, which may use these medications as an energy source after the first exposure.

Investigations have demonstrated that an initial dose of praziquantel at 2 mg/L degraded below detectable limits in a naïve recirculating saltwater system in less than 9 days; however, 2 subsequent treatments at that same dose resulted in nondetectable levels in less than 3 days.[20] In a clinical setting, praziquantel was observed to reach nondetectable levels in as little as 8 hours in a freshwater aquarium when dosed at 5 mg/L (Hyatt M, personal communication, February 27, 2017) and to reach nondetectable levels in as little as 4 to 6 hours in a saltwater aquarium when dosed at 14 mg/L (Boylan S, personal communication, February 27, 2017). Similarly, a recent study reported an initial dose of formalin at 25 mg/L reached below therapeutic levels in a recirculating saltwater system after 14 hours. The rate of removal continued to increase over the course of 5 days with concentrations regularly decreasing from 25 mg/L to 0 mg/L in less than 5 hours.[19] These investigations emphasize the significance of monitoring drug concentrations throughout treatment to determine appropriate dosage frequencies and to ensure that therapeutic levels are maintained. Removing fish from an experienced system into a naïve system or enclosure for each treatment may help to minimize rapid degradation but is more labor intensive and possibly more stressful for the fish.

Mycobacterial Infections

Nontuberculous mycobacteria infections of fish are common, usually resulting in an acute or chronic systemic granulomatous disease. Clinical signs are variable and nonspecific including but not limited to emaciation, skin ulceration or hemorrhages, exophthalmos, skeletal deformities, and ascites. Predisposing environmental factors for the disease include low dissolved oxygen, low pH, high organic loads, and increased stocking densities. It is believed that there are no effective treatments that eliminate mycobacteria in fish; therefore, depopulation of the entire fish stock and appropriate disinfection of the entire system are typically recommended.[8] However, where individual and/or highly valuable fish are infected, management of the disease may be possible. Correcting abnormal environmental factors, maintaining oxygen near saturation, avoiding acidic and organically rich environments, and providing ultraviolent filtration or ozone may reduce bacterial numbers and enhance quality of life for the fish.[5] A combination of depopulation, isolation, maintaining appropriate water quality, repeated testing, and triple therapy with oral rifampin, doxycycline, and enrofloxacin for 8 months were recently reported to have managed a polymycobacterial outbreak in a collection of Australian lungfish (*Neoceratodus fosteri*).[27]

SUMMARY AND DISCUSSION

Prevention and early diagnosis of infectious diseases are recommended by establishing a thorough quarantine and preventative medicine protocol whenever possible. There are a multitude of published and unpublished protocols that have been used for the treatment and management of infections in fish with variable success; therefore, the reader is strongly encouraged to use caution and perform a thorough literature search and discuss treatment options with experienced colleagues to select the treatment protocol that is best suited for each specific situation. The relationship between and among water quality parameters, targeted pathogens, aquarium species, and medications should be investigated thoroughly before selecting a treatment regimen. The reader is encouraged to monitor drug concentrations throughout treatment to determine appropriate dosage frequencies and ensure that therapeutic levels are maintained. Further pharmacokinetic research evaluating the effects and safety of medications in various species of fish are greatly needed in the available peer-reviewed literature.

REFERENCES

1. Harms CA. Treatments for parasitic diseases of aquarium and ornamental fish. Seminars in Avian and Exotic Pet Medicine 1996;5:54–63.
2. Harms CA. Fish. In: Fowler ME, Miller RE, editors. Zoo and wild animal medicine. 5th edition. St Louis (MO): Elsevier; 2003. p. 2–20.
3. Hadfield CA, Clayton LA. Fish quarantine: current practices in public zoos and aquaria. J Zoo Wildl Med 2011;42:641–50.
4. Hadfield CA. Quarantine of fish and aquatic invertebrates in public display aquaria. In: Miller RE, Fowler ME, editors. Zoo and wild animal medicine: current therapy. 7th edition. St Louis (MO): Elsevier; 2012. p. 202–9.
5. Francis-Floyd R. Aquatic systems. In: Aiello SE, Moses MA, editors. The Merck veterinary manual. 11th edition. Kenilworth (NJ): Merck & Co., Inc; 2016.
6. Petty BD. In: Basic water quality for fish. In: Proceedings of The North American Veterinary Conference: Small Animal Edition, 20 2006. Available at: http://www.ivis.org/proceedings/navc/2006/SAE/549.pdf?LA=1. Accessed November 20, 2017.
7. Noga EJ. Fish disease: diagnosis and treatment. 2nd edition. Ames (IA):: Wiley-Blackwell; 2010.
8. Petty BD, Francis-Floyd R. Aquarium fishes. In: Aiello SE, Moses MA, editors. The Merck veterinary manual. 11th edition. Kenilworth (NJ): Merck & Co., Inc; 2016.
9. Yanong RPE. Fungal diseases of fish. Vet Clin North Am Exot Anim Pract 2003;6: 377–400.
10. Crow GM, Brock JA, Kaiser S. *Fusarium solani* fungal infection of the lateral line canal system in captive scalloped hammerhead sharks (*Sphyma lewini*) in Hawaii. J Wildl Dis 1995;31:562–5.
11. Garner MM. A retrospective study of disease in elasmobranchs. Vet Pathol 2013; 50:377–89.
12. Morris AL, Stremme DW, Sheppard BJ, et al. The onset of goiter in several species of sharks following the addition of ozone to a touch pool. J Zoo Wildl Med 2012;43:621–4.
13. Morris AL, Hamlin HJ, Francis-Floyd R, et al. Nitrate-induced goiter in captive whitespotted bamboo sharks *Chiloscyllium plagiosum*. J Aquat Anim Health 2011;23:92–9.
14. Anderson PA, Huber DR, Berzins IK. Correlations of capture, transport, and nutrition with spinal deformities in sandtiger sharks, *Carcharias taurus*, in public aquaria. J Zoo Wildl Med 2012;43:750–8.

15. Tate EE, Anderson PA, Huber DR, et al. Correlations of swimming patterns with spinal deformities in the sand tiger shark, *Carcharias taurus*. Int J Comp Psychol 2013;26:75–82.

16. Jones R, Gilchrist S. Botox as a possible treatment for spinal problems in sand tiger sharks (Carcharias taurus). In: The Regional Aquatics Workshop Proceedings. 2016.

17. Yanong RPE, Francis-Floyd R. Aquaculture. In: Aiello SE, Moses MA, editors. The Merck veterinary manual. 11th edition. Kenilworth (NJ): Merck & Co., Inc; 2016.

18. Yanong RPE. Use of antibiotics in ornamental fish aquaculture. Program in fisheries and aquatic sciences, SFRC, Florida Cooperative Extension Service, Institute of Food and Agricultural Sciences. Gainesville (FL): University of Florida; 2016. Available at: http://edis.ifas.ufl.edu/fa084. Accessed November 20, 2017.

19. Knight SJ, Boles L, Stamper MA. Response of recirculating saltwater aquariums to long-term formalin treatment. J Zoo Aquarium Res 2016;4:77–84.

20. Thomas A, Dawson MR, Ellis H, et al. Praziquantel degradation in marine aquarium water. Peer J 2016;4:e1857.

21. Quick desk reference guide to approved drugs for use in aquaculture, 2nd edition. US Fish and Wildlife Services Aquatic Animal Drug Approval Partnership Program, American Fisheries Society's Fish Culture and Fish Health Sections, and Association of Fish and Wildlife Agencies-Fisheries and Water Resources Policy Committee's Drug Approval Working Group. 2015. Available at: https://www.fws.gov/fisheries/aadap/PDF/2nd-Edition-FINAL.pdf. Accessed November 20, 2017.

22. Larrat S, Marvin J, Lair S. Low sensitivity of antemortem gill biopsies for the detection of subclinical *Pseudodactylogyrus bini* infestations in American eels (*Anguilla rostrata*). J Zoo Wildl Med 2012;43:190–2.

23. Stoskopf MK. Fish pharmacotherapy. In: Fowler ME, Miller RE, editors. Zoo and wild animal medicine. 4th edition. Philadelphia: WB Saunders; 1999. p. 182–90.

24. Yanong RPE. Use of vaccines in finfish aquaculture. Program in Fisheries and Aquatic Sciences, SFRC, Florida Cooperative Extension Service, Institute of Food and Agricultural Sciences. Gainesville (FL): University of Florida; 2014. Available at: http://edis.ifas.ufl.edu/fa156. Accessed November 20, 2017.

25. Marancik DP, Dove AD, Camus AC. Experimental infection of yellow stingrays *Urobatis jamaicensis* with the marine leech *Branchellion torpedinis*. Dis Aquat Organ 2012;101:51–60.

26. Kuemmerer K. Antibiotics in the aquatic environment: a review. Part II. Chemosphere 2009;75:435–41.

27. Strike TB, Feltrer Y, Flach E, et al. Investigation and management of an outbreak of multispecies mycobacteriosis in Australian lungfish (*Neoceratodus fosteri*) including the use of triple antibiotic treatment. J Fish Dis 2017;40:557–70.

28. Clinicians are recommended to visit the following website for up-to-date information regarding medications approved for use in select aquaculture species: Available at: https://www.fda.gov/animalveterinary/developmentapprovalprocess/aquaculture/. Accessed November 20, 2017.

Therapeutic Contraindications in Exotic Pets

Olivia A. Petritz, DVM, DACZM[a],*, Sue Chen, DVM, DABVP (Avian)[b]

KEYWORDS

- Ivermectin • Fipronil • Benzimidazoles • Glucocorticoids
- Antibiotic-associated dysbiosis • Ibuprofen • Ketoprofen

KEY POINTS

- Veterinarians who treat exotic pets are often forced to prescribe drugs to a particular species without any knowledge of the pharmacokinetics or safety of that drug in that species; a drug may cause no problems in certain species but lead to death in another, sometimes closely related species.
- Ivermectin, even at low doses, has led to flaccid paralysis and death in many chelonians, and this drug should not be used in any of these species.
- When applied topically to rabbits, fipronil can lead to seizures and death and is not recommended for use in this species.
- Benzimidazoles can negatively affect rapidly growing cells, leading to pancytopenia in many species.
- β-Lactam and macrolide antibiotics often lead to a fatal dysbiosis if given orally to hind-gut fermenters, such as rabbits, guinea pigs, and chinchillas.

INTRODUCTION

Many of the drugs used in exotic pets have never been pharmacologically evaluated in the species of interest, and doses are sometimes extrapolated from nonrelated animal species. In addition, many of these drugs have no safety data in anything other than common domestic species. A drug may cause no problems in certain species but lead to death in other—sometimes closely related—species. Widespread death of Old World *Gyps* vultures after ingestion of cattle carcasses treated with diclofenac is an example of this phenomenon, because no apparent toxicity is seen in certain

Disclosure Statement: The authors have nothing to disclose.
[a] Department of Clinical Sciences, North Carolina State University, College of Veterinary Medicine, 1060 William Moore Drive, Raleigh, NC 27607, USA; [b] Gulf Coast Avian and Exotics, Gulf Coast Veterinary Specialists, 3800 Southwest Freeway, Houston, TX 77027, USA
* Corresponding author.
E-mail address: Olivia.dvm@gmail.com

other vulture species when treated directly with various nonsteroidal anti-inflammatory drugs (NSAIDs).[1,2] The purpose of this review is to provide a brief overview of drugs that have documented contraindications in certain exotic pet species but could be administered in other species without apparent complications. Specific toxins (ie, lead), drugs that have known complications in all species (ie, renal toxicity of aminoglycosides), and drugs that are contraindicated for regulatory reasons are not discussed, because they are outside the scope of this review.

ANTIPARASITIC MEDICATIONS
Ivermectin

Ivermectin is a macrocyclic lactone that targets the ivermectin-sensitive glutamate-gated chloride channel receptors, only found in invertebrates, and the γ-aminobutyric acid (GABA) receptors.[3] In many species of animals, it does not cross the blood-brain barrier; however, in certain species, neurologic signs can occur after ivermectin administration, even at recommended doses. Ivermectin toxicity in chelonian species was first described in 1983 by Teare and Bush[4] Five red-footed tortoises (*Chelonoidis carbonarius*) received a single intramuscular (IM) injection of ivermectin (0.4 mg/kg) and developed paresis or flaccid paralysis. Additional studies in the red-footed tortoise showed that paresis occurred with dosages as low as 0.05 mg/kg. These investigators found several other species of chelonians were considered susceptible to ivermectin toxicosis at dosages of 0.1 mg/kg or less. The leopard tortoise (*Stigmochelys pardalis*) seemed the most susceptible of the species tested, and they consistently developed paresis with a dosage of as low as 0.025 mg/kg and death with dosages as low as 0.3 mg/kg. Based on these and other published data, the use of ivermectin in any chelonian species is not recommended. Treatment of ivermectin toxicity is largely supportive, and respiratory support must be maintained for at least the duration of action of ivermectin at the neurotransmitter site (7 days).[5] Anecdotal reports of full recoveries after 4 weeks to 6 weeks of supportive care have been reported in tortoises.[6] Aside from reported toxicities in tortoises, ivermectin toxicosis has also been suspected in a chameleon (*Chamaeleo senegalensis*), which received a single dose of 0.2 mg/kg IM of ivermectin. This animal's clinical signs resolved within a week with supportive care.[7] In addition, there are conflicting reports of toxicity in prehensile-tailed skinks (*Corucia zebrata*)—1 reported death 24 hours after an oral dose of ivermectin at 0.2 mg/kg[8] and a second report of the same dose administered up to 6 times IM with no apparent adverse effects.[9] Nevertheless, several investigators advise against the use of ivermectin in skinks. Similarly, specific recommendations to avoid the use of ivermectin in crocodilians and indigo snakes have also been previously published.[10]

Ivermectin toxicosis in birds has been reported sporadically. There are several toxicity studies, which examined the histologic effects of feeding high levels of avermectins to pigeons.[11,12] The purpose of those studies, however, was to examine the potential negative effects of avermectin residues in the environment rather than for use in the clinical setting. Additionally, there are anecdotal reports of ivermectin toxicity in finches.[10]

Fipronil

Fipronil is a phenylpyrazole insecticide used for the treatment of fleas, ticks, pediculosis, sarcoptic mange, and cheyletiellosis in dogs and cats.[13] Fipronil blocks GABA receptors in the central nervous system by preventing chloride ion uptake. This results in excessive central nervous system stimulation. Fipronil has a greater binding affinity for insect GABA receptors than mammalian receptors; however, rabbits seem more sensitive to fipronil compared with other mammals. Dermal absorption is 0.07%, but oral absorption is 30% to 50% if a rabbit licks off product after topical applica- tion.[14] The narrow safety margin in rabbits makes them susceptible to the neurologic effects of this drug.

Seizures, tremors, anorexia, and lethargy are the most commonly seen clinical signs of toxicity and can develop within a few hours up to a few weeks after exposure. Other clinical signs commonly encountered include hypothermia, gastrointestinal stasis, diarrhea, emaciation, ptyalism, and sudden death. Diagnosis is generally made based on the history with corresponding clinical signs; however, other causes of seizures, such as hypoglycemia, hypocalcemia, and lead toxicity, should be ruled out.

Affected rabbits should be bathed if exposure was within 48 hours to remove any residual drug from the surface of the skin. Light sedation with midazolam may be warranted in nervous rabbits. Bathe with a mild puppy/kitten shampoo in warm water to prevent hypothermia. Wash to the level of the skin to remove all toxin.[15] Activated charcoal may be considered to limit additional absorption of the drug if ingestion is suspected. If seizures are present, midazolam (1–2 mg/kg IM or intravenous [IV]) can be administered to control seizures. Continued seizures can be treated with lev- etiracetam (20 mg/kg orally every 8 h).[16] Parental fluids and nutritional support should be administered to anorectic rabbits. The prognosis is guarded for rabbits that are seizing.

Benzimidazoles

Benzimidazoles are used widely as an anthelmintic for a variety of domestic species, including dogs, cats, cattle, horses, swine, and birds. In rabbits, they have also been used in treatment protocols for *Encephalitozoon cuniculi*. This class of drugs binds to β-tubulin and thus inhibits microtubule formation in parasitic intestinal cells. This in turn decreases glucose uptake and effectively starves the parasite, which results in death.[17] Their binding affinity is greater to parasitic tubulin, which interferes with the parasite cyto- skeleton. Vertebrate tubulin can also be affected, especially in rapidly dividing cells, including bone marrow and the cells lining the intestinal tract. Consequently, this medi- cation can result in radiomimetic lesions, such as depletion of the myeloid, erythroid, and megakaryocytic cell lines.[18] This pancytopenia can lead to severe immunosuppres- sion and subsequent bacterial and/or fungal infections, which may be fatal. Additionally, gastrointestinal erosion and crypt necrosis can contribute to generalized septicemia. Benzimidazoles undergo extensive hepatic metabolism (by cytochrome P450 and others) after oral administration; therefore, if hepatic disease is present, a patient may be at greater risk for toxicosis. Toxicity associated with benzimidazole anthelmintic has been reported in avian,[19–23] reptile,[24] elasmobranch,[25] and several exotic/zoo mammalian species including rabbits and North American porcupines.[18,26]

A study was performed in 6 Hermann tortoises (*Testudo hermanni*) to evaluate hema- tologic parameters after administration of a standard fenbendazole treatment (two 5-day courses of fenbendazole, 2 weeks apart, at a dosage of 50 mg/kg).[24] The tortoises remained clinically healthy during the 125-day study; however, there were significant biochemical changes considered to be in response to fenbendazole administration, including an extended heteropenia with transient hypoglycemia, hyperuricemia, hyperphosphatemia, and equivocal hyperproteinemia/hyperglobulinemia.

Benzimidazole toxicosis or suspected toxicosis has been reported in 2 vulture spe- cies,[19] 2 stork species,[19,22] columbiformes,[20,21] and pelicans.[23] Nonspecific clinical signs are typically seen within 48 hours of drug administration, and clinicopathologic findings include heteropenia to agranulocytosis and sometimes anemia. Additionally, feather abnormities have been noted in birds treated with fenbendazole during active molt. The resulting bone marrow dysplasia, primarily of the myeloid series, can result in peracute bacteriemia and sepsis.[23,27]

Various benzimidazoles are also used in the treatment of E cuniculi in rabbits. A retrospective study compiled 13 cases of benzimidazole toxicosis in rabbits.[19] Rabbits presented for signs of anorexia, lethargy, diarrhea, pale mucous membranes, epistaxis, petechial to ecchymotic hemorrhage, abdominal hemorrhage, gastrointestinal stasis, fever, and acute death.[18] If considering the use of a benzimidazole for the treatment of E cuniculi, it is highly advisable to have pretreatment serology, biochemical profiles, and complete blood cell count performed. Serologic testing for E cuniculi could help determine if a rabbit is strongly seropositive and likely to have an active E cuniculi infection. A biochemical profile is used to screen for hepatic disease, because decreased hepatic function may predispose a rabbit to toxicosis. Complete blood cell counts should be performed prior to treatment as well as weekly throughout treatment to assess for anemia, thrombocytopenia, and/or leukopenia.

Immediate cessation of benzimidazoles is recommended if signs of lethargy or significant decreases in the complete blood cell count are noted. Sucralfate and acid reducers, such as famotidine and omeprazole, can be used to treat and prevent gastrointestinal ulceration. If septicemia is suspected, antibiotics and fluid therapy are recommended. Blood transfusions should be performed in patients with severe anemia and may need to be repeated until the bone marrow is functional. Medications to support anemia, such as iron dextran and vitamin B_{12}, may be beneficial. Based on these studies and several anecdotal reports of toxicity in these various species, clinicians should carefully consider the risk of mortality of an individual from a parasitic infection compared with the risk of septicemia after damage to hematopoietic and gastrointestinal systems from fenbendazole therapy. Despite reported side effects, fenbendazole has been used safely in many species kept as pets and in zoos.

ANTI-INFLAMMATORY MEDICATIONS
Glucocorticoids

Glucocorticoids are used in veterinary and human medicine for a variety of maladies but most commonly for their anti-inflammatory, immunosuppressive, and antineoplastic effects and as replacement therapy in patients with adrenal insufficiency and associated endogenous glucocorticoid deficiency.[13] Glucocorticoids exert their anti-inflammatory effects by inhibiting both the cyclooxygenase-mediated and lipoxygenase-mediated arachidonic acid inflammatory pathways.[28] The mechanisms of their immunosuppressive effects are less well understood but seems related to effects on leukocyte kinetics, phagocytic immunity, cell-mediated immunity, and humoral immunity.[28] Glucocorticoids also increase the secretion of gastric acid, pepsin, and trypsin as well as decrease mucosal cell proliferation, thus increasing the risk for gastrointestinal ulceration in susceptible species.[13]

Birds and certain mammalian species, such as mouse, rat, and rabbit, are considered steroid-sensitive species, whereas dogs, ferrets, and guinea pigs are considered steroid-resistant species.[28,29] When exposed to exogenous glucocorticoids, steroid-sensitive species exhibit an immediate and profound lymphopenia due to lymphocytolysis induced by activation of a resident endonuclease.[28] Lymphocytes of steroid-resistant species, in contrast, do not succumb to the same lytic effects and, instead, their circulating lymphocytes redistribute to the lymph nodes, spleen, and bone marrow. This is not to say, however, that steroid-resistant species are not susceptible to the adverse effects of steroid administration, especially with high doses and/or chronic use.

Clinical recommendations for corticosteroid administration to steroid-sensitive species (including birds) include using lower doses than in steroid-resistant species and ideally using a short treatment time of no more than 5 consecutive days.[30] The most common uses of glucocorticoids in exotic animal medicine include palliative treatment of systemic neoplasia, treatment of ocular disease, or postoperative cataract therapy. In 1 exotic animal formulary, there are several references for use of glucocorticoids for treatment of shock conditions in a variety of avian species.[10] The use of glucocorticoids in certain emergencies (acute lung injury, acute spinal cord injury, anaphylaxis, and so forth) of domestic mammalian species is controversial. Based on information from human medicine, however, the routine use of glucocorticoids for treatment of traumatic brain injury is not recommended.[31]

Systemic administration of steroids as an adjunct to chemotherapy for treatment of hematopoietic neoplasia in several avian species have been previously described.[32–35] Prednisone has also been used as a sole palliative treatment after radiation for periorbital lymphoma in a blue-and-gold macaw (*Ara ararauna*).[36] Prednisolone has been used in conjunction with radiation therapy for the treatment of lymphocytic thymomas in rabbits.[37] In the clinic of 1 author (Chen), prednisolone has also been used solely as a palliative measure. In these rabbits, clinical signs improved and radiographic evidence of a significant decrease in the size of their thymomas was noted after receiving oral prednisolone alone. Adverse effects, including mild to moderate pododermatitis and mild upper respiratory infections, did develop in some but not all rabbits (Sue Chen, DVM, unpublished data, 2017).

Topical therapy with prednisolone acetate for uveitis secondary to multicentric lymphoma has been associated with transient improvement in ocular disease in a macaw.[38] To reduce the risks of systemic side effects of the corticosteroid, the clinicians used a 0.12% prednisolone acetate ophthalmic medication for that patient rather than the more commonly prescribed 1% solution. According to a recent review of cataract management in avian species in zoologic collections, a majority (72%) of birds that underwent cataract surgery received a topical antibiotic-steroid ophthalmic solution postoperatively. In addition, some birds also received preoperative and intraoperative topical steroid ophthalmic solutions.[39] Bilateral phacoemulsification and intraocular lens implantation were performed in a great horned owl, and an antibiotic-steroid ophthalmic solution was applied topically at a tapering frequency for 5 weeks postoperatively.[40] An immunosuppressive dose of prednisolone was prescribed for 40 days in a case of presumed immune-mediated hemolytic anemia in a conure.[41] After discontinuation of the medication, the clinical signs returned and the patient died; however, the association between dosage discontinuation and return of clinical signs may or may not have been directly correlated.

In rabbits, most adverse effects are secondary to the immunosuppressive effects of steroids, such as mucopurulent ocular and nasal discharge associated with an upper respiratory infection. Pododermatitis, progressing to hock abscesses, may be due to a combination of immunosuppression and thinning of the skin that occur with administration of long-term glucocorticoids. The investigators have seen a case of severe otitis externa and pinna abscessation in a rabbit after a short course of topical otic medication containing a steroid (**Fig. 1**). In birds, there is limited peer-reviewed literature to document the adverse effects of steroids, which reportedly include immunosuppression and secondary bacterial and fungal infections, delayed wound healing, diabetes mellitus, hepatic disease, and gastrointestinal ulceration.[42] Involution of the cloacal bursa, thymus, and spleen with resulting suppression of both

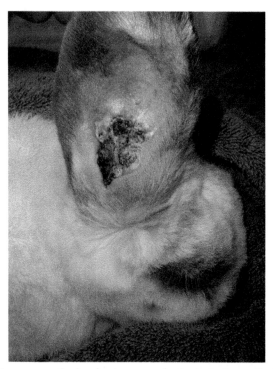

Fig. 1. This rabbit was prescribed a short course of a topical otic medication containing a steroid for mild otitis externa. After less than a week of treatment, the rabbit was evaluated by the authors for severe otitis externa and pinna abscessation. Although progression of otic disease cannot be definitively ruled out, the authors strongly suspect that the steroid greatly exacerbated the existing otitis, especially due to the short clinical progression.

cell-mediated and humoral immunity has been reported after corticosteroid use in birds.[43,44] Pigeons were found to react to exogenous glucocorticoids by early delayed feedback and were overall more sensitive to suppression of the hypothalamic-pituitary-adrenal system by glucocorticoids compared with mammals.[45] In humans, the function of respiratory macrophages is negatively impacted by exposure to systemic corticosteroids.[46] Because these immune cells provide the initial defense against *Aspergillus* infections in avian species and humans, immunocompromised patients are predisposed to fungal disease.[27] A published case series described severe mycotic airsacculitis after accidental prolonged corticosteroid treatment in 7 blue-fronted Amazon parrots. These birds also had a history of smoke inhalation and dyspnea 14 days to 20 days prior, which further complicated the suspected association between prolonged corticosteroid use and development of fungal disease.[47] Caution should also be taken with use of topical corticosteroids, because adverse effects have also been reported in some species.[30] A study in pigeons found a single ocular application of a glucocorticoid caused suppression of the pituitary-adrenocortical system, and the duration of suppression was comparable to that of a comparable single IV dose of glucocorticoids, which exceeded 24 hours in some cases.[48]

Although there are numerous studies evaluating steroid-induced immunosuppression in animal models for experimental purposes, unfortunately, there are no pharmacokinetic, efficacy, or safety studies of the use of any steroid for treatment of any disease in any exotic companion species to date. In disease conditions where the use of steroid therapy is indicated and the benefits outweigh the negative, clinicians should closely monitor patients' white cell count by checking a complete blood cell count prior to and during treatment. A biochemical profile is also recommended to evaluate for hyperglycemia and hepatic dysfunction. Administration of antibiotics or antifungals may be necessary if a concurrent bacterial or fungal infection develops during the course of treatment. In several avian patients[34,40] that received steroids long term (ie, greater than 1 week), an antifungal medication was prescribed concurrently to help reduce the risk of systemic aspergillosis. This is clinician preference, and to the authors' knowledge, there are no studies that have evaluated the efficacy of antifungal medication(s) during treatment with topical or systemic steroid administration in birds. Antifungal medications are used in human medicine for specific, high-risk immunosuppressed patients, including those with acute myelogenous leukemia and bone marrow transplant recipients.[49] There is concern within the medical community, however, about increasing antifungal resistance due to widespread use, in particular, of voriconazole and the increasing incidence of other fungal infections in immunosuppressed populations, such as mucormycosis.[50,51]

Acid reducers, such as H_2-blockers and proton pump inhibitors, can be administered to reduce the risk of gastrointestinal ulceration. Concurrent use of other drugs and the complicated nature of the underlying disease also hamper interpretation of presumed efficacy from these published case reports. Moreover, concurrent administration of certain medications, such as NSAIDs, may exacerbate adverse reactions associated with steroid administration and are not recommended. Therefore, exotic animal and zoo clinicians must extrapolate what is known for other domestic animals and assume some degree of risk when prescribing steroids to their patients, especially if the steroid sensitivity of that species is unknown.

There is no right or wrong answer to the question, Should glucocorticoids be used in avian and exotic species?[52,53] Many opinions are forged after apparent success or failure of a glucocorticoid in patients with a variety of clinical syndromes. Although formation of these opinions is inevitable in the exotic and zoo animal community due to a paucity of scientific data, clinicians should critically evaluate case outcome with as much evidence-based medicine as possible. Was the positive case outcome directly related to the use of a steroid, or were there other factors involved? Was the deterioration of a case related to the use of a steroid, or was that simply the natural progression secondary to severity of the patient's disease? There is universal agreement that corticosteroids, as in all species, have well-documented side effects in exotic companion animals, and these risks should be weighed against their potential benefits for each patient.

Ibuprofen in Ferrets

Ibuprofen is a widely used NSAID used in human medicine for its analgesic, anti-inflammatory, and antipyretic effects. Despite its therapeutic effects in people, its use is not recommended in certain species due to its narrow safety margin in dogs, cats, and ferrets. Ibuprofen is consistently one of the most common toxicoses reported to the American Society for the Prevention of Cruelty to Animals (ASPCA) Animal Poison Control Center.[54] Various over-the-counter formulations exist, including 200-mg tablets/capsules, pediatric suspensions of 20 mg/mL and 40 mg/mL, and prescription-strength tablets as high as 800 mg per tablet. Because of a ferret's small size, even a single 200-mg tablet can result in a toxic dose of 100 mg/kg to 400 mg/kg in a ferret.

Ibuprofen nonselectively inhibits cyclooxygenase enzymes by blocking the conversion of arachidonic acid into various prostaglandins that mediate pain and inflammation, regulating mucus and bicarbonate synthesis, maintaining water homeostasis, stimulating repair of gastrointestinal epithelia cells, and controlling blood flow to the stomach and kidneys.[55,56] Inhibition of cyclooxyegenase-1 enzymes seems to target the prostaglandins that have a cytoprotective effect on the stomach and the regulation of gastric and renal blood flow. The conversion of arachidonic acid to thromboxane A_2 is also blocked, which can lead to impaired platelet aggregation and clot formation. As a group, NSAIDs are also recognized to have direct cytotoxic effects on the gastric mucosa, which can subsequently lead to gastrointestinal upset, ulceration, and hemorrhage, especially in cases of overdosage and/or chronic usage.[56] In dogs, doses as low as 8 mg/kg every 24 hours for 30 days have resulted in gastric ulceration, and single, acute overdoses as low as 25 mg/kg can result in vomiting.[54] Renal effects are attributed to disruption of vasodilatory prostaglandins that maintain blood flow to the kidneys, and the effects are exacerbated in patients that are dehydrated or have underlying renal or cardiovascular disease.[56] Central nervous symptoms are well documented in people and dogs with overdoses of greater than 400 mg/kg, with neurologic symptoms ranging from drowsiness to coma. Additionally, overdoses in children and dogs have resulted in seizures and episodes of apnea associated with metabolic acidosis.[54,56] The pharmacokinetics and pathophysiology of ibuprofen toxicosis in ferrets are unknown.[55]

Ferrets are especially sensitive to the toxic effects of ibuprofen. The first case of toxicosis was reported in 2000, in a 20-month-old ferret that presented for gastrointestinal signs and acute lethargy of 2 hours' duration.[57] In that case, the patient's clinical signs progressed quickly from being lethargic to being semicomatose shortly after presentation and eventually going into cardiopulmonary arrest 8 hours later despite supportive measures. In a retrospective study of 43 cases reported to the ASPCA, 93% of ferrets developed neurologic signs, including depression, ataxia, tremors, weakness, and being comatose.[55] Gastrointestinal signs, such as vomiting, anorexia, diarrhea, and melena, were noted in 55% of the ferrets. Renal dysfunction as evidenced by polyuria, polydipsia, and dysuria were noted in 13% of the cases. Other reported clinical signs included weight loss, shallow breathing, metabolic acidosis, dehydration, hypothermia, and death. In that study, the minimum lethal dose was 220 mg/kg. More than half of the ferrets developed clinical signs within 8 hours of ingestion, with many developing signs within 4 hours.[55]

Biochemical analysis should be performed to assess for renal and hepatic function. Elevated blood urea nitrogen, creatinine, and hyperphosphatemia may be noted on biochemical analysis if renal compromise is present but may be normal early in the course of disease. The urine specific gravity should also be assessed and the urine should be monitored for tubular casts, which can be seen within 18 hours of exposure.[54,55] In cases of gastrointestinal bleeding, anemia may be noted on a complete blood cell count. Metabolic acidosis may be noted on analysis of venous blood gas.[56] Toxicologic analyses for ibuprofen can be performed on serum, urine, and hepatic samples using gas chromatography and mass spectrophotometry.

If ingestion of ibuprofen occurred within 2 hours of presentation to a veterinarian, consider induction of emesis if the ferret is not showing neurologic signs or vomiting.[54,55] Activated charcoal should be administered every 6 to 8 hours to prevent enterohepatic recirculation. Gastroprotectants, such as sucralfate, and acid reducers, such as famotidine and omeprazole, should be administered to treat and prevent gastric ulcers. Misoprostol, a synthetic prostaglandin E1 analog, has a cytoprotective effect on the gastric mucosa and also inhibits gastric acid secretion.[13] Although there are no pharmacokinetic or safety studies for the use of misoprostol in ferrets, anecdotal dosage, 1 μg/kg to 5 μg/kg orally every 8 hours, has been suggested.[55] Diuresis with IV fluids is strongly recommended for a minimum of 48 hours and should be continued until renal values are back to normal. Patients that are severely anemic from gastrointestinal bleeding benefit from whole-blood transfusions. Reports of IV lipid infusion has been described in a dog with ibuprofen toxicosis,[58] but use of this therapeutic modality has not been reported in a ferret. Seizures can be controlled with diazepam, midazolam, phenobarbital, or other anticonvulsants; however, once a patient develops seizures, the prognosis is guarded.

Ketoprofen in Rats

Like ibuprofen, ketoprofen is a nonselective NSAID used for its analgesic, anti-inflammatory, and antipyretic effects in a variety of veterinary species. Ketoprofen has been used in a variety of zoo and exotic species, including ferrets, birds, reptiles, and other small mammals.[10] A prospective study by Shientag and colleagues[59] evaluated a single dose of ketoprofen (5 mg/kg) in rats, a dose previously found safe and effective for postoperative pain in this species.[60,61] Those investigators found significant mucosal damage in the intestinal tract within 24 hours of administration. The rats administered ketoprofen (with and without anesthesia) had significant drops in their packed cell volume, positive fecal occult blood tests, and varying grades of intestinal ulcers on necropsy compared with control rats. The severity of the lesions was exacerbated when ketoprofen was administered in conjunction with anesthesia.[59]

Rats with ketoprofen toxicosis have clinical signs related to ulceration of the gastrointestinal tract and include lethargy, pale mucous membranes, abdominal pain, and melena. Rats that survive the acute gastrointestinal ulceration may die 1 week to 2 weeks later possibly due to bacterial translocation and sepsis. Necropsy findings have included intestinal ulcers, diffuse bleeding into the intestinal lumen, adhesions, fibrosis, and ascites secondary to peritonitis. Treatment should center around treating and protecting the gastrointestinal mucosa by administering gastroprotectants, such as sucralfate, and acid-reducers, such as famotidine, omeprazole, and raniditine. Antibiotic therapy and supportive measures, such as parental fluids and nutritional support, may also be beneficial, especially in cases of possible sepsis. Based on the findings of Shientag and colleagues' study,[59] the standard dosing of 5 mg/kg of ketoprofen cannot be recommended for pain control in rats and additional toxicity and safety studies need to be performed.

CONTRAINDICATED ANTIBIOTICS IN HERBIVOROUS RODENTS AND RABBITS

Although any antibiotic can potentially cause disruption of the cecum's microbial flora, antibiotics that target primarily gram-positive flora can lead to fatal dysbiosis and should not be used in rabbits and rodents, such as guinea pigs, chinchillas, and hamsters. These species have a diverse gut microflora that is adversely impacted by those particular antibiotics. Antibiotics, such as penicillins, cephalosporins, clindamycin, lincomycin, erythromycin, and tylosin, have been implicated in the eradication in these species' normal gastrointestinal flora, allowing for the overgrowth of pathogenic bacteria, such as *Clostridium difficile*. Exotoxins produced by *C difficile* causes hyperactivity of the secretory neurons, which leads to secretory diarrhea, mucosal damage, and hemorrhagic typhlitis.[62] The adverse effects seem most commonly associated with oral administration of these antibiotics, but there is a peer-reviewed report of lethal hemorrhagic typhlitis in guinea pigs administered penicillin parenterally.[63] In contrast, parental administration of penicillin and cephalosporins do not seem to affect the rabbit gastrointestinal tract in the same manner and have been used successfully for β-lactam–sensitive bacterial infections or abscesses in rabbits.[64]

Rabbits, guinea pigs, chinchillas, and hamsters may present with profuse and watery diarrhea, although they sometimes are brought in for generalized signs of gastrointestinal stasis, such as anorexia, lethargy, and diminished fecal production. A distended abdomen and perineal fecal staining are common findings. Animals may exhibit signs of abdominal pain, including a hunched posture, reluctance to move, and resistance to abdominal palpation. Varying levels of dehydration is common, and hypovolemic shock may be present in severely affected animals.

Diagnosis is usually based on clinical signs and history of recent administration of one of the offending antibiotics. A complete blood cell count and biochemical profile should be performed to evaluate for underlying metabolic and systemic disorders that may or may not be associated with the gastrointestinal tract. Radiographs may be unremarkable or have signs of ileus and gas dissension. Gram stains of the diarrhea may reveal large numbers of spore-forming bacteria as well as yeast overgrowth. The presence of toxin A, an enterotoxin, and toxin B, a cytotoxin, can be detected by enzyme immunoassay in fecal samples. Confirming the presence of cytotoxin is considered the gold standard in diagnosing enterotoxemia caused by C difficile,[62] although this test is not commonly performed in clinical practice.

Administration of an antibiotic should be discontinued immediately in any small herbivorous mammal presenting with diarrhea. Treatment is geared toward supportive measures to keep patients from becoming fluid and electrolyte depleted. If a patient is still bright and alert, subcutaneous fluids may be adequate to treat dehydration and electrolyte imbalances. IV fluids, however, are recommended if a patient is lethargic, hypothermic, and showing signs of hypovolemic shock. Pain medication may be beneficial for patients exhibiting signs of acute abdomen (hunched behavior, bruxism, and reluctance to move). Buprenorphine can be administered in patients with severe pain. One study found cholestyramine, an ion exchange resin that binds to clostridial iota toxins, effective in preventing deaths in rabbits challenged with acute clostridial enterotoxemia when given at 2 g in 20 mL water by mouth once daily for 18 days to 21 days.[65] Anecodotal experience with this medication, however, has been equivocal. Metronidazole (20 mg/kg orally or IV every 12 h) can be administered for clostridial overgrowth and has been reported to reduce the number of mortalities associated with enterotoxemia.[66] The re-establishment of normal colonic microbiome through fecal microbiota transplantation has an inhibitory effect against pathogenic bacteria and is now considered a standard treatment of recurrent C difficile infections in humans.[67] Based on this principle, anecdotal reports of transfaunation with cecotrophes from a healthy conspecific show that this treatment may be of benefit in rabbits with antibiotic-associated dysbiosis.[68]

ITRACONAZOLE IN AFRICAN GRAY PARROTS (PSITTACUS ERITHACUS)

Anecdotally, African gray parrots (Psittacus erithacus timneh) are more sensitive to itraconazole than other species, and adverse clinical signs, including anorexia, depression, and even death, have been reported.[10,69,70] Similar to the experience of many exotic animal clinicians, the authors have seen similar adverse effects in this species, even with doses as low as 2.5 mg/kg orally once daily. To the authors' knowledge, however, there are no safety studies or even published case reports of itraconazole toxicity in African gray parrots. Because of toxicity concerns, despite the paucity of published information, itraconazole should be used with caution in this species. The pharmacokinetics of voriconazole in African gray parrots has been evaluated, and this may be a more suitable alternative for susceptible fungal diseases in this species.[71]

REFERENCES

1. Green RE, Taggart MA, Das D, et al. Collapse of Asian vulture populations: risk of mortality from residues of the veterinary drug diclofenac in carcasses of treated cattle. J Appl Ecol 2006;43:949–56.
2. Rattner BA, Whitehead MA, Gasper G, et al. Apparent tolerance of turkey vultures (Cathartes aura) to the non-steroidal anti-inflammatory drug diclofenac. Environ Toxicol Chem 2008;27:2341–5.
3. Peterson M, Talcott P. Small animal toxicology. St Louis (MO): Elsevier Saunders; 2006.
4. Teare JA, Bush M. Toxicity and efficacy of ivermectin in chelonians. J Am Vet Med Assoc 1983;183(11):1195–7.
5. Bennett R, Mehler S. Neurology. In: Mader D, editor. Reptile medicine and surgery. 2nd edition. St Louis (MO): Saunders/Elsevier; 2006. p. 239–50.
6. Fitzgerald KT, Newquist KL. Poisonings in reptiles. Vet Clin North Am Exot Anim Pract 2008;11:327–57.
7. Széll Z, Sréter T, Varga I. Ivermectin toxicosis in a chameleon (Chamaeleo senegalensis) infected with Foleyella furcata. J Zoo Wildl Med 2001;32:115–7.
8. Boyer D. Adverse ivermectin reaction in the prehensile-tailed skink, Corucia zebrata. Bulletin of the Association of Reptilian and Amphibian Veterinarians 1992;2:6.
9. Stahl S. Use of ivermectin in the prehensile-tailed skink, Corucia zebrata. Bulletin of the Association of Reptilian and Amphibian Veterinarians 1992;2:6–7.
10. Carpenter JW. Exotic animal formulary. 4th edition. St Louis (MO): Elsevier Health Sciences; 2012.
11. Chen L-J, Sun B-H, Qu JP, et al. Avermectin induced inflammation damage in king pigeon brain. Chemosphere 2013;93:2528–34.
12. Qu J, Li M, Zhao F, et al. Autophagy is upregulated in brain tissues of pigeons exposed to avermectin. Ecotoxicol Environ Saf 2015;113:159–68.
13. Plumb DC. Plumb's veterinary drug handbook. 7th edition. Ames (IA): Wiley, John & Sons, Inc; 2011.
14. Stern LA. Fipronil toxicosis in rabbits. 2015. Available at: http://veterinarymedicine.dvm360.com/fipronil-toxicosis-rabbits. Accessed October 27, 2017.
15. Johnston MS. Clinical toxicoses of domestic rabbits. Vet Clin North Am Exot Anim Pract 2008;11:315–26.
16. Strolin Benedetti M, Coupez R, Whomsley R, et al. Comparative pharmacokinetics and metabolism of levetiracetam, a new anti-epileptic agent, in mouse, rat, rabbit and dog. Xenobiotica 2004;34:281–300.
17. Martin R. Modes of action of anthelmintic drugs. Vet J 1997;154:11–34.
18. Graham JE, Garner MM, Reavill DR. Benzimidazole toxicosis in rabbits: 13 cases (2003 to 2011). Journal of Exotic Pet Medicine 2014;23:188–95.
19. Bonar CJ, Lewandowski AH, Schaul J. Suspected fenbendazole toxicosis in 2 vulture species (Gyps africanus, Torgos tracheliotus) and marabou storks (Leptoptilos crumeniferus). J Avian Med Surg 2003;17:16–9.
20. Howard LL, Papendick R, Stalis IH, et al. Fenbendazole and albendazole toxicity in pigeons and doves. J Avian Med Surg 2002;16:203–10.

21. Gozalo AS, Schwiebert RS, Lawson GW. Mortality associated with fenbendazole administration in pigeons (Columba livia). J Am Assoc Lab Anim Sci 2006;45: 63–6.
22. Weber MA, Terrell SP, Neiffer DL, et al. Bone marrow hypoplasia and intestinal crypt cell necrosis associated with fenbendazole administration in five painted storks. J Am Vet Med Assoc 2002;221:417–9.
23. Lindemann DM, Eshar D, Nietfeld JC, et al. Suspected fenbendazole toxicity in an american white pelican (pelecanus erythrorhynchos). J Zoo Wildl Med 2016;47: 681–5.
24. Neiffer DL, Lydick D, Burks K, et al. Hematologic and plasma biochemical changes associated with fenbendazole administration in Hermann's tortoises (Testudo hermanni). J Zoo Wildl Med 2005;36:661–72.
25. Garner M. A retrospective study of disease in elasmobranchs. Vet Pathol 2013; 50:377–89.
26. Weber MA, Miller MA, Neiffer DL, et al. Presumptive fenbendazole toxicosis in North American porcupines. J Am Vet Med Assoc 2006;228:1240–2.
27. Pendl H, Tizard I. Immunology. In: Speer B, editor. Current therapy in avian medicine and surgery. St Louis (MO): Elsevier; 2016. p. 400–32.
28. Cohn LA. The influence of corticosteroids on host defense mechanisms. J Vet Intern Med 1991;5:95–104.
29. O'Malley B. Clinical anatomy and physiology of exotic species. Edinburgh (Scotland): Elsevier Saunders; 2005.
30. Hess L. Corticosteroid synthesis and metabolism in birds. Seminars in Avian and Exotic Pet Medicine 2002;11(2):65–70.
31. Aharon MA, Prittie JE, Buriko K. A review of associated controversies surrounding glucocorticoid use in veterinary emergency and critical care. J Vet Emerg Crit Care 2017;27:267–77.
32. Newell SM, McMillan MC, Moore FM. Diagnosis and treatment of lymphocytic leukemia and malignant lymphoma in a Pekin duck (Anas platyrhynchos domesticus). J Assoc Avian Vet 1991;5:83–6.
33. Yu PH, Chi CH. Long-term management of thymic lymphoma in a java sparrow (Lonchura oryzivora). J Avian Med Surg 2015;29:51–4.
34. Sinclair KM, Hawkins MG, Wright L, et al. Chronic T-cell lymphocytic leukemia in a black swan (Cygnus atratus): diagnosis, treatment, and pathology. J Avian Med Surg 2015;29:326–35.
35. Hammond EE, Guzman DS-M, Garner MM, et al. Long-term treatment of chronic lymphocytic leukemia in a green-winged macaw (Ara chloroptera). J Avian Med Surg 2010;24:330–8.
36. Alexander AB, Griffin L, Johnston MS. Radiation therapy of periorbital lymphoma in a Blue-and-Gold Macaw (Ara ararauna). J Avian Med Surg 2016;31:39–46.
37. Huston S, Lee P, Quesenberry K, et al. Cardiovascular disease, lymphoproliferative disorders, and thymomas. In: Quesenberry K, Carpenter JW, editors. Ferrets, rabbits, and rodents: clinical medicine and surgery. St Louis (MO): Elsevier Saunders; 2012. p. 265–6.
38. Hausmann JC, Mans C, Gosling A, et al. Bilateral Uveitis and Hyphema in a Catalina Macaw (Ara ararauna × Ara macao) With Multicentric Lymphoma. J Avian Med Surg 2016;30:172–8.
39. Rainwater KL, Sykes JM, Sapienza JS. Retrospective investigation of cataract management in avian species in a zoologic collection. J Zoo Wildl Med 2015; 46:858–69.

40. Carter RT, Murphy CJ, Stuhr CM, et al. Bilateral phacoemulsification and intraocular lens implantation in a great horned owl. J Am Vet Med Assoc 2007;230:559–61.

41. Jones JS, Thomas JS, Bahr A, et al. Presumed immune-mediated hemolytic anemia in a Blue-Crowned Conure (Aratinga acuticaudata). J Avian Med Surg 2002; 16:223–9.

42. Rosenthal KL. Therapeutic contraindications in exotic pets. Seminars in Avian and Exotic Pet Medicine 2004;13:44–8.

43. Leili S, Scanes CG. The effects of glucocorticoids (dexamethasone) on insulin-like growth factor-I, IGF-binding proteins, and growth in chickens. Proc Soc Exp Biol Med 1998;218:329–33.

44. Lumeij J. Endocrinology. In: Ritchie B, Harrison G, Harrison L, editors. Avian medicine; principles and application. Lake Worth (FL): Wingers Publishing; 1994. p. 599–601.

45. Westerhof I, Van den Brom WE, Mol JA, et al. Sensitivity of the hypothalamic-pituitary-adrenal system of pigeons (Columba livia domestica) to Suppression by Dexamethasone, Cortisol, and Prednisolone. Avian Dis 1994;38:435–45.

46. Safdar A. Immunotherapy for invasive mold disease in severely immunosuppressed patients. Clin Infect Dis 2013;57:94–100.

47. Verstappen FALM, Dorrestein GM. Aspergillosis in Amazon parrots after corticosteroid therapy for smoke-inhalation injury. J Avian Med Surg 2005;19:138–41.

48. Westerhof I, Pellicaan CHP. Effects of different application routes of glucocorticoids on the pituitary-adrenocortical axis in pigeons (Columba livia domestica). J Avian Med Surg 1995;9:175–81.

49. Perfect JR, Hachem R, Wingard JR. Update on epidemiology of and preventive strategies for invasive fungal infections in cancer patients. Clin Infect Dis 2014; 59:S352–5.

50. van der Linden JWM, Arendrup MC, Warris A, et al. Prospective multicenter international surveillance of azole resistance in Aspergillus fumigatus. Emerg Infect Dis 2015;21:1041–4.

51. Benedict K, Richardson M, Vallabhaneni S, et al. Emerging issues, challenges, and changing epidemiology of fungal disease outbreaks. Lancet Infect Dis 2017;17(12):e403–11.

52. Flinchum G. Corticosteroids may have some use in birds. Exotic DVM 2001;3(5):43.

53. Orcutt CJ. Risks of corticosteriod use in birds. Exotic DVM 2001;3(5):42.

54. Dunayer E. Toxicology of ferrets. Vet Clin North Am Exot Anim Pract 2008;11: 301–14.

55. Richardson JA, Balabuszko RA. Ibuprofen ingestion in ferrets: 43 cases January 1995–March 2000. J Vet Emerg Crit Care 2001;11:53–8.

56. Hunter LJ, Wood DM, Dargan PI. The patterns of toxicity and management of acute nonsteroidal anti-inflammatory drug (NSAID) overdose. Open Access Emerg Med 2011;3:39.

57. Cathers TE, Isaza R, Oehme F. Acute ibuprofen toxicosis in a ferret. J Am Vet Med Assoc 2000;216:1426–8.

58. Bolfer L, McMichael M, Ngwenyama TR, et al. Treatment of ibuprofen toxicosis in a dog with IV lipid emulsion. J Am Anim Hosp Assoc 2014;50:136–40.

59. Shientag LJ, Wheeler SM, Garlick DS, et al. A therapeutic dose of ketoprofen causes acute gastrointestinal bleeding, erosions, and ulcers in rats. J Am Assoc Lab Anim Sci 2012;51:832–41.

60. Flecknell R, Orr H, Roughan J, et al. Subcutaneous carprofen or ketoprofen in rats undergoing laparotomy. Vet Rec 1999;144:65–7.

61. Roughan JV, Flecknell PA. Behavioural effects of laparotomy and analgesic effects of ketoprofen and carprofen in rats. Pain 2001;90:65–74.
62. Perkins SE, Fox JG, Taylor NS, et al. Detection of Clostridium difficile toxins from the small intestine and cecum of rabbits with naturally acquired enterotoxemia. Lab Anim Sci 1995;45:379–84.
63. Lowe B, Fox J, Bartlett J. Clostridium difficile-associated cecitis in guinea pigs exposed to penicillin. Am J Vet Res 1980;41:1277–9.
64. Gardhouse S, Guzman DS-M, Cox S, et al. Pharmacokinetics and safety of ceftiofur crystalline free acid in New Zealand White rabbits (Oryctolagus cuniculus). Am J Vet Res 2017;78:796–803.
65. Lipman N, Weischedel A, Connors M, et al. Utilization of cholestyramine resin as a preventive treatment for antibiotic (clindamycin) induced enterotoxaemia in the rabbit. Lab Anim 1992;26:1–8.
66. Oglesbee B, Jenkins J. Gastrointestinal diseases. Ferrets, rabbits, and rodents: clinical medicine and surgery. St Louis, MO: Elsevier Health Sciences; 2012. p. 193.
67. Chen B, Avinashi V, Dobson S. Fecal microbiota transplantation for recurrent Clostridium difficile infection in children. J Infect 2017;74:S120–7.
68. Fann MK, O'Rourke D. Normal bacterial flora of the rabbit gastrointestinal tract: a clinical approach. Seminars in Avian and Exotic Pet Medicine 2001;10(1):45–7.
69. Orosz SE, Frazier DL. Antifungal agents: a review of their pharmacology and therapeutic indications. J Avian Med Surg 1995;9(1):8–18.
70. Orosz SE, Frazier DL, Schroeder EC, et al. Pharmacokinetic properties of itraconazole in blue-fronted Amazon parrots (Amazona aestiva aestiva). J Avian Med Surg 1996;10(3):168–73.
71. Flammer K, Osborne JAN, Webb DJ, et al. Pharmacokinetics of voriconazole after oral administration of single and multiple doses in African grey parrots (Psittacus erithacus timneh). Am J Vet Res 2008;69:114–21.

Prudent Use of Antimicrobials in Exotic Animal Medicine

Els M. Broens, PhD, DVM[a],
Ingeborg M. van Geijlswijk, PhD, PharmD[b],*

KEYWORDS

- Antimicrobial stewardship • Use • Resistance • Monitoring • Policy

KEY POINTS

- Awareness starts with monitoring: knowing what resistant bacteria are emerging in patients and the environment and which and how frequently antimicrobials are being prescribed and used by veterinarians in specified animal species.
- The next step is to choose effective therapy strategies of active substances, doses, and duration that result in minimal selection of resistance.
- The recognition of the nonrenewable nature of the available antimicrobials in animal medicine stimulates the prudent use of antimicrobial medicines.
- Antimicrobial stewardship consists of a coherent set of actions that promote prudent use of antimicrobials with an emphasis on societal responsibility.

INTRODUCTION

Antimicrobial use (AMU) in veterinary medicine is considered a potential threat for public health. Overuse and misuse of antimicrobials in animals and humans are contributing to the rising threat of antimicrobial resistance (AMR). AMR is the ability of microorganisms, such as bacteria, to become increasingly resistant to an antimicrobial to which they were previously susceptible. Any use of antimicrobials favors the survival and spread of resistant bacteria or genes. This selection pressure applies to pathogenic bacteria, but also to commensal bacteria (eg, gut flora). Longer treatments automatically result in more selection of AMR, underdosing or poor client compliance results in therapy failure and therefore futile application of antimicrobials. Over time, this makes antimicrobials less effective and ultimately useless. To reduce

The authors have nothing to disclose.
[a] Department of Infectious Diseases and Immunology, Clinical Infectiology, Utrecht University, Yalelaan 106, Utrecht 3584 CM, The Netherlands; [b] IRAS Veterinary Pharmacology and Therapeutics Group, Pharmacy Department, Utrecht University, Yalelaan 106, Utrecht 3584 CM, The Netherlands
* Corresponding author.
E-mail address: I.M.vanGeijlswijk@uu.nl

Vet Clin Exot Anim 21 (2018) 341–353
https://doi.org/10.1016/j.cvex.2018.01.014
1094-9194/18/© 2018 Elsevier Inc. All rights reserved.

the burden of AMR, prudent use of antimicrobials should be promoted. In 2015, the World Health Organization (WHO) endorsed a global action plan to tackle AMR[1] and recently it recommended banning the prophylactic use of antimicrobials in healthy animals.[2] The WHO also compiled a list of critically important antimicrobials for human medicine for risk management of AMR because of nonhuman use (**Table 1**).

Most action plans are primarily focusing on AMU in food-producing animals, but recommendations are also applicable for other animal species, including exotic animals. In response to publications from WHO, the European Commission (making the European Union a best practice region[3]), other international organizations, and several national and international veterinary associations have developed recommendations and policies on prudent use of antimicrobials, not only for food-producing animals, but also for companion animals[4] and horses.[5] In exotic animals, such recommendations and policies seem to be lacking. A search on Web sites of various exotic animal–related veterinary associations (eg, Association of Exotic Mammal Veterinarians [AEMV], European College of Zoological Medicine [ECZM], European Association of Zoo and Wildlife Veterinarians [EAZWV]) revealed no documents on prudent use of antimicrobials. Evaluation of overuse or misuse in exotic animals is hard because little to no information is available on AMU and AMR in these animals. In general, it seems that there is plenty of room for improvement in AMU and AMR in exotic animal medicine. This article discusses different actions in veterinary medicine on prudent AMU, and addresses the applicability of these actions in exotic animal medicine.

MONITORING OF ANTIMICROBIAL USE

Any plan to promote prudent use has to start with monitoring AMU: the numbers tell the tale. Implementation of monitoring programs is crucial to reduce AMU and AMR. National programs monitoring AMU and AMR in animals have been established in several

Table 1	
List and classification of antimicrobials important for human medicine	
Antimicrobial Class	**Example of Drugs**
Aminoglycosides	Gentamicin
Ansamycins	Rifampicin
Carbapenems and other penems	Meropenem
Cephalosporins (third, fourth, and fifth generation)	Ceftazidime, cefepime
Glycopeptides	Vancomycin
Glycylcyclines	Tigecycline
Lipopeptides	Daptomycin
Macrolides and ketolides	Erythromycin, azithromycin
Monobactams	Aztreonam
Oxazolidinones	Linezolid
Penicillins (natural, aminopenicillins, and antipseudomonal)	Ampicillin
Phosphonic acid derivatives	Fosfomycin
Polymyxins	Colistin
Quinolones	Ciprofloxacin
Drugs used solely to treat tuberculosis or other mycobacterial diseases	Isoniazid

Data from World Health Organization. Critically important antimicrobials for human medicine. 5th revision. 2017. Available at: http://www.who.int/foodsafety/publications/antimicrobials-fifth/en/. Accessed December 17, 2017.

countries (eg, DANMAP,[6] SWEDRES,[7] MARAN,[8] AMCRA[9]). The methodologies among countries might differ, making direct comparisons or conclusions difficult.[10,11] Most monitoring programs are based on the total mass of active substances sold per year. However, the comparison of use in mass neglects the dosing differences between different antimicrobial agents, dosing regimens, and animal species.

The European Medicines Agency started the European Surveillance of Veterinary Antimicrobial Consumption (ESVAC) project in 2010 to harmonize data collection and analysis methodologies for AMU across the European Union. ESVAC has established standardized ways to calculate the animal population (ie, population correction unit).[12,13] This methodology is mainly based on production parameters and therefore needs additional refinement for application in non-food-producing animals. Ideally, calculation of the potentially exposed population of companion animals, such as exotics, should mimic the method applied in human AMU calculations (eg, by the European Surveillance of Antimicrobial Consumption[14]). This requires that the number of animals is known, so some kind of registration of animals is needed. In the Netherlands this method was applied for measuring AMU in dogs, cats, and rabbits,[15] which also showed the limitations of this system when an official registration of number of animals is missing, and no standard weight (like in humans) is available.

ESVAC has also established standardized units of measurement for reporting antimicrobial consumption in specific animal species, called the defined daily dose.[16] The defined daily dose will enable a better analysis over time and a comparison among species at the European level in time, but currently animal species specified sales data are available for only a few countries on a national level, because the attribution to species level of sales data is not possible within the current data collection system. Most of the monitoring programs focus on AMU in livestock; data on AMU in companion animals (eg, dogs, cats, horses, and rabbits) are scarce and data specifically on exotic animals are absent.

The seventh ESVAC report presents data on the sales of veterinary antimicrobial agents from 30 European countries in 2015 and trends in consumption of veterinary antimicrobials for the years 2010 to 2015.[17] In this report, the sales of tablets, in tons of active ingredient, by antimicrobial class and country, was used to estimate AMU in companion animals. The data might be slightly biased, because the assumption was that tablets are used almost solely for companion animals and tablets marketed for human use and injectables were not included. Especially in minor species, such as exotic animals, the use of human or injectable products might be high compared with its use in dogs and cats. In Europe, aminopenicillins combined with β-lactamase inhibitors (mainly amoxicillin/clavulanic acid) and first- and second-generation cephalosporins (mainly cephalexin) account for 65% of the total mass of active substance of sold antimicrobial tablets for companion animals. In some countries, fluoroquinolones represent more than 50% of the active substance mass in tablets.[17] The comparison of use in mass neglects the dosing differences between antimicrobials. For example, fluoroquinolones (2–6 mg/kg/d) require lower dosing in comparison with aminopenicillins (25–50 mg/kg/d), which implies that 50% in mass means that far more than 50% of the oral treatments consist of treatment with fluoroquinolones.

In the United States pharmaceutical companies selling veterinary antimicrobial products (called antimicrobial drug sponsors) are obliged by Section 105 of the Animal Drug User Fee Amendments of 2008 to report their sales data of all veterinary antimicrobial products to the US Food and Drug Authority. Starting with calendar year 2016, additionally species-specific sales estimates as a percentage of total domestic sales and distribution for each product was required. Of the 2016 sales, 4% was reported intended for use in species other than cattle, swine, chickens, and turkeys or unknown uses. The report does not specify this "other use" further.[18]

The Netherlands Veterinary Medicines Institute (SDa) has been monitoring the amounts of antibiotics used at Dutch livestock farms since 2011. After rigorous measures taken in livestock during 2009 to 2016 resulting in a 60% reduction of use, monitoring of AMU was extended to companion animals.[19] In 2016, a survey was performed by the SDa to assess AMU in companion animals (dogs, cats, and rabbits). The survey, which included data from 10% of Dutch veterinary practices, revealed a large variation in AMU between practices, but overall usage levels were low. Results showed that amoxicillin (either alone or combined with a β-lactamase inhibitor) and first-generation cephalosporins accounted for 51% of the treatment days in 2012, and fluoroquinolones and third-generation cephalosporins for 21%. In 2014, these numbers were, respectively, 51% and 6.9%.[15] In Australia in 2011, treatment incidences were estimated with a questionnaire, and overall, the most common antimicrobial classes were potentiated aminopenicillins (36%), fluoroquinolones (15%), first- and second-generation cephalosporins (14%), and tetracyclines (11%). In cats, third-generation cephalosporins were overrepresented.[20] In New Zealand, Canada, and the United Kingdom similar figures were found.[21–23] These figures indicate that fluoroquinolones, potentiated aminopenicillins, and cephalosporins are among the most used antimicrobial agents in companion animals, despite it being common knowledge that these agents select for multidrug resistant bacteria (eg, methicillin-resistant staphylococci and extended-spectrum β-lactamase-producing Enterobacteriaceae).[24]

The only published data on AMU in exotic animals came from a study at the Zoologic Medicine Service of the Veterinary Teaching Hospital at the University of Georgia. Although this study did not provide information on the amount or type of antimicrobials used, it did indicate that most antimicrobial prescriptions were unnecessary or inappropriate.[25] Most antimicrobial prescriptions seemed to be empiric and not based on proper diagnostics. The occurrence of multidrug-resistant bacteria has been reported in several exotic animal species, such as methicillin-resistant staphylococci in birds and rabbits, and extended-spectrum β-lactamase-producing Enterobacteriaceae in wild birds and turtles.[26–30]

RECOMMENDATIONS AND POLICIES

Several international and national organizations have developed recommendations and policies to promote prudent use of antimicrobials in veterinary and human medicine. The WHO list of critically important antimicrobials for human medicine contains several antimicrobial classes used in animals. The antimicrobial classes with the highest priority are quinolones, third- and fourth-generation cephalosporins, macrolides, and glycopeptides.[31] Except for the latter, all classes are authorized in animals, and especially in exotic animals, quinolones and macrolides are used often. The guidelines for the prudent use of antimicrobials in veterinary medicine composed by the European Commission in 2015 state: "The off-label (cascade) use of antimicrobials not authorized in veterinary medicine to treat non-food-producing animals should be avoided, especially when the drugs are of critical importance for human health (eg, carbapenems and tigecycline). Their use should only be considered in very exceptional cases, for example, when laboratory susceptibility testing has confirmed that no other antimicrobials will be effective and where there are ethical reasons to justify such a course of treatment."[32] In the Netherlands, the use of carbapenems, glycopeptides, oxazolidones, daptomycin, mupirocin, and tigecyclin in animals is prohibited.[33] The use of fluoroquinolones and third- and fourth-generation cephalosporins is by

Dutch law restricted to infections caused by bacteria with susceptibility results indicating that all other options are ineffective.[34,35] In other countries no such legislations are implemented yet, but empiric or prophylactic use of these antimicrobials should be avoided whenever possible.

Although the European Commission guidelines mainly focus on food-producing animals, these also address clinical infections with methicillin-resistant *Staphylococcus aureus* or methicillin-resistant *Staphylococcus pseudintermedius* in horses and companion animals. The guidelines state that these infections should be monitored and transmission should be minimized.

In countries where a substantial reduction in AMU was achieved, a decline in AMR in commensal bacteria, such as *Escherichia coli*, was seen in the following years.[36,37] The second Joint Interagency Antimicrobial Consumption and Resistance Analysis report of July 2017 confirms the positive association between AMU and AMR in humans and food-producing animals and underlines the need to ensure prudent use of antimicrobials in food-producing animals and humans.[14] The WHO guidelines on use of medically important antimicrobials in food-producing animals[2] is based on a meta-analysis by Tang and colleagues[38] concluding that reduction of AMU in food-producing animals was associated with a reduction in AMR in food-producing animals and in humans in direct contact with these animals. These results provide evidence for an association between reduction of AMU and reduction of AMR and confirm that prudent use of antimicrobials should be promoted or even enforced in veterinary (and human) medicine.

ANTIMICROBIAL STEWARDSHIP

In human medicine, the term antimicrobial stewardship was introduced a few decades ago and describes the multifaceted approach considering the long-term effects of antimicrobial selection, dosage, and duration of treatment on resistance development.[39] Antimicrobial stewardship focuses on the reduction of resistance selection and the preservation of effective antimicrobials for future generations. It consists of a coherent set of actions that promote responsible use of antimicrobials with an emphasis on the societal responsibility.[40] During the 1990s and 2000s antimicrobial stewardship programs were implemented in human hospitals in many countries. The primary goal of these programs was to optimize clinical outcomes while minimizing unintended consequences of AMU, including toxicity, the selection of pathogenic organisms, and the emergence of resistance. Antimicrobial stewardship involves coordinated approaches and interventions; it is not only about reducing AMU, but also about infection control, clinical microbiology, surveillance of AMU and AMR, education, guidelines, and regulations. Nowadays, antimicrobial stewardship programs are up and running in most human hospitals. Multidisciplinary teams are formed, the so-called A(ntibiotic) teams, monitoring all aspects of AMU and AMR, including the implementation of and compliance with guidelines.

Most veterinarians are aware of AMR, but antimicrobial stewardship is new to veterinary medicine. Few papers have been published on veterinary antimicrobial stewardship, mainly focusing on companion animals[4] and horses.[5] National organizations of veterinarians (eg, Royal Netherlands Veterinary Association [RNVA], British Small Animal Veterinary Association [BSAVA]), and international organizations specialized in companion animals (Federation of Companion Animal Veterinary Associations [FECAVA]) and horses (British Equine Veterinary Association [BEVA]) initiated programs to stimulate awareness and provide guidelines for veterinarians and pet owners. A recent paper provides an overview on antimicrobial stewardship in laboratory animals, mainly focusing on rodents and rabbits.[41] Experts in veterinary antimicrobial steward-ship suggest to add two Rs to the well-known three Rs frequently used in laboratory animals. Antimicrobial stewardship not only requires reduction, refinement, and replacement, but also responsibility and review.[42] The establishment of an antimicrobial stewardship program in a veterinary hospital or clinic requires a comprehensive list of components, such as knowledge, guidelines, surveillance, diagnostic tools, collabora-tion, commitment, finances, and willingness of all involved parties including the pet owner. Considering all these components, one might be discouraged before even start-ing. However, not all components have to be in place at the start of implementing an antimicrobial stewardship program. Every clinic can start with minor steps, such as re-sponsibility by awareness and recognition of the problem, reduction by shortening the duration of antimicrobial therapy, refinement by using narrow-spectrum antimicrobials when possible, replacement by introducing alternative (nonantimicrobial) treatment when available, and review by implementation of therapy evaluation.

CHALLENGES FOR RESPONSIBLE ANTIMICROBIAL USE IN EXOTIC ANIMALS

Data estimating AMU and AMR in exotic animals are lacking. The options in available antimicrobials for the different exotic animal species are often limited. Potentially toxic or adverse effects of some antimicrobials in specific animal species and the formula-tion make the range of available products even smaller.

In exotic animals, several challenges complicate antimicrobial treatment, and may result in practical arguments to choose certain veterinary medicinal products or prod-ucts authorized for human use, compromising the choice for the right antimicrobial drug in this patient at this time. Challenges comprise the right formulation (liquids are preferred over tablets), the right concentration, and the acceptance of the animal (taste). In veterinary practice this means that in birds liquid oral forms of aminopenicil-lins for human use are attractive, because these substances are dosed much higher in most birds, so even doses for a small exotic animal are measurable, and the liquid has an acceptable taste for most birds. The same arguments are applicable for azithromy-cin, of which the liquid formula authorized for human use is convenient for dosing in small birds and rodents.[43] In rabbits, guinea pigs, and other herbivorous rodents, antimicrobial treatment options are limited because oral treatment with several antimi-crobial agents (ie, penicillin, lincomycin, amoxicillin, ampicillin, cephalosporins, clinda-mycin, erythromycin, streptomycin) may result in dysbiosis and enterotoxaemia. This results in generic advices comprising fluoroquinolones, such as respiratory infections and abscesses of odontogenic origin.[44,45] In reptiles, infections are often associated with *Pseudomonas* spp, resulting in the application of ceftazidime. Although ceftazi-dime has great antipseudomonal activity, it is a third-generation cephalosporin autho-rized for human use only, and classified as highest priority critically important for human medicine.[31]

Another challenge is the availability of literature concerning the dosing of antibiotics in exotics. Controversially, more dosing information is available about newer antimi-crobial substances, such as fluoroquinolones.[46–48] As a result, in the Netherlands, four enrofloxacin-containing veterinary medicinal products are authorized for exotic animals including rodents, in addition to two trimethoprim/sulfonamide-containing drugs. No other antimicrobial products are authorized, making off-label use common practice in exotic animal medicine.

In addition, information on common bacterial pathogens to be encountered in spe-cific locations in the different species is not always readily available. Without this knowledge, choosing the right antimicrobial drug becomes more difficult, thereby rendering it more likely for the veterinarian to make decisions based on empiric evidence and pragmatic arguments.

GUIDELINES FOR RESPONSIBLE ANTIMICROBIAL USE IN EXOTICS

Several factors should be considered when prescribing and selecting an antimicrobial agent (**Fig. 1**). First, antimicrobials should only be used when a primary bacterial infection or secondary bacterial involvement is proven or highly likely. If other, nonbacterial causes (eg, parasitic, viral, or mycotic infection, noninfectious disease) are more likely, diagnosis and treatment should primarily focus on those causes. The need for AMU to prevent infection is debatable, and should be reserved for those cases where occurrence of an infection is likely to occur and result in life-threatening disease (eg, sepsis in severely immunocompromised patients). Other considerations that should be taken

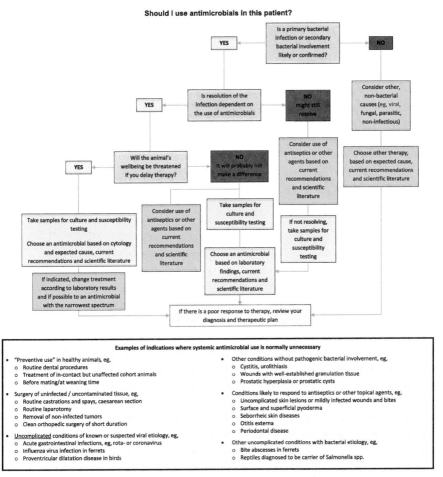

Fig. 1. Flow diagram to support the decision-making process and prevent unnecessary use of antimicrobials in exotic patients. (*Adapted from* FECAVA Advice on responsible use of antimicrobials. FECAVA working group on hygiene and the use of antimicrobials in veterinary practice. 2014; with permission. Available at: http://www.fecava.org/sites/default/files/files/2014_12_fecava_responsible%20use%20AM.pdf.)

Table 2
Antimicrobial classes and agents and their antimicrobial activity against common veterinary pathogens

Antimicrobial Class	Antimicrobial Agents	Susceptible Pathogens	Resistance
Penicillins (narrow-spectrum)	Benzylpenicillin, procaïnepenicillin	Many gram positives; most anaerobes; Pasteurellaceae; *Mannheimia* spp; *Actinobacillus* spp; *Haemophilus* spp; *Histophilus* spp	Most gram negatives; mycoplasmata; methicillin-resistant staphylococci
Penicillins (broad-spectrum)	Ampicillin, amoxicillin, amoxicillin/ clavulanic acid	See penicillin (narrow-spectrum); many gram negatives	*Pseudomonas* spp; *Klebsiella* spp; *Enterobacter* spp; *Citrobacter* spp; *Acinetobacter* spp; *Yersinia enterocolitica*; mycoplasmata; methicillin-resistant staphylococci
Penicillins (antipseudomonal)	Ticarcillin,[a] piperacillin[a]	See penicillin (broad-spectrum); *Pseudomonas* spp	Mycoplasmata; methicillin-resistant staphylococci
Cephalosporins	First-generation cephalosporins (eg, cephalexin, cefazolin[a])	Many gram positives; most *Enterobacteriaceae*; most anaerobes; Pasteurellaceae; *Mannheimia* spp; *Haemophilus* spp	*Enterobacter* spp; *Pseudomonas* spp; *Citrobacter* spp; *Acinetobacter* spp; *Y enterocolitica*; methicillin-resistant staphylococci; enterococci
	Third- and fourth-generation cephalosporins (eg, ceftiofur, cefquinome, ceftazidime[a])	See first-generation cephalosporins; *Pseudomonas* spp (fourth and ceftazidime)	Some *Pseudomonas* spp (third); methicillin-resistant staphylococci; enterococci
Lincosamides	Lincomycin, clindamycin	Gram-positive aerobes; anaerobes; mycoplasmata	Gram-negative aerobes; enterococci
Macrolides/azalides	Erythromycin, tylosin, spiramycin, azithromycin[a]	Many gram positives; most mycoplasmata; *Chlamydia* spp; *Mycobacterium* spp; *Campylobacter* spp	Many gram negatives; enterococci
Aminoglycosides	Gentamicin, neomycin, amikacin[a]	Some gram positives; most gram negatives	Streptococci; anaerobes

(continued on next page)

Table 2
(continued)

Antimicrobial Class	Antimicrobial Agents	Susceptible Pathogens	Resistance
Tetracyclins	Doxycycline, tetracycline	Many gram positives; many gram negatives; mycoplasmata; *Chlamydia* spp	*Pseudomonas* spp; *Proteus* spp
Phenicols	Chloramphenicol, florfenicol	Many gram positives; many gram negatives; anaerobes; mycoplasmata; *Chlamydia* spp	*Pseudomonas* spp
Diaminopyrimidines	Trimethoprim	Many gram positives; many gram negatives	*Pseudomonas* spp; anaerobes
Sulfonamides	Sulfadiazine, sulfamethoxazole	Many gram positives; many gram negatives	*Pseudomonas* spp
Fluoroquinolones	Enrofloxacin, marbofloxacin	Most gram negatives; mycoplasmata; *Chlamydia* spp; *Mycobacterium* spp; *Campylobacter* spp	Less active against gram positives; anaerobes
Nitroimidazoles	Metronidazole	Anaerobes	Aerobes

[a] Authorized for human use only.

into account are the likelihood of the bacterial infection to resolve without the use of antibiotics and the disease severity. Antimicrobials are preferably reserved for those cases where no other options (eg, use of antiseptics) are available and delay of therapy will result in a compromised well-being of the animal.

If the use of antibiotics is deemed appropriate, the selection of a therapy should ideally be based on an accurate diagnosis and antimicrobial susceptibility testing. However, in several situations (eg, seriously ill animal requiring immediate therapy, no representative sample obtainable, no routine susceptibility testing available) empirical therapy is the next best thing. When prescribing antimicrobials based on empiricism, knowledge of the most common pathogens causing certain infections and of antimicrobial spectrum of antimicrobial agents is indispensable. For certain bacteria (eg, β-hemolytic streptococci, Pasteurellaceae, and Chlamydiaceae) susceptibilities are predictable. Other, mostly gram-negative bacteria rapidly acquire resistance genes, making susceptibility patterns hard to predict. Additional factors to consider when prescribing and selecting antimicrobials are pharmacokinetic and pharmacodynamics properties, potential toxicities or adverse effects, the route of administration, and costs of the selected antimicrobial agent.[42] To avoid disturbance of the normal gut flora and to minimize selection of antimicrobial resistant organisms, local treatment with antiseptic drugs and narrow-spectrum antimicrobials are preferable to systemic treatment and broad-spectrum antimicrobials, respectively.

Table 2 presents a concise overview of veterinary important antimicrobial agents and their activity against common veterinary pathogens.

RECOMMENDATIONS

In exotic animals, evidence-based treatment guidelines for infections, including anti-microbial stewardship considerations, are not yet available. Common practice is based on personal experiences of successful strategies by individual veterinary specialists because of absence of suitable veterinary medicinal products, or on literature aiming at 100% susceptibility of all suspected pathogens.[42] This results in frequent (off label) application of antimicrobials categorized as critically important antimicrobials by the WHO, such as fluoroquinolones, aminopenicillins, third-generation cephalosporins, and macrolides. The most important consideration in case of an acute infection in exotic animal should be what pathogen is most likely causing the symptoms, and whether antimicrobial therapy is needed. A list of appropriate antimicrobials is needed for empiric therapy, and consensus on the right dose and preferable length of therapy. For these antimicrobials, adequate pharmaceutical formulations should be developed. Until then, antimicrobial stewardship in exotic animals will be hampered by the un-availability of treatment options.

ACKNOWLEDGMENTS

We would like to thank Dr. Y.R.A. van Zeeland for proofreading of and valuable contribution to the article.

REFERENCES

1. World Health Organization. Global action plan on antimicrobial resistance. At the Sixty-Eight World Health Assembly in May 2015. 2015. Available at: http://www.who.int/antimicrobial-resistance/global-action-plan/en/. Accessed December 17, 2017.
2. World Health Organization. WHO guidelines on use of medically important antimicrobials in food-producing animals. Available at: http://apps.who.int/iris/bitstream/10665/258970/1/9789241550130-eng.pdf?ua=1. Accessed December 17, 2017.
3. European Commission. A European one health action plan against antimicrobial resistance (AMR). 2017. Available at: https://ec.europa.eu/health/amr/sites/amr/files/amr_action_plan_2017_en.pdf. Accessed December 17, 2017.
4. Weese JS, Giguère S, Guardabassi L, et al. ACVIM consensus statement on therapeutic antimicrobial use in animals and antimicrobial resistance. J Vet Intern Med 2015;29(2):487–98.
5. Johns I. Antimicrobial stewardship in the treatment of equine bacterial infections. Vet J 2017;219:4–5.
6. DANMAP. 1996–2016. Use of antimicrobial agents and occurrence of antimicrobial resistance in bacteria from food animals, food and humans in Denmark. Available at: https://www.danmap.org/Downloads/Reports.aspx. Accessed December 17, 2017.
7. SWEDRES/SVARM. 2000–2016. Consumption of antibiotics and occurrence of antibiotic resistance in Sweden. Available at: http://www.sva.se/en/antibiotika/svarm-reports. Accessed December 17, 2017.
8. NETHMAP/MARAN. 2012–2017. NethMap: Consumption of antimicrobial agents and antimicrobial resistance among medically important bacteria in the Netherlands/MARAN: Monitoring of antimicrobial resistance and antibiotic usage in animals in the Netherlands in 2016. Available at: http://www.swab.nl/swab/cms3.

nsf/viewdoc/20BCD3983B5C390AC12575850031D33D. Accessed December 17, 2017.

9. BelVet-SAC. Belgian veterinary surveillance of antibacterial consumption. National consumption report. 2013–2016. Available at: http://www.amcra.be/nl/rapporten-publicaties-en-wetgeving/nationale-rapporten. Accessed December 17, 2017.

10. Taverne F, Jacobs J, Heederik D, et al. Influence of applying different units of measurement on reporting antimicrobial consumption data for pig farms. BMC Vet Res 2015;11:250, 9.

11. Postma M, Sjölund M, Collineau L, et al. MINAPIG consortium. Assigning defined daily doses animal: a European multi-country experience for antimicrobial products authorized for usage in pigs. J Antimicrob Chemother 2015;70(1):294–302.

12. Grave K, Torren-Edo J, Mackay D. Comparison of the sales of veterinary antibacterial agents between 10 European countries. J Antimicrob Chemother 2010;65: 2037–40.

13. European Medicines Agency. Revised ESVAC reflection paper on collecting data on consumption of antimicrobial agents per animal species, on technical units of measurement and indicators for reporting consumption of antimicrobial agents in animals. 2013. Available at: http://www.ema.europa.eu/docs/en_GB/document_library/Scientific_guideline/2012/12/WC500136456.pdf. Accessed December 17, 2017.

14. ECDC (European Centre for Disease Prevention and Control), EFSA (European Food Safety Authority), EMA (European Medicines Agency). ECDC/EFSA/EMA second joint report on the integrated analysis of the consumption of antimicrobial agents and occurrence of antimicrobial resistance in bacteria from humans and food-producing animals–Joint Interagency Antimicrobial Consumption and Resistance Analysis (JIACRA) Report. EFSA Journal 2017;15:4872, 135.

15. Netherlands Veterinary Medicines Institute, Expert panel. Usage of antimicrobial drugs in companion animals 2012 – 2014 results of a survey of veterinary practices in the Netherlands. 2017. Available at: http://www.autoriteitdiergeneesmiddelen.nl/en/publications. Accessed December 17, 2017.

16. European Medicines Agency. Standardised units of measurement for veterinary antimicrobials. 2016. Available at: http://www.ema.europa.eu/ema/index.jsp?curl=pages/regulation/general/general_content_001493.jsp&mid=WC0b01ac0580a2fcf5. Accessed December 17, 2017.

17. European Medicines Agency, European Surveillance of Veterinary Antimicrobial Consumption. Sales of veterinary antimicrobial agents in 30 European countries in 2015 (EMA/184855/2017). Available at: http://www.ema.europa.eu/docs/en_GB/document_library/Report/2017/10/WC500236750.pdf. Accessed December 17, 2017.

18. U.S. Food and Drug Administration FDA. Annual summary report on antimicrobials sold or distributed in 2016 for use in food-producing animals. 2017. Available at: https://www.fda.gov/downloads/ForIndustry/UserFees/AnimalDrugUserFeeActADUFA/UCM588085.pdf. Accessed January 1, 2018.

19. Netherlands Veterinary Medicines Institute, Expert panel. Usage of antibiotics in agricultural livestock in the Netherlands in 2016. Trends and benchmarking of livestock farms and veterinarians. 2017. Available at: http://www.autoriteitdiergeneesmiddelen.nl/Userfiles/Eng%20rapport%20AB%202016/engels-def-rapportage-2016-deel-1-en-2-22-09-2017.pdf. Accessed December 17, 2017.

20. Hardefeldt LY, Holloway S, Trott DJ, et al. Antimicrobial prescribing in dogs and cats in Australia: results of the Australasian infectious disease advisory panel survey. J Vet Intern Med 2017;31:1100–7.
21. Pleydell EJ, Souphavanh K, Hill KE, et al. Descriptive epidemiological study of the use of antimicrobial drugs by companion animal veterinarians in New Zealand. N Z Vet J 2012;60:115–22.
22. Murphy CP, Reid-Smith RJ, Boerlin P, et al. Out-patient antimicrobial drug use in dogs and cats for new disease events from community companion animal practices in Ontario. Can Vet J 2012;53(3):291–8.
23. Buckland EL, O'Neill D, Summers J, et al. Characterisation of antimicrobial usage in cats and dogs attending UK primary care companion animal veterinary practices. Vet Rec 2016;179:489.
24. Guardabassi L, Prescott JF. Antimicrobial stewardship in small animal veterinary practice: from theory to practice. Vet Clin North Am Small Anim Pract 2015;45: 361–76.
25. Divers SJ, Sladakovic I, Mayer J, et al. Development of an antibiotic policy in a zoological medicine service and approach to antibiotic dosing using mic data. In: 3rd International Conference on Avian herpetological and Exotic mammal medicine PROCEEDINGS 2017. Available at: https://distribuzione.evsrl.it/ArticleDetail.aspx?lang=en&from=HP&id=4822. Accessed December 17, 2017.
26. Briscoe JA, Morris DO, Rankin SC, et al. Methicillin-resistant *Staphylococcus aureus*-associated dermatitis in a Congo African grey parrot (Psittacus erithacus erithacus). J Avian Med Surg 2008;22:336–43.
27. Loncaric I, Künzel F. Sequence type 398 methicillin-resistant *Staphylococcus aureus* infection in a pet rabbit. Vet Dermatol 2013;24:370–2.
28. Sousa M, Silva N, Igrejas G, et al. Genetic diversity and antibiotic resistance among coagulase-negative staphylococci recovered from birds of prey in Portugal. Microb Drug Resist 2016;22:727–30.
29. Yilmaz ES, Dolar A. Detection of extended-spectrum β-lactamases in *Escherichia coli* from cage birds. J Exotic Pet Med 2017;26:13–8.
30. Cortés-Cortés G, Lozano-Zarain P, Torres C, et al. Detection and molecular characterization of *Escherichia coli* strains producers of extended-spectrum and CMY-2 type beta-lactamases, isolated from turtles in Mexico. Vector Borne Zoonotic Dis 2016;16:595–603.
31. World Health Organization. Critically important antimicrobials for human medicine. 5th revision. 2017. Available at: http://www.who.int/foodsafety/publications/antimicrobials-fifth/en/. Accessed December 17, 2017.
32. European Commission. Commission Notice. Guidelines for the prudent use of antimicrobials in veterinary medicine. Official Journal of the European Union 2015; C 299/04. Available at: https://ec.europa.eu/health/sites/health/files/antimicrobial_resistance/docs/2015_prudent_use_guidelines_en.pdf. Accessed December 17, 2017.
33. Werkgroep Veterinair Antibiotica Beleid (Working Party for Policy on Veterinary Antimicrobials). WVAB –richtlijn classificatie van veterinaire antimicrobiële middelen. Available at: http://wvab.knmvd.nl/media/default.aspx/emma/org/10886458/170201%20wvab%20richtlijn%203.2%20definitief.pdf. Accessed December 17, 2017.
34. Anonymus (Dutch legislation). Besluit Diergeneeskundigen art 5.7 Gevoeligheidsbepaling bij toepassing aangewezen diergeneesmiddelen. Available at: http://wetten.overheid.nl/jci1.3:c:BWBR0035091&hoofdstuk=5&artikel=5.7&z=2016-09-01&g=2016-09-01. Accessed December 17, 2017.

35. Anonymus (Dutch legislation). Regeling Diergeneeskundigen art. 5.8 Gevoeligheidsbepaling bij toepassing aangewezen diergeneesmiddelen. Available at: http://wetten.overheid.nl/jci1.3:c:BWBR0035238&hoofdstuk=5&paragraaf=2&artikel=5.8&z=2017-01-01&g=2017-01-01. Accessed December 17, 2017.
36. Netherlands Veterinary Medicines Institute, Expert panel. Association between antimicrobial use and the prevalence of resistant micro-organisms. SDa-report. 2016. Available at: http://www.autoriteitdiergeneesmiddelen.nl/en/publications. Accessed December 17, 2017.
37. ECDC (European Centre for Disease Prevention and Control), EFSA (European Food Safety Authority), EMA (European Medicines Agency). ECDC/EFSA/EMA first joint report on the integrated analysis of the consumption of antimicrobial agents and occurrence of antimicrobial resistance in bacteria from humans and food producing animals. Stockholm/Parma/London: ECDC/EFSA/EMA, 2015. EFSA Journal 2015;13:4006, 114.
38. Tang KL, Caffrey NP, Nóbrega DB, et al. Restricting the use of antibiotics in food-producing animals and its associations with antibiotic resistance in food-producing animals and human beings: a systematic review and meta-analysis. Lancet Planet Health 2017;1:e316–27.
39. McGowan JE Jr, Gerding DN. Does antibiotic prevent resistance? New Horiz 1996;4:370–6.
40. Dyar OJ, Huttner B, Schouten J, et al. ESGAP (ESCMID Study Group for Antimicrobial stewardshiP). What is antimicrobial stewardship? Clin Microbiol Infect 2017;23:793–8.
41. Narver HL. Antimicrobial stewardship in laboratory animal facilities. J Am Assoc Lab Anim Sci 2017;56:6–10.
42. Weese JS, Page SW, Prescott JF. Antimicrobial stewardship in animals. In: Giguère S, Prescott J, Dowling PM, editors. Antimicrobial therapy in veterinary medicine. Hoboken (NJ): John Wiley and Sons; 2013. p. 117–32.
43. Padovan J, Ralić J, Letfus V, et al. Investigating the barriers to bioavailability of macrolide antibiotics in the rat. Eur J Drug Metab Pharmacokinet 2012;37: 163–71.
44. Rougier S, Galland D, Boucher S, et al. Epidemiology and susceptibility of pathogenic bacteria responsible for upper respiratory tract infections in pet rabbits. Vet Microbiol 2006;115:192–8.
45. Minarikova A, Hauptman K, Knotek Z, et al. Microbial flora of odontogenic abscesses in pet guinea pigs. Vet Rec 2016;179:331, 4.
46. Watson MK, Wittenburg LA, Bui CT, et al. Pharmacokinetics and bioavailability of orbifloxacin oral suspension in New Zealand white rabbits (Oryctolagus cuniculus). Am J Vet Res 2015;76:946–51.
47. Marín P, García-Martínez F, Hernándis V, et al. Pharmacokinetics of norfloxacin after intravenous, intramuscular and subcutaneous administration to rabbits. J Vet Pharmacol Ther 2018;41:137–41.
48. Abo-el-Sooud K, Goudah A. Influence of pasteurella multocida infection on the pharmacokinetic behavior of marbofloxacin after intravenous and intramuscular administrations in rabbits. J Vet Pharmacol Ther 2010;33:63–8.

Antifungal Therapy in Birds
Old Drugs in a New Jacket

Gunther Antonissen, DVM, MSc, PhD[a,b,*],
An Martel, DVM, MSc, PhD, DECZM (Wildlife Population Health)[b]

KEYWORDS

- Amphotericin B • Antifungal • Drug formulation • Itraconazole • Nanoparticles
- Nebulization • Terbinafine • Voriconazole

KEY POINTS

- Large interspecies and interindividual variability can be found in the pharmacokinetics of antifungal drugs in birds, which can significantly affect drug safety and efficacy.
- The absorption of antifungals is affected by numerous factors, including drug formulation and gastrointestinal anatomy and physiology.
- New antifungal drug delivery systems enhance drug stability, reduce off-target side effects, prolong residence time in the blood, and improve drug efficacy, and should therefore be considered in the treatment of mycoses.
- Nebulization seems to be a promising method to deliver antifungals in the respiratory tract of birds; however, therapeutic output is influenced by drug formulation and nebulizer type.

INTRODUCTION

The early diagnosis of systemic fungal diseases in birds, especially aspergillosis, remains challenging because the clinical signs are usually nonspecific and there still is no single reliable noninvasive diagnostic test available in birds.[1–3] Consequently, antifungal therapy is frequently administered empirically for presumptive invasive fungal infections in these patients without a definitive diagnosis being made. However, different factors need to be considered in the rational drug selection of antifungal therapy. First, the selected antifungal drug must be able to penetrate the center of infection in a concentration to which the fungus is susceptible. However, fungi, in

Disclosure Statement: The authors have nothing to disclose.
G. Antonissen is supported by a postdoctoral fellowship from the Research Foundation, Flanders (12V6418N).
^a Department of Pharmacology, Toxicology and Biochemistry, Faculty of Veterinary Medicine, Ghent University, Salisburylaan 133, Merelbeke 9820, Belgium; ^b Department of Pathology, Bacteriology and Avian Diseases, Faculty of Veterinary Medicine, Ghent University, Salisburylaan 133, Merelbeke 9820, Belgium
* Corresponding author. Department of Pharmacology, Toxicology and Biochemistry, Faculty of Veterinary Medicine, Ghent University, Merelbeke, Belgium.
E-mail address: Gunther.Antonissen@UGent.be

contrast with bacteria, are eukaryotes, and consequently most antifungal agents are also toxic to the eukaryotic host cells. Therefore, taking into account their (often narrow) therapeutic index, no perfect antifungal agent exists. Nevertheless, in the last decades, newer and less toxic antifungals, including the azoles and echinocandins, have been developed for use in human medicine. Aside from the chemical structure, the impact of antifungal drug formulation and route of administration on treatment safety and efficacy have been investigated as well.[4]

Because knowledge of avian antifungal treatment is limited, treatment protocols are often developed empirically, based on case reports, or extrapolated from humans or other animal species. Because of the narrow therapeutic index, the dosing of antifungal drugs should be done carefully, with dose extrapolation preferably based on more advanced allometric and physiologically based pharmacokinetic (PK) modeling.[5] In avian medicine, different antifungal agents are being used, but most of these substances have not been approved for administration in birds.[6] However, recently (2014) the first antifungal product (itraconazole 10 mg/mL oral solution; Fungitraxx, Avimedical, Hengelo, The Netherlands) was registered for ornamental birds in Europe (EMA/698698/2013). The purpose of this review is to describe the interrelation of antifungal drug formulation, administration route, therapeutic–toxic range, and treatment outcome in fungal diseases, with a particular emphasis on aspergillosis in companion birds.

MECHANISM OF ACTION

In general, the main targets for antifungal drug development are cell wall polymer (glucans, chitin, mannoproteins), cell membrane (especially ergosterol) biosynthesis, DNA and protein synthesis (topoisomerases, nucleases, elongation factors and myristoylation), and signal transduction pathways (protein kinases and protein phosphatases).[7,8] The 3 major groups of antifungal agents in clinical use, that is, polyenes, azole derivatives, and allylamines, all owe their antifungal activities to the inhibition of synthesis or direct interaction with ergosterol (the predominant component of the fungal cell membrane).[8,9]

Amphotericin B and nystatin are polyene macrolides that act by binding to ergosterol. This binding alters the membrane permeability, causing leakage of sodium, potassium, and hydrogen ions, which eventually leads to cell death. Polyenes have a broad antifungal spectrum, including a variety of yeasts (eg, *Candida* spp) and molds (eg, *Aspergillus* spp).[9]

Azoles inhibit the enzyme cytochrome P450-dependent 14-α-sterol demethylase, which is required for the conversion of lanosterol to ergosterol. Exposed fungi become depleted of ergosterol and accumulate 14-α-methylated sterols. This action causes disruption of membrane structure and function, thereby inhibiting fungal growth.[9,10] Azoles are classified as imidazoles (including clotrimazole, miconazole, enilconazole, and ketoconazole) or triazoles (including itraconazole, fluconazole, and voriconazole) based on possessing 2 or 3 nitrogen atoms in the 5-membered azole ring, respectively. Depending on the particular compound, azole antifungal agents have fungistatic and broad-spectrum activity against most yeasts and filamentous fungi.[9] With the exception of voriconazole, azoles are known to be fungistatic at the doses used in birds and need several days to reach steady-state concentrations.[11]

Finally, allylamines (eg, terbinafine) act by a reversible, noncompetitive inhibition of the squalene epoxidase, a key enzyme in the cyclization of squalene to lanosterol, resulting in an ergosterol depletion and squalene accumulation. The antifungal spectrum of terbinafine includes yeast (fungistatic) as well as dermatophytes and molds (fungicidal).[6,9,12]

TOXICITY

The clinical use of amphotericin B has been associated with a dose-dependent nephrotoxicity in mammals. Because amphotericin B binds to mammalian sterols, including cholesterol, renal toxicity is related to binding of the drug to the sterol rich cell membranes in kidney tubules. As a result, amphotericin B affects the ionic permeability of the renal brush border cells, releasing mediators that cause an abrupt decrease in renal blood flow. However, no evidence of nephrotoxicity has been observed in birds, which might be associated with the shorter elimination half-life ($T_{1/2el}$) in birds compared with mammals after intravenous (IV) administration.[11,13] Nevertheless, clinicians are advised to monitor the renal function of their avian patients.

The relative toxicity of azoles depends on the specificity for binding to the fungal cytochrome P450 enzyme, instead of the avian/mammalian cytochrome P450 enzymes. The most common adverse side effects associated with azole administration in birds are gastrointestinal (GI) signs, such as anorexia and vomiting, and alterations in liver function.[14,15] In general itraconazole, is well-tolerated; however, caution should be used when considering the use of this drug in African or timneh gray parrots, because they are more sensitive to itraconazole present in the form of distinct anorexia and depression.[6,11] Remarkably, PK studies explaining this higher sensitivity in African or timneh gray parrots are still lacking (**Table 1**). The apparent sensitivity to azoles experienced by different bird species may be explained in part by the drug's PK and metabolism. In humans, cytochrome P450 isoenzyme CYP2C19 genotypic polymorphism has been linked to differential sensitivity to voriconazole toxicity.[16,17] Although undocumented in avian species, similar polymorphisms could be responsible for the wide variability in avian voriconazole PK properties. After a single oral administration of voriconazole, a 4 to 5 times longer $T_{1/2el}$ was observed in pigeons (*Columba livia domestica*) and African penguins (*Spheniscus demersus*), compared with Hispaniolan Amazon parrots (*Amazona ventralis*), timneh gray parrots (*Psittacus erithacus timneh*), mallard ducks (*Anas platyrhynchos*), and red-tailed hawks (*Buteo jamaicensis*; **Table 2**).[18–23] This prolonged $T_{1/2el}$ in pigeons and penguins presents a potential for drug accumulation with extended dosing and toxicity. After oral administration of voriconazole (10 and 20 mg/kg body weight [BW] twice a day) to pigeons, Beernaert and colleagues[19] observed hepatic changes, such as hepatomegaly and miliary hepatic necrosis and, on histology, vacuolization up to apoptosis of hepatocytes and heterophilic and lymphocytic infiltration. Similarly, Hyatt and colleagues[24] demonstrated signs indicative of toxicity in multiple penguin species after administering voriconazole (6.1–22.2 mg/kg BW once or twice a day), which ranged in severity and included anorexia, lethargy, weakness, change in mentation, ataxia, paresis, apparent vision changes, seizurelike activity, and generalized seizures. The toxicity and efficacy of all azole derivatives can furthermore be influenced by drug–drug interactions that are based on the mechanism of action of these drugs being potent cytochrome P450 inhibitors. Consequently, caution should be taken when azoles are coadministered with other drugs, such as midazolam, enrofloxacin, and clindamycin.[6,24]

Finally, terbinafine is generally associated with a low index of toxicity and few adverse effects. In humans, only mild GI toxicity and hepatobiliary dysfunction are reported. In red-tailed hawks, oral administration of a high dose of terbinafine (120 mg/kg BW) was furthermore demonstrated to induce regurgitation.[25] Anecdotally, some mild GI toxicity and hepatobiliary dysfunction were observed in some psittacine species including an African gray parrot, a blue-fronted Amazon parrot

Table 1
Plasma and lung itraconazole and hydroxyitraconazole concentrations after single bolus and steady-state pharmacokinetic studies of itraconazole in different bird species

Animal Species	BW (g)	Dosage Itraconazole (mg/kg BW)	Drug Formulation	Frequency of Administration	Feed	Itraconazole (ng/mL)			Hydroxyitraconazole (ng/mL)			Reference
						C_{min}	C_{max}	C_{lung}	C_{min}	C_{max}	C_{lung}	
PK single bolus												
Pigeon	488	10.3	ITRA-LAC	Single bolus	—	—	1130	250	—	—	—	Lumeij et al,[55] 1995
		5	ITRA-LAC + orange juice	Single bolus	No	—	100–200[a]	339	—	—	—	Orosz et al,[53] 1995
		5	ITRA-LAC + orange juice + 0.1 N HCl	Single bolus	Yes	—	100–200[a]	476	—	—	—	
Blue-fronted Amazon parrot	306–424	5	ITRA-LAC + orange juice + 0.1 N HCl	Single bolus	Yes	—	1743	—	—	247	—	Orosz et al,[57] 1996
		10	ITRA-LAC + orange juice + 0.1 N HCl	Single bolus	Yes	—	2312	—	—	1976	—	
Red-tailed hawks		5	ITRA-LAC + orange juice + 0.1 N HCl	Single bolus	Yes	—	50–300[a]	—	—	50–150[a]	—	Jones et al,[56] 2000
		10	ITRA-LAC + orange juice + 0.1 N HCl	Single bolus	Yes	—	250–300[a]	—	—	200–250[a]	—	
Mallard Duck	979–1442	20	ITRA-LAC + orange juice + 0.1 N HCl	Single bolus	Yes	—	1070	730	—	340	275	Tell et al,[49] 2005
Black-footed penguin	2600–4400	20	ITRA-CD	Single bolus	Yes	—	1350	796	—	270	313	Smith et al,[80] 2010
		7	ITRA-GEN	Single bolus	Yes	—	350	—	—	—	—	
		7	ITRA-CD	Single bolus	Yes	—	750	—	—	—	—	

PK at steady state

	BW	Dose	Formulation	Regimen	Detected						Reference
Pigeon	488	10.3	ITRA-LAC	QID, 3 d	—	—	3875	—	—	—	Lumeij et al,[55] 1995
		5	ITRA-LAC + orange juice	SID, 14 d	No	—	100–200[a]	250	—	3206	Orosz et al,[53] 1995
		5	ITRA-LAC + orange juice + 0.1 N HCl	SID, 14 d	Yes	—	500–600[a]	359	—	79,876	
Blue-fronted Amazon parrot	306–424	5	ITRA-LAC + orange juice + 0.1 N HCl	SID, 14 d	Yes	—	1437	197	309	—	Orosz et al,[57] 1996
		10	ITRA-LAC + orange juice + 0.1 N HCl	SID, 14 d	Yes	—	3434	92	1976	—	
Red-tailed hawks		5	ITRA-LAC + orange juice + 0.1 N HCl	SID, 14 d	Yes	—	300–360[a]	2598	150–360[a]	1750	Jones et al,[56] 2000
		10	ITRA-LAC + orange juice + 0.1 N HCl	SID, 14 d	Yes	—	150–500[a]	2941	120–480[a]	2113	
Humboldt penguin	3420–5760	6	ITRA-GEN	SID, 14 d	Yes	—	ND	30	248	—	Bunting et al,[51] 2009
		12	ITRA-GEN	SID, 14 d	Yes	—	52	55	331	—	
		6	ITRA-CD	SID, 14 d	Yes	—	10–100[a]	166	829	—	
		12	ITRA-CD	SID, 14 d	Yes	—	175	525	2335	—	
		7	ITRA-CD	BID, 14 d	Yes	104	262	673	994	—	

Abbreviations: BID, twice a day; BW, bodyweight; C_{lung}, concentration in lung; C_{max}, maximum plasma concentration; C_{min}, minimal plasma concentration in multiple doses PK; ITRA-CD, itraconazole + hydroxypropyl-β-cyclodextrin; ITRA-GEN, generic bulk compounded itraconazole powder; ITRA-LAC, itraconazole-coated lactose granules; ND, not detected; PK, pharmacokinetic; QID, 4 times a day; SID, once a day.

[a] Estimated concentration based on graph or table in original study.

Table 2
PK characteristics of voriconazole after single bolus and multiples doses administration in different bird species

	Animal Species	BW (g)	Dosage Voriconazole (mg/kg BW)	Frequency of Administration	Feed	F (%)	C_{min} (ng/mL)	T_{max} (h)	C_{max} (ng/mL)	V_d (IV) V_d/F (Oral) (mL/kg)	$T_{1/2el}$ (h)	Cl (IV) Cl/F (Oral) (mL/h·kg)	C_{lung} (ng/g)	C_{liver} (ng/g)	Reference
PK IV bolus	Chicken: layers	740–1110	10[b]	Single	No	100	—	—	7400	1681	1.99	586	—	—	Burhenne et al,[59] 2008
	Pigeon	400–500	2.5[a]	Single	Yes	100	—	—	—	1110	6.62	120	—	—	Beernaert et al,[19] 2009
	Mallard duck	1060 ± 110	5[a]	Single	Yes	100	—	—	—	1410	11.33	86	—	—	Kline et al,[22] 2011
			10[a]	Single	Yes	100	—	—	5576	1790	16.25	76	—	—	
			10[a]	Single	No	100	—	—	—	1440	1.34	530	ND	ND	
PK oral bolus	Chicken: layers	740–1106	5	Single	No	—	—	0.83	350	—	1.35	—	—	—	Burhenne et al,[59] 2008
			7.5	Single	No	—	—	2.00	410	—	2.40	—	—	—	
			10	Single	No	—	—	0.83	440	—	1.23	—	—	—	
			10	Single	No	16	—	1.50	700	—	—	—	—	—	
			10	Single	No	20	—	0.75	880	—	1.45	—	—	—	
			15	Single	No	—	—	1.50	510	—	1.77	—	—	—	
	Pigeon	400–500	10[b]	Single	No	44	—	2.15	3317	2600	10.32	176	—	—	Beernaert et al,[19] 2009
	Japanese quail	104–179	20	Single	Yes	—	—	2.00	5800	1770	—	—	—	—	Tell et al,[60] 2010
			40[b]	Single	Yes	—	—	2.00	6900	6100	—	—	—	—	

	Body weight	Dose	Regimen										Reference
Hispaniolan Amazon parrot	260–320	12[c]	Single	No	—	1.00	2490	2054	0.90	1576	—	—	Guzman et al,[20] 2010
Timneh gray parrot	290–339	24[c]	Single	No	—	2.00	5080	2349	1.25	1306	—	—	Flammer et al,[21] 2008
		6[b]	Single	—	—	2.00	540	3498	1.11	2185	—	—	
		12[b]	Single	—	—	4.00	1890	2634	1.59	1151	—	—	
		12[c]	Single	—	—	2.00	3020	1051	1.07	679	—	—	
		18[c]	Single	—	—	2.00	5670	1200	1.59	521	—	—	
Mallard duck	1060 ± 110	10[b]	Single	No	61	0.77	3940	1504	—	—	ND	ND	Kline et al,[22] 2011
		10[b]	Single	Yes	—	1.50	7350	—	1.00	—	ND	0.04–0.06	
		20[b]	Single	Yes	—	1.50	10,600	—	1.75	—	ND-0.16	0.04–0.47	
		40[b]	Single	Yes	—	2.00	24,443	—	1.37	—	ND	0.06–0.17	
Red-tailed hawks	926–1410	15[b]	Single	No	—	2.29	7230	1180	2.04	431	—	—	Parsley et al,[23] 2017
African penguin	2200–3400	15[b]	Single	Yes	—	4.86	6180	1349	2.29	485	—	—	Hyatt et al,[18] 2017
		5[c]	Single	No	—	0.40	1890	—	10.92	—	—	—	
Multiple doses PK — Chicken: layers	1030–1770	10[b]	SID, 10 d	Yes	—	1.00	280	—	—	—	ND	140	Burhenne et al,[59] 2008
		10[b]	SID, 20 d	Yes	—	3.00	1590	—	—	—	765	5360	
		10[b]	SID, 30 d	Yes	—	3.00	400	—	—	—	255	817	
		10[b]	SID, 3 d	Yes	134–418	2.00	2417–3683	—	—	—	ND-598	—	
Pigeon	400–500	20[b]	SID, 10 d	Yes	154–1516	2.00	5352–9183	—	—	—	—	—	Beernaert et al,[19] 2009
		10[b]	BID, 4 d	Yes	ND-3500[d]	2.00	3350–8000[d]	—	1.60	—	100	—	
		20[b]	BID, 4 d	Yes	5847	2.00	15,876	—	—	—	ND-1241	—	

(continued on next page)

Table 2
(continued)

Animal Species	BW (g)	Dosage Voriconazole (mg/kg BW)	Frequency of Administration	Feed	F (%)	C_{min} (ng/mL)	T_{max} (h)	C_{max} (ng/mL)	V_d (IV) V_d/F (Oral) (mL/kg)	$T_{1/2el}$ (h)	CI (IV) CI/F (Oral) (mL/h·kg)	C_{lung} (ng/g)	C_{liver} (ng/g)	Reference
Hispaniolan Amazon parrot	260–320	18[c]	TID, 11 d	Yes	—	—	2.00	790	—	1.29	—	—	—	Guzman et al,[20] 2010
Timneh gray parrot	290–339	18[c]	BID, 9 d	—	—	58–63	—	2600–2800	—	—	—	—	—	Flammer et al,[21] 2008
Mallard duck	1060 ± 110	20[b]	SID, 21 d	No	—	—	1.00	9960	904	0.72	—	ND-0.19	ND-0.06	Kline et al,[22] 2011
African penguin	220–3400	20[b]	SID, 21 d	Yes	—	—	1.08	8090	1624	1.11	—	ND	ND-0.12	Hyatt et al,[18] 2017
		5[b]	SID, 8 d	Yes	—	500–3250	1.53	3640–5640	1193[e]	—	64[e]	—	—	

Abbreviations: BID, twice a day; BW, bodyweight; CI or CI/F, clearance; C_{liver} voriconazole concentration in liver; C_{lung} voriconazole concentration in lung; C_{max} maximum plasma concentration; C_{min} minimal plasma voriconazole concentration in multiple doses PK; F, absolute bioavailability; IV, intravenous; ND, not detected; PK, pharmacokinetic; SID, once a day; $T_{1/2el}$, elimination half-life; TID, 3 times a day; T_{max}, time point of maximum plasma concentration; V_d or V_d/F, volume of distribution.

[a] Voriconazole sulfobutylether-β-cyclodextrin was suspended in 0.9% NaCl.
[b] Water.
[c] Commercial suspending agent.
[d] Estimated concentration based on graph in original study.
[e] Calculated based on average bodyweight.

(*Amazona aestiva*), and a Senegal parrot (*Poicephalus senegalus*) after long-term administration of terbinafine (10–15 mg/kg BW, twice a day) alone or in combination with itraconazole or voriconazole (van Zeeland, personal communication, 2017).

DRUG RESISTANCE

Antifungal susceptibility testing is a useful tool to provide information to clinicians to help guide therapy. The European Committee on Antimicrobial Susceptibility Testing and the Clinical and Laboratory Standards Institute have developed a standardized in vitro antifungal susceptibility testing method for yeasts and molds, whereby the minimum inhibitory concentration (MIC) is measured and referenced to a clinical breakpoint. However, in birds, the interpretation of the MICs of different antifungal agents remains uncertain, because of lack of correlation of in vitro resistance with clinical outcome.[26,27] Although information on antifungal resistance in avian medicine is very limited, human medicine shows that antifungal resistance is increasing and is an emerging threat to patient management and clinical success. Beernaert and colleagues[28] reported an acquired resistance of *Aspergillus fumigatus* strains, isolated from companion and wild birds, to both itraconazole and voriconazole. However, current in vitro antifungal susceptibility tests do not (yet) take the impact of drug formulation into account. Consequently, interpretation of MICs of amphotericin B against *Aspergillus* spp remains uncertain because of lack of correlation of in vitro resistance with clinical outcome. For example, differences in PK characteristics (eg, tissue concentration of free drug in the site of infection) or immunomodulating properties between, for example, amphotericin B deoxycholate and liposomal amphotericin B, might be more important determinants of outcome of amphotericin B-based therapy than the MIC. In a murine model of disseminated invasive aspergillosis, treatment with liposomal amphotericin B resulted in a better outcome than treatment with amphotericin B deoxycholate, despite no differences in the MIC being observed between the drug formulations.[27]

DRUG FORMULATION

Several antifungal drugs are characterized by their insolubility in water at physiologic pH, poor oral bioavailability, and limited formulation approaches. In addition, a narrow therapeutic–toxic range and drug–drug interactions of systemic antifungal agents are other major problems that compromise optimal treatment.[29,30] Therefore, there is a strong need to develop innovative drug formulations to address these issues.

In an attempt to decrease the intrinsic toxicity and enhance the efficacy of amphotericin B, 3 lipid-associated formulations were developed and approved for use in human medicine in the 1990s, that is, amphotericin B lipid complex, liposomal amphotericin B, and amphotericin B colloidal dispersion. Amphotericin B lipid complex (Abelcet, Cephalon, Inc., Fraser, PA) forms ribbonlike particles of dimyristoyl phosphatidyl choline and dimyristoyl phosphatidyl glycerol with amphotericin B; liposomal amphotericin B (AmBisome, Gilead Sciences International Ltd., Cambridge, UK; and Fungisome, Lifecare Innovations Pvt Ltd, Gurgaon, India) is a true unilamellar liposome composed of a mixture of phosphatidyl choline:distearoyl:phosphatidylglycerol:cholesterol; and amphotericin B colloidal dispersion (Amphotec of Amphocil, Sequus Pharmaceuticals, Menlo Park, CA) is a formulation in which amphotericin B is complexed to cholesterol sulfate resulting in the formation of disclike structures. Knowledge based on in vitro and in vivo studies in rodents, dogs, and humans suggest that these lipid formulations of amphotericin B generally have a slower onset of action, because of the required dissociation of free amphotericin B from the lipid vehicle.

Moreover, incorporation of amphotericin B into the lipid vesicle will enhance drug uptake by the liver and spleen, and cause accumulation of the drug by the mononuclear phagocyte system and at sites of capillary damage and inflammation. Consequently, the PK characteristics of lipid-based amphotericin is strongly determined by its physicochemical properties. Amphotericin B lipid complex is the largest compound of the lipid preparations (diameter of 1600–11,000 nm), resulting in a fast recognition in the blood by activated monocytes/macrophages, which subsequently transport the drug to the site of infection, where phospholipases release the free drug. In addition, this compound is sequestered to a high extent in the tissues of the mononuclear phagocyte system (liver and spleen), including the lungs. This rapid and extensive distribution, predominantly to the liver, spleen, and lungs, is reflected in the PK characteristics by a very large volume of distribution and a low area under the plasma concentration time curve. Lung levels are considerably higher than those achieved with other lipid-associated preparations and amphotericin B deoxycholate. The small size of liposomal amphotericin B (diameter of 60–80 nm) and negative charge tend to result in a prolonged circulation in plasma, because these compounds are not readily recognized and taken up by the mononuclear phagocyte system. However, the clinical relevance of these PK differences between liposomal amphotericin B and amphotericin B lipid complex remains unknown. After IV infusion, amphotericin B colloidal dispersion (disks of 122 nm diameter and 4 nm thickness) is rapidly removed from the circulation by the mononuclear phagocyte system, predominantly by Kupffer cells of the liver, and to a lesser extent in the spleen and bone marrow. These differences in PK and pharmacodynamic characteristics are reflected in the dose recommendations in human medicine: amphotericin B deoxycholate 0.25 to 1.5 mg/kg once a day, amphotericin B lipid complex 5 mg/kg BW once a day, liposomal amphotericin B 1 to 5 mg/kg BW once a day, and amphotericin B colloidal dispersion 3 to 5 mg/kg once a day.[31] However, the impact of these differences in PK/pharmacodynamics on clinical efficacy in birds is still unclear. Comparatively, amphotericin B deoxycholate is administered at a dose of 1 to 1.5 mg/kg BW 3 times a day to birds.[3]

In humans, the superior safety profile of lipid-associated formulations is characterized by decreased acute infusion-related reactions and dose-related nephrotoxicity, allowing the administration of larger doses and therefore similar efficacy with fewer administrations. In vitro studies and human clinical data suggest that amphotericin B lipid complex and liposomal amphotericin B induce a Toll-like receptor 4 reaction instead of a Toll-like receptor 2 reaction, as observed with amphotericin deoxycholate, causing attenuation of the characteristic proinflammatory response. Unlike the other lipid-associated amphotericin B preparations, the amphotericin B colloidal dispersion is associated with a higher frequency of infusion-related reactions associated with an inflammatory gene upregulation similar as amphotericin B deoxycholate. The pathophysiology of amphotericin B–induced nephrotoxicity is associated with a vasoconstrictive effect on the afferent renal arterioles, decreasing the glomerular filtration rate and inducing tubular dysfunction. Complexation with lipids seems to stabilize amphotericin B in a self-associated state so that it is not available to interact with cholesterol in mammalian or avian cellular membranes, which is the presumed major site of toxicity. Moreover, amphotericin B alone binds preferentially to low-density lipoproteins and can be internalized into renal cells that express low-density lipoprotein receptors, resulting in toxicity. Amphotericin B from lipid-associated formulations binds preferentially to high-density lipoproteins, which reduces nephrotoxicity by decreasing the uptake of amphotericin B by renal cells because of their low level of high-density lipoprotein receptors.[32] Recently, Phillips and colleagues[33] demonstrated that a single dose (3 mg/kg BW) of liposomal amphotericin B delivered by aerosol to healthy mallard ducks resulted in minimal systemic distribution of the drug after administration, characterized by low plasma and kidney amphotericin B concentrations and no signs of drug-associated damage on histopathologic examination of renal, hepatic, or cardiac tissue samples. Similarly, based on clinical examination and plasma uric acid levels, no signs of nephrotoxicity were observed in a goliath heron (*Ardea goliath*) with a deep infection with *Aspergillus* species of its pectoral muscle topically treated with liposomal amphotericin B (1.35 mg/kg, once a day) mixed with sterile, water-soluble, gelatin lubricant for more than 1 month.[34]

Studies in mouse and rabbit models of fungal infection and human metaanalyses have shown the liposomal formulation of amphotericin B to be at least as effective as amphotericin B deoxycholate in improving survival and resolving the infection.[35–37] After intratracheal aerosol administration of liposomal amphotericin B to healthy mallard ducks, drug concentrations in pulmonary parenchyma reached above the targeted MIC for avian isolates of *Aspergillus* species of 1 µg/mL.[33] Although these lipid formulations are reported to have excellent safety and efficacy, the high price of these drugs may currently preclude their use in veterinary medicine compared with the conventional form.

Among many new antifungal drug delivery systems currently under investigation, nanoparticles (NPs) have emerged as an innovative and promising platform able to enhance drug stability, reduce off-target side effects, prolong residence time in the blood, and improve drug efficacy. NPs are characterized by their small particle size ranging from 1 to 1000 nm.[30] Liposomal amphotericin is the first and most successful commercial NP of antifungal drugs in humans.[38] NPs used in drug delivery can be classified into phospholipid vesicles (eg, liposomes), nonphospholipid vesicles, polymeric NPs, polymeric micelles, solid lipid NPs, nanostructured lipid carriers, nanoemulsions, and dendrimers.[30] For example, liposomal nystatin allowed the IV administration of nystatin, increased the maximum tolerated dose in mice from 4 to 16 mg/kg BW, and increased the survival rate of mice infected with *Candida albicans*.[39] Itraconazole incorporated into poly(lactide-co-glycolide) (PLGA) resulted in a sustained-release formulation for IV administration with plasma itraconazole levels for more than 3 times longer than the commercial formulation.[40] PLGA containing voriconazole was detectable in lungs until 5 to 7 days after pulmonary disposition in mice via an inhalation chamber.[41] Recently, Pardeike and colleagues[42] demonstrated that nebulized itraconazole-loaded nanostructured lipid carriers penetrate deeply into the lungs and air sacs of a falcon, being a prerequisite for pulmonary treatment of aspergillosis.

Administration Route

The route of administration of antifungals will depend on the drug, available drug formulation, condition of the bird, ability of the owner and/or veterinary staff to deliver the drug, and the financial and emotional commitment of the bird's owner. Taking into account the narrow therapeutic–toxic range of all commercially available antifungal drugs, selecting the most optimal route of administration of a certain compound, in a certain patient, helps to decrease toxicity and to quickly establish effective local drug concentration.

Systemic Treatment

Most systemic fungal infections require long-term therapy that often extends for weeks to months.[3,6] Treatment protocols should not merely include drugs for IV administration because of problems related to maintaining a permeable venous pathway for long periods of time in birds. Nevertheless, vascular access devices have been suggested to be useful for cases that require long-term, frequent venipuncture.[43] Despite these possibilities, the IV administration of antifungals (predominantly amphotericin B) in birds is only performed in rare cases, for example, in the initial treatment of acute aspergillosis, or in severely debilitated birds. IV administration should always be combined with an oral antifungal drug, which is often administered for at least several weeks to months.[6] PK studies of IV-administered amphotericin B deoxycholate in turkeys (*Meleagris gallapavo*), red-tailed hawks, broad-winged hawks (*Buteo platypterus*), and great horned owls (*Bubo virginianus*) have reported that the $T_{1/2el}$ for avian species is much shorter than that for mammals, suggesting that twice daily dosing is appropriate.[11,13] Amphotericin B can be administered IV under the form of amphotericin B deoxycholate or in a lipid-associated formulation. Standardized electrolyte supplementation and fluid management improve clinical amphotericin B efficacy by minimizing toxicity.[44] Voriconazole and fluconazole have the advantage compared with amphotericin B that, in addition to an IV formulation, an oral formulation is commercially available as well, rendering these drugs suitable for long-term use in birds.[45–47]

Recently, Souza and colleagues[48] assessed the efficacy of itraconazole, voriconazole and terbinafine containing implants in Japanese quails (*Coturnix japonica*). These implants were administered subcutaneously over the dorsum and between the scapulae. Targeted plasma terbinafine concentrations were achieved in some birds at various time points; however, concentrations were inconsistent. Itraconazole and voriconazole concentrations were also inconsistent and below the minimal MIC. Similarly, after subcutaneous administration of 2 itraconazole controlled release gel formulations, only very low or undetectable plasma and tissue concentrations of itraconazole and hydroxyitraconazole were found.[49] Consequently, the administration of an impregnated subcutaneous implant is not (yet) an effective method to treat a fungal infection in birds.

Oral dosing of antifungal drugs is the most common route of administration in systemic fungal diseases. However, oral drug absorption is a complex process affected by numerous factors associated with the drug's formulation characteristics and the GI anatomy and physiology of the target species.[50] Bunting and colleagues[51] demonstrated that the maximum itraconazole and hydroxyitraconazole plasma concentrations after oral administration of the commercially available itraconazole with hydroxypropyl-β-cyclodextrin were much higher compared with generic bulk compounded itraconazole powder in Humboldt penguins (see **Table 1**). In addition, factors such as GI pH and transit time are characterized by considerable variability between and within types of birds. Many azoles are highly lipophilic and poorly water soluble at a neutral pH; however, they are soluble in acidic solutions. The pH of the crop and stomach of birds is considerably less acidic than the mammalian stomach, possibly because of the rapid digestive transit time, which negatively affect antifungal drug solubility and absorption.[52] Further adding to the complexity of absorption is the coadministration of food. Concurrent administration of itraconazole with an intracrop feed bolus and dissolving itraconazole-lactose granules in 0.1 N hydrochloric acid (HCl) before oral administration to pigeons (5 mg/kg BW, once a day for 14 days) increased the maximum plasma concentration of itraconazole and the concentration of its metabolite hydroitraconazole in the lung (see **Table 1**).[53] The relative bioavailability of voriconazole administered orally (20 mg/kg BW, once a day) in mallard ducks with a bolus of liquid feed was slightly higher compared with birds that were not being fed at the time of drug administration (see **Table 2**).[22] In contrast, in falcons, it was observed that, by administering voriconazole in meat, the median peak plasma concentrations were reduced by 21% to 26%.[54]

Several PK studies have reported plasma and lung itraconazole and hydroxyitraconazole concentrations after a single bolus and steady-state PK studies in different bird species (see **Table 1**). Because of the extended time to reach steady state, in cases of acute aspergillosis or in severely diseased birds, itraconazole should initially be combined with amphotericin B (IV) or voriconazole (IV or by mouth) for 3 to 5 days. In the different studies, steady-state concentrations after oral administration were reached within 3 to 14 days.[51,53,55–57] Steady-state plasma concentrations itraconazole plus hydroxyitraconazole above the MIC of 500 to 1000 ng/mL were achieved in pigeons, blue-fronted Amazon parrots, red-tailed hawks, and Humboldt penguins administered itraconazole (see **Table 1**).[28,51,53,55–57] Unfortunately, concentration of itraconazole and its active metabolite in the lung and other target organs were only measured in pigeons and red-tailed hawks.[53,55,56] After oral administration of itraconazole to pigeons and red-tailed hawks in a dosage of 5 mg/kg BW, once a day for 14 days, the sum of the mean lung concentration of itraconazole and hydroxyitraconazole was above the MIC in both species, 3456 to 80,235 ng/g and 4348 ng/g, respectively (see **Table 1**). However, a high interindividual variability of itraconazole and hydroxyitraconazole concentrations was observed in all tissues.[53,56] Based on these studies, the following dosing regimens have been suggested for itraconazole: pigeons, 6 to 26 mg/kg BW twice a day; blue-fronted Amazon parrot, 5 mg/kg BW once a day; red-tailed hawks, 10 mg/kg once a day; and Humboldt penguins, 8.5 mg/kg twice a day or 20 mg/kg once a day.[51,53,56,57] Recently, it was demonstrated in rats that the oral bioavailability of an experimental liposomal formulation of itraconazole-containing sodium deoxycholate was 1.67-fold higher than that of the commercially available itraconazole formulation containing hydroxypropyl-β-cyclodextrin.[58] However, whether this new experimental liposomal formulation can also improve the oral bioavailability of itraconazole in birds, and decrease the high interindividual variability of itraconazole and hydroxyitraconazole concentrations in the target organs, needs further investigation. In addition, an increased oral bioavailability might also lower the GI toxicity of itraconazole; however, systemic toxicity (eg, hepatotoxicity) might increase.

Voriconazole is increasingly used to treat invasive aspergillosis in birds, given the broad antifungal spectrum, which includes molds (fungicidal) and yeasts (fungistatic), and its fast bioavailability.[6,19,22,59] Beernaert and colleagues[45] demonstrated that administering voriconazole (10 mg/kg BW twice a day) orally in pigeons reduced clinical signs and eliminated *A fumigatus* in racing pigeons experimentally infected with *A fumigatus*. Similarly, Tell and colleagues[60] showed that oral administration of voriconazole (20 and 40 mg/kg BW once a day) reduced mortality rate in Japanese quails after experimental *A fumigatus* infection.

The clinical efficacy of voriconazole was also demonstrated in falcons with aspergillosis. Complete clinical resolution occurred in 70% of the birds, partial response in 25%, and 1 bird (5%) died during treatment.[61] However, interspecies and interindividual variability in this drug's PK profile necessitates species-specific PK studies. The average oral voriconazole bioavailability for pigeons and mallard ducks, 44% and 61%, respectively, is much higher compared with chickens, at 16% to 20% (see **Table 2**).[19,22,59] After a single oral voriconazole administration, the $T_{1/2el}$ was longer in pigeons and African penguins, at 10.32 and 10.92 hours, respectively, compared with other bird species (range, 0.90–2.29 hours), which presents the potential for drug accumulation with extended dosing.[18–22,59] In pigeons, the administration of 20 mg voriconazole/kg BW twice daily maintained plasma concentrations of greater than the MIC of 500 ng/mL for 4 days, but induced hepatotoxicity.[19,28] Furthermore, voriconazole concentrations in the lung were only above the MIC in a few pigeons.[19]

In contrast, lung levels were above this MIC value in chickens after oral administration of voriconazole (10 mg/kg BW, once a day) for 20 to 30 days (see **Table 2**).[28,59] Based on these studies, the following dosing regimens have been suggested for voriconazole: pigeons, 10 mg/kg BW twice a day or 20 mg/kg once a day; chicken, 10 mg/kg BW once a day; Hispaniolan Amazon parrot, 18 mg/kg BW 3 times a day; timneh gray parrot, 12 to 18 mg/kg BW twice a day; African penguin, 5 mg/kg once a day; mallard duck, 20 mg/kg BW twice a day-3 times a day; and falcons, 12.5 mg/kg BW once or twice a day.[18–22,54,59]

On contrast with other azoles, fluconazole is highly water soluble. Consequently, the drug can also be administered in the drinking water. Ratzlaff and colleagues[47] demonstrated that, by administering fluconazole-mediated drinking water at a concentration of 100 mg/L for 8 days to cockatiels (*Nymphicus hollandicus*), fluconazole plasma concentrations could be maintained above the MIC for most strains of *C albicans* (based on susceptibility data from humans). After oral administration of 10 mg fluconazole/kg BW to cockatiels and timneh gray parrots, a similar relative bioavailability was observed in both species; the area under the plasma concentration time curve was 149.28 versus 154.55 h·μg/mL, respectively. However, the maximum plasma concentration was lower and the $T_{1/2el}$ longer in the cockatiel compared with timneh African gray parrot (4.94 μg/mL vs 7.45 μg/mL, and 19.01 hours vs 9.22 hours, respectively).[21,47] Based on these studies, the following dosing regimens have been suggested: cockatiels 5 to 10 mg/kg BW orally every 24 to 48 hours, drinking water 100 mg/L, and timneh gray parrots 10 to 20 mg/kg BW orally every 24 to 48 hours. However, clinical studies are needed to verify the efficacy.

Beside the azoles, polyene macrolide antifungal agents are also frequently used in avian medicine. Oral administration of amphotericin B is used widely to treat *Macrorhabdus ornithogaster*, at a recommended dosage of 25 to 100 mg/kg BW twice a day.[2] However, amphotericin B deoxycholate is amphipathic and exhibits low solubility and permeability, resulting in negligible absorption when administered orally. Consequently, oral application to treat systemic aspergillosis is not recommended.[6] Advances in drug delivery systems have overcome some of the solubility issues that prevent oral bioavailability by improving drug stability in the GI tract environment, providing opportunities for targeting specific sites in the GI tract, increasing drug solubility and bioavailability, and providing sustained release in the GI tract. However, unknown in birds, poly(ethylene glycol)ylated PLGA NPs formulation of amphotericin B increased the oral bioavailability of amphotericin B from 1.5% to 10.5% when compared with the commercially available amphotericin B deoxycholate in rats by increasing amphotericin B solubility.[62] Similar to amphotericin, oral administration of nystatin was shown to be effective in the treatment of *M ornithogaster*.[2] A flock of budgerigars was successfully treated with nystatin at 3,500,000 IU/L drinking water for 2 days, followed by 2,000,000 IU/L for 28 days.[63]

Terbinafine hydrochloride, an allylamine, can be given orally or topically. The administration of terbinafine hydrochloride (15 mg/kg, once a day) for 2 days in a multiple-dose PK trial in African penguins provided plasma levels approaching the MIC of 1000 ng/mL against *Aspergillus fumigatus* (**Table 3**).[64] Based on these PK parameters of terbinafine, steady-state trough levels in African penguins are predicted to occur in 2 weeks at 1200 ng/mL, using 15 mg/kg BW once a day.[64] Unfortunately, no PK parameters could be calculated after multiple oral administration of terbinafine in red-tailed hawks (50–120 mg/kg BW; see **Table 3**), because most of the birds regurgitated within a few hours after administration.[25] As a result, additional multiple dose and clinical trials are needed to demonstrate the actual efficacy and safety of long-term treatment with terbinafine against aspergillosis in birds.

Table 3
PK characteristics of terbinafine hydrochloride after single bolus and multiples doses administration in different bird species

	Animal Species	BW (g)	Dosage Terbinafine Hydrochloride (mg/kg BW)	Frequency of Administration	Feed	C_{min} (ng/mL)	T_{max} (h)	C_{max} (ng/mL)	V_d/F (mL/kg)	$T_{1/2}$ (h)	Cl/F (mL/h·kg)	C_{lung} (ng/g)	C_{liver} (ng/g)	Reference
PK oral bolus	African penguins	2700–3300	3	Single	Yes	—	2.70	100	37,000	—	867[a]	—	—	Bechert et al,[64] 2010
	Red-tailed hawks	1070–1670	7	Single	Yes	—	1.60	200	37,000	—	633[a]	—	—	
			15	Single	Yes	—	2.40	200	68,000	—	933[a]	—	—	Bechert et al,[25] 2010
			15	Single	No	—	5.40	300	72,000	15.00	2300	—	—	
	Hispaniolan Amazon parrot	274–329	30	Single	No	—	3.40	1200	50,100	18.20	1400	—	—	
			60	Single	No	—	5.10	2000	45,500	13.30	1400	—	—	Evans et al,[81] 2013
			60	Single	Yes	—	6.40	353	—	8.71	—	—	—	
Multiple doses PK	African penguins	2700–3300	15	SID, 4 d	Yes	400	0.80	2100	—	16.00	500	—	—	Bechert et al,[64] 2010
	Red-tailed hawks	1070–1670	120	SID, 2 d	Yes	—	—	—	—	—	—	—	—	Bechert et al,[25] 2010
			Day 1: 60; d 2: 50	SID, 2 d	Yes	—	—	—	—	—	—	ND	270	

Abbreviations: BW, bodyweight; Cl/F, clearance; C_{liver}, terbinafine concentration in liver; C_{lung}, terbinafine concentration in lung; C_{max}, maximum plasma concentration; C_{min}, minimal plasma terbinafine concentration in multiple doses PK; F, absolute bioavailability; ND, not detected; PK, pharmacokinetic; SID, once a day; $T_{1/2el}$, elimination half-life; T_{max}, time point of maximum plasma concentration; Vd or Vd/F, volume of distribution.
[a] Calculated based on average bodyweight.

Topical Treatment

Inhalation is a very common technique of drug administration to patients with a variety of lung diseases in humans. The treatment of respiratory fungal infections in avian patients requires currently the use of oral or systemic agents; however, aerosolized delivery (**Fig. 1**) is an attractive option because the lag time of the action onset of the drug is short, less drug substance is needed, systemic side effects are reduced, and nebulization is achieved with only minor patient stress.[6,65] Pressurized metered dose inhalers and dry powder inhalers systems might be difficult to use in avian patients because of practical difficulties. In contrast, nebulization is frequently used in avian medicine, and administered to birds in a closed cage, induction chamber, or by means of a face mask.[43] Tell and colleagues[66] showed that, with an increasing time of exposure to aerosolized particles, the degree of particle deposition into the avian respiratory system could be enhanced, until an equilibrium is established with approximately uniform particle deposition/translocation to each of the air sacs of the respiratory system.

Nebulizers convert a liquid in solution or suspension into small droplets. Two basic types of nebulizers are frequently used, that is, the jet and the ultrasonic nebulizer. In jet nebulizers, compressed air/oxygen passes through a capillary tube, trespasses the entrained drug solution, and droplets suitable for inhalation are formed (**Fig. 2**). In an ultrasonic nebulizer, an electronic oscillator generates a high-frequency ultrasonic wave, and an aerosol is generated by the ultrahigh-frequency vibration of a piezoelectric crystal at the bottom of a liquid (**Fig. 3**).[65,67] Particles of the nebulized drug should preferably have a mass median aerodynamic diameter between 1 and 5 μm, to reach the lower respiratory tract, which is needed in case of aspergillosis.[42,65] The newer generation vibrating mesh nebulizers use electricity to vibrate a piezo element that moves liquid formations through a fine mesh to generate aerosol.[67] Mesh nebulizers generate aerosols either passively with a transducer horn vibrating ultrasonically against a static mesh or actively with a mesh mounted in an ultrasonically vibrating piezo ring. These nebulizers have several distinct advantages over jet or ultrasonic

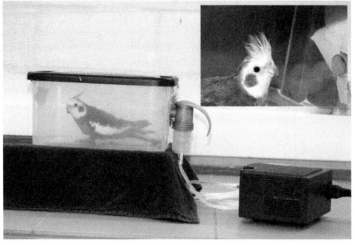

Fig. 1. Aerosol therapy in a cockatiel via a jet nebulizer. Nebulization is a drug delivery method used to administer medication in the form of a mist (*insert*) inhaled into the respiratory tract.

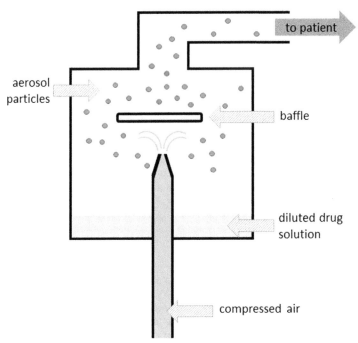

Fig. 2. Jet nebulizer working scheme. Compressed air/oxygen passes through a capillary tube, trespasses the entrained drug solution, and droplets suitable for inhalation are formed.

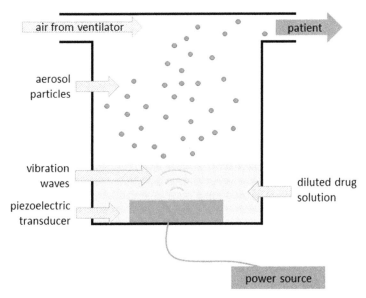

Fig. 3. Ultrasonic nebulizer working scheme. An electronic oscillator generates a high-frequency ultrasonic wave, and an aerosol is generated by the ultrahigh- frequency vibration of a piezoelectric crystal at the bottom of a liquid.

devices, such as having a higher respiratory tract deposition, negligible residual volumes, minimizing drug loss to evaporation, a fast rate of nebulization, and the possibility to nebulize a wider variability of drug compounds.[68] Additionally, liposomes can be delivered using a mesh and jet nebulizer, whereas an ultrasonic nebulizer is less suitable for delivering these particles, because they only deposit a very small proportion of phospholipids in the lower respiratory tract.[67,69]

Currently, there are no antifungal drugs on the market that have been developed specifically to administer by nebulization. Consequently, in different avian studies and clinical cases, birds are nebulized with the off-label use with antifungal drug formulations that were developed for IV or oral administration. Nebulization of a Hispaniolan Amazon parrot with terbinafine (crushed 250 mg terbinafine HCl tablet, Camber Pharmaceuticals Inc, Piscataway, NJ; and raw terbinafine HCl powder) dissolved in sterile water (1 mg/mL) for 15 minutes resulted in therapeutic plasma concentrations (above MIC of A fumigatus and A fluvus) for 0.5 to 4.0 hours after administration.[70] However, because the lung levels were not assessed in this study, clinical efficacy of this protocol in cases of avian aspergillosis still needs to be elucidated.

After 15 minutes of nebulization of a commercially available IV formulation of voriconazole (Vfend, Pfizer Global Pharmaceuticals, Ixelles, Belgium) dissolved in 0.9% NaCl (10 mg/mL) with a jet nebulizer in pigeons, only low plasma and lung concentrations (below the MIC of 0.5 mg/L) could be achieved for less than 1 hour.[19] In contrast, high and clinically relevant lung and plasma levels were found in mice after nebulization with an aqueous solution of the IV voriconazole formulation (Vfend, 6.25 mg voriconazole/mL in sterile water for injection, for 20 minutes) with an active mesh nebulizer.[71] In this study, the commercially available IV formulation was adjusted to ensure that the osmolality (293.2 mOsm/kg) and pH (6.4–6.8) were within the physiologically acceptable ranges for pulmonary delivery by adding sulfobutylether-β-cyclodextrin up to a concentration of 100 mg/mL.[71,72] The addition of this substance helps to increase the water solubility of voriconazole in the commercial IV formulation via complexation with sulfobutylether-β-cyclodextrin.[73] Inhaled voriconazole significantly improved the severity and survival of invasive pulmonary aspergillosis in mice compared with control and treatment with intraperitoneal amphotericin B.[72] Therefore, the impact of adding extra sulfobutylether-β-cyclodextrin to the commercially available IV voriconazole formulation, and the use of a mesh nebulizer instead of a jet nebulizer, on the PK/pharmacodynamic aspects of voriconazole aerosol therapy in birds needs to be investigated.

In contrast with the older antifungal drug formulations, promising results are observed when nebulizing antifungal NPs. A single intratracheal aerosol administration of liposomal amphotericin B (AmBisome; 3 mg/kg BW) with a jet nebulizer in mallard ducks resulted in drug concentrations above the MIC (1 μg/mL) in lung tissue for up to 9 days after administration. However, the drug distribution was uneven, with the majority of the drug concentrated in 1 lung lobe.[33] Nebulized liposomal amphotericin B showed an improved survival rate of rats with pulmonary aspergillosis compared with animals treated with amphotericin deoxycholate IV.[74] Similarly, once daily nebulization with a 10% itraconazole NP suspension for 30 minutes was capable of alleviating an acute A fumigatus infection in quails.[75] High lung itraconazole concentrations, well above the MIC for A fumigatus, were achieved after a single-dose inhalation of itraconazole NP suspension (1% and 10% dissolved in distilled water with addition of a 1.4% polysorbate 80 solution) to Japanese quails via a jet nebulizer for 30 minutes. Drug clearance from the lungs was slow, with a $T_{1/2el}$ of 19.7 and 35.8 hours after inhalation of 1% and 10% suspension, respectively. Even after 5-day repeated administration, no adverse clinical reactions were observed. Moreover, serum concentrations were low (only 0.1% of the lung tissue concentration).[76]

In rare cases of fungal dermatologic infections in birds, the topical application of miconazole, enilconazole, or clotrimazole might be used, whether or not combined with systemic treatment.[3,77] Oral candidiasis, which is most often seen in lorikeets and associated with vitamin A deficiency, responds well to therapy with topical nystatin, ketoconazole, fluconazole, miconazole, or itraconazole.[78,79] Furthermore, wound aspergillosis was successfully treated in a goliath heron (A goliath) with topical liposomal amphotericin B, after well-established therapies with surgical debridement followed by topical povidone-iodine in conjunction with oral itraconazole, and also topical miconazole, failed.[34]

In conclusion, because the conventional treatment options have limitations such as restricted efficacy, limited biodistribution, and toxicity, the use of newer antifungal drug delivery methods should be considered by clinicians to overcome these limitations and drawbacks in cases of treatment failure and toxicity.

SUMMARY

This review article aimed to provide insight into the interrelation of antifungal drug formulation, administration route, therapeutic–toxic range, and treatment outcome in fungal diseases, focusing in particular on aspergillosis in birds. The major antifungal agents used in avian medicine are azole derivatives, polyenes, and allylamines, which all owe their antifungal activities to inhibition of synthesis, or direct interaction with ergosterol. Antifungal pharmacokinetics in birds are characterized by a large interspecies and even interindividual variability. Consequently, conventional antifungal therapies in avian medicine are frequently associated with a lack of efficacy and high toxicity. Innovative drug formulations such as NPs can help to reduce the intrinsic toxicity and enhance efficacy of antifungal agents in birds. Because the majority of systemic fungal infections require long-term therapy, oral administration of antifungal drugs is preferred, with IV administration being reserved for the initial phase of treatment in cases of acute aspergillosis or severely debilitated birds. Finally, topical administration of antifungals through nebulization shows promising results in birds; however, because drug formulations and type of nebulizer are found to highly influence the therapeutic output, clinicians are recommended to take these factors into account when considering to use this administration route in their patients.

REFERENCES

1. Fischer D, Lierz M. Diagnostic procedures and available techniques for the diagnosis of aspergillosis in birds. J Exot Pet Med 2015;24:283–95.
2. Phalen DN. Update on the diagnosis and management of Macrorhabdus ornithogaster (formerly megabacteria) in avian patients. Vet Clin North Am Exot Anim Pract 2014;17:203–10.
3. Beernaert LA, Pasmans F, Van Waeyenberghe L, et al. Aspergillus infections in birds: a review. Avian Pathol 2010;39:325–31.
4. Hamill RJ. Amphotericin B formulations: a comparative review of efficacy and toxicity. Drugs 2013;73(9):919–34.
5. Blanchard OL, Smoliga JM. Translating dosages from animal models to human clinical trials-revisiting body surface area scaling. FASEB J 2015;29:1629–34.
6. Krautwald-Junghanns ME, Vorbruggen S, Bohme J. Aspergillosis in birds: an overview of treatment options and regimens. J Exot Pet Med 2015;24:296–307.

7. Ostrosky-Zeichner L, Casadevall A, Galgiani JN, et al. An insight into the antifungal pipeline: selected new molecules and beyond. Nat Rev Drug Discov 2010;9:719–27.

8. Sant DG, Tupe SG, Ramana CV, et al. Fungal cell membrane-promising drug target for antifungal therapy. J Appl Microbiol 2016;121:1498–510.

9. Ghannoum MA, Rice LB. Antifungal agents: mode of action, mechanisms of resistance, and correlation of these mechanisms with bacterial resistance. Clin Microbiol Rev 1999;12(4):501–17.

10. Van den Bossche H, Willemsens G, Cools W, et al. Hypothesis on the molecular basis of the antifungal activity of N-substituted imidazoles and triazoles. Biochem Soc Trans 1983;11:665–7.

11. Orosz SE. Overview of aspergillosis: pathogenesis and treatment options. In: Seminars in Avian and Exotic Pet Medicine. WB Saunders; 2000. p. 59–65.

12. Ryder NS. Terbinafine - mode of action and properties of the squalene epoxidase inhibition. Br J Dermatol 1992;126:2–7.

13. Redig PT, Duke GE. Comparative Pharmacokinetics of antifungal drugs in domestic turkeys, red-tailed hawks, broad-winged hawks, and great-horned owls. Avian Dis 1985;29:649–61.

14. Flammer K. An overview of antifungal therapy in birds. Paper presented at: Proc Annu Conf Assoc Avian Vet, Nashville, TN, August 31 - September 4, 1993.

15. Keller KA. Itraconazole. J Exot Pet Med 2011;20:156–60.

16. Scholz I, Oberwittler H, Riedel KD, et al. Pharmacokinetics, metabolism and bioavailability of the triazole antifungal agent voriconazole in relation to CYP2C19 genotype. Br J Clin Pharmacol 2009;68:906–15.

17. Wang G, Lei HP, Li Z, et al. The CYP2C19 ultra-rapid metabolizer genotype influences the pharmacokinetics of voriconazole in healthy male volunteers. Eur J Clin Pharmacol 2009;65:281–5.

18. Hyatt MW, Wiederhold NP, Hope WW, et al. Pharmacokinetics of orally administered voriconazole in African penguins (*Spheniscus demersus*) after single and multiple doses. J Zoo Wildl Med 2017;48:352–62.

19. Beernaert LA, Baert K, Marin P, et al. Designing voriconazole treatment for racing pigeons: balancing between hepatic enzyme auto induction and toxicity. Med Mycol 2009;47:276–85.

20. Guzman DSM, Flammer K, Papich MG, et al. Pharmacokinetics of voriconazole after oral administration of single and multiple doses in Hispaniolan Amazon parrots (*Amazona ventralis*). Am J Vet Res 2010;71:460–7.

21. Flammer K, Osborne JAN, Webb DJ, et al. Pharmacokinetics of voriconazole after oral administration of single and multiple doses in African grey parrots (*Psittacus erithacus timneh*). Am J Vet Res 2008;69:114–21.

22. Kline Y, Clemons KV, Woods L, et al. Pharmacokinetics of voriconazole in adult mallard ducks (*Anas platyrhynchos*). Med Mycol 2011;49:500–12.

23. Parsley RA, Tell LA, Gehring R. Pharmacokinetics of a single dose of voriconazole administered orally with and without food to red-tailed hawks (*Buteo jamaicensus*). Am J Vet Res 2017;78:433–9.

24. Hyatt MW, Georoff TA, Nollens HH, et al. Voriconazole toxicity in multiple penguin species. J Zoo Wildl Med 2015;46:880–8.

25. Bechert U, Christensen JM, Poppenga R, et al. Pharmacokinetics of terbinafine after single oral dose administration in red-tailed hawks (*Buteo jamaicensis*). J Avian Med Surg 2010;24:122–30.

26. Albataineh MT, Sutton DA, Fothergill AW, et al. Update from the laboratory clinical identification and susceptibility testing of fungi and trends in antifungal resistance. Infect Dis Clin North Am 2016;30:13–35.

27. Chamilos G, Kontoyiannis DP. Update on antifungal drug resistance mechanisms of *Aspergillus fumigatus*. Drug Resist Updat 2005;8:344–58.

28. Beernaert LA, Pasmans F, Van Waeyenberghe L, et al. Avian *Aspergillus fumigatus* strains resistant to both itraconazole and voriconazole. Antimicrob Agents Chemother 2009;53:2199–201.

29. Lewis RE. Current concepts in antifungal pharmacology. Mayo Clin Proc 2011;86: 805–17.

30. Soliman GM. Nanoparticles as safe and effective delivery systems of antifungal agents: achievements and challenges. Int J Pharm 2017;523:15–32.

31. Steinbach WJ, Stevens DA. Review of newer antifungal and immunomodulatory strategies for invasive aspergillosis. Clin Infect Dis 2003;37(Suppl 3):S157–87.

32. Ramaswamy M, Peteherych KD, Kennedy AL, et al. Amphotericin B lipid complex or amphotericin B multiple-dose administration to rabbits with elevated plasma cholesterol levels: pharmacokinetics in plasma and blood, plasma lipoprotein levels, distribution in tissues, and renal toxicities. Antimicrob Agents Chemother 2001;45:1184–91.

33. Phillips A, Fiorello CV, Baden RM, et al. Amphotericin B concentrations in healthy mallard ducks (*Anas platyrhynchos*) following a single intratracheal dose of liposomal amphotericin B using an atomizer. Med Mycol 2017. https://doi.org/10.1093/mmy/myx049.

34. Bonar CJ, Lewandowski AH. Use of a liposomal formulation of amphotericin B for treating wound aspergillosis in a goliath heron (*Ardea goliath*). J Avian Med Surg 2004;18:162–6.

35. Clemons KV, Schwartz JA, Stevens DA. Therapeutic and toxicologic studies in a murine model of invasive pulmonary aspergillosis. Med Mycol 2011;49:834–47.

36. Al-Nakeeb Z, Petraitis V, Goodwin J, et al. Pharmacodynamics of amphotericin B deoxycholate, amphotericin B lipid complex, and liposomal amphotericin B against *Aspergillus fumigatus*. Antimicrob Agents Chemother 2015;59:2735–45.

37. Steimbach LM, Tonin FS, Virtuoso S, et al. Efficacy and safety of amphotericin B lipid-based formulations-A systematic review and meta-analysis. Mycoses 2017; 60:146–54.

38. Hiemenz JW, Walsh TJ. Lipid formulations of amphotericin B: recent progress and future directions. Clin Infect Dis 1996;22(Suppl 2):S133–44.

39. Mehta RT, Hopfer RL, McQueen T, et al. Toxicity and therapeutic effects in mice of liposome-encapsulated nystatin for systemic fungal infections. Antimicrob Agents Chemother 1987;31:1901–3.

40. Patel NR, Damann K, Leonardi C, et al. Itraconazole-loaded poly(lactic-co-glycolic) acid nanoparticles for improved antifungal activity. Nanomedicine (Lond) 2010;5:1037–50.

41. Sinha B, Mukherjee B, Pattnaik G. Poly-lactide-co-glycolide nanoparticles containing voriconazole for pulmonary delivery: *in vitro* and *in vivo* study. Nanomedicine 2013;9:94–104.

42. Pardeike J, Weber S, Zarfl HP, et al. Itraconazole-loaded nanostructured lipid carriers (NLC) for pulmonary treatment of aspergillosis in falcons. Eur J Pharm Biopharm 2016;108:269–76.

43. Powers LV. Techniques for drug delivery in psittacine birds. J Exot Pet Med 2006; 15:193–200.

44. Holler B, Omar SA, Farid MD, et al. Effects of fluid and electrolyte management on amphotericin B-induced nephrotoxicity among extremely low birth weight infants. Pediatrics 2004;113:E608–16.

45. Beernaert LA, Pasmans F, Baert K, et al. Designing a treatment protocol with voriconazole to eliminate *Aspergillus fumigatus* from experimentally inoculated pigeons. Vet Microbiol 2009;139:393–7.

46. Flammer K, Papich M. Pharmacokinetics of fluconazole after oral administration of single and multiple doses in African grey parrots. Am J Vet Res 2006;67:417–22.

47. Ratzlaff K, Papich MG, Flammer K. Plasma concentrations of fluconazole after a single oral dose and administration in drinking water in cockatiels (*Nymphicus hollandicus*). J Avian Med Surg 2011;25:23–31.

48. Souza MJ, Redig P, Cox SK. Plasma concentrations of itraconazole, voriconazole, and terbinafine when delivered by an impregnated, subcutaneous implant in Japanese quail (*Coturnix japonica*). J Avian Med Surg 2017;31:117–22.

49. Tell LA, Craigmill AL, Clemons KV, et al. Studies on itraconazole delivery and pharmacokinetics in mallard ducks (*Anas platyrhynchos*). J Vet Pharmacol Ther 2005;28:267–74.

50. Abuhelwa AY, Williams DB, Upton RN, et al. Food, gastrointestinal pH, and models of oral drug absorption. Eur J Pharm Biopharm 2017;112:234–48.

51. Bunting EM, Abou-Madi N, Cox S, et al. Evaluation of oral itraconazole administration in captive Humboldt penguins (*Spheniscus humboldti*). J Zoo Wildl Med 2009;40:508–18.

52. Denbow DM. Gastrointestinal anatomy and physiology. In: Scanes CG, editor. Sturkie's avian physiology. 6th edition. Waltham (MA): Academic Press; 2015. p. 337–66.

53. Orosz SE, Schroeder EC, Cox SK, et al. The effects of formulation on the systemic availability of itraconazole in pigeons. J Avian Med Surg 1995;9(4):255–62.

54. Schmidt V, Demiraj F, Di Somma A, et al. Plasma concentrations of voriconazole in falcons. Vet Rec 2007;161:265–8.

55. Lumeij J, Gorgevska D, Woestenborghs R. Plasma and tissue concentrations of itraconazole in racing pigeons (*Columba livia domestica*). J Avian Med Surg 1995;9(1):32–5.

56. Jones MP, Orosz SE, Cox SK, et al. Pharmacokinetic disposition of itraconazole in red-tailed hawks (*Buteo jamaicensis*). J Avian Med Surg 2000;14:15–22.

57. Orosz SE, Frazier DL, Schroeder EC, et al. Pharmacokinetic properties of itraconazole in blue-fronted Amazon parrots (*Amazona aestiva aestiva*). J Avian Med Surg 1996;10(3):168–73.

58. Li ZB, Zhang MY, Liu C, et al. Development of Liposome containing sodium deoxycholate to enhance oral bioavailability of itraconazole. Asian J Pharm Sci 2017;12:157–64.

59. Burhenne J, Haefeli WE, Hess M, et al. Pharmacokinetics, tissue concentrations, and safety of the antifungal agent voriconazole in chickens. J Avian Med Surg 2008;22:199–207.

60. Tell LA, Clemons KV, Kline Y, et al. Efficacy of voriconazole in Japanese quail (*Coturnix japonica*) experimentally infected with *Aspergillus fumigatus*. Med Mycol 2010;48:234–44.

61. Di Somma A, Bailey T, Silvanose C, et al. The use of voriconazole for the treatment of aspergillosis in falcons (*Falco species*). J Avian Med Surg 2007;21:307–16.

62. Radwan MA, AlQuadeib BT, Siller L, et al. Oral administration of amphotericin B nanoparticles: antifungal activity, bioavailability and toxicity in rats. Drug Deliv 2017;24:40–50.

63. Kheirandish R, Salehi M. Megabacteriosis in budgerigars: diagnosis and treatment. Comp Clin Path 2011;20:501–5.
64. Bechert U, Christensen JM, Poppenga R, et al. Pharmacokinetics of orally administered terbinafine in African penguins (*Spheniscus demersus*) for Potential Treatment of Aspergillosis. J Zoo Wildl Med 2010;41(2):263–74.
65. Le Brun PPH, de Boer AH, Heijerman HGM, et al. A review of the technical aspects of drug nebulization. Pharm World Sci 2000;22:75–81.
66. Tell LA, Stephens K, Teague SV, et al. Study of nebulization delivery of aerosolized fluorescent microspheres to the avian respiratory tract. Avian Dis 2012;56: 381–6.
67. Dolovich MB, Dhand R. Aerosol drug delivery: developments in device design and clinical use. Lancet 2011;377:1032–45.
68. Hatley R, Hardaker L. Mesh nebulizer capabilities in aerosolizing a wide range of novel pharmaceutical formulations. Eur Respiratory Soc 2016;48:PA967.
69. Rudokas M, Najlah M, Alhnan MA, et al. Liposome delivery systems for inhalation: a critical review highlighting formulation issues and anticancer applications. Med Princ Pract 2016;25(Suppl 2):60–72.
70. Emery LC, Cox SK, Souza MJ. Pharmacokinetics of nebulized terbinafine in hispaniolan amazon parrots (*Amazona ventralis*). J Avian Med Surg 2012;26(3): 161–6.
71. Tolman JA, Nelson NA, Son YJ, et al. Characterization and pharmacokinetic analysis of aerosolized aqueous voriconazole solution. Eur J Pharm Biopharm 2009; 72:199–205.
72. Tolman JA, Wiederhold NP, McConville JT, et al. Inhaled voriconazole for prevention of invasive pulmonary aspergillosis. Antimicrob Agents Chemother 2009;53: 2613–5.
73. Vyas A, Saraf S, Saraf S. Cyclodextrin based novel drug delivery systems. J Incl Phenom Macro 2008;62:23–42.
74. Gavalda J, Martin MT, Lopez P, et al. Efficacy of nebulized liposomal amphotericin B in treatment of experimental pulmonary aspergillosis. Antimicrob Agents Chemother 2005;49:3028–30.
75. Rundfeldt C, Wyska E, Steckel H, et al. A model for treating avian aspergillosis: serum and lung tissue kinetics for Japanese quail (*Coturnix japonica*) following single and multiple aerosol exposures of a nanoparticulate itraconazole suspension. Med Mycol 2013;51:800–10.
76. Wlaz P, Knaga S, Kasperek K, et al. Activity and safety of inhaled itraconazole nanosuspension in a model pulmonary *Aspergillus fumigatus* infection in inoculated young quails. Mycopathologia 2015;180:35–42.
77. Abrams GA, Paul-Murphy J, Ramer JC, et al. Aspergillus blepharitis and dermatitis in a peregrine falcon-gyrfalcon hybrid (*Falco peregrinus* X *Falco rusticolus*). J Avian Med Surg 2001;15:114–20.
78. Koski MA. Dermatologic diseases in psittacine birds: an investigational approach. Semin Avian Exot Pet 2002;11:105–24.
79. Velasco MC. Candidiasis and cryptococcosis in birds. Semin Avian Exot Pet 2000;9(2):75–81.
80. Smith JA, Papich MG, Russell G, et al. Effects of compounding on pharmacokinetics of itraconazole in black-footed penguins (Spheniscus demersus). J Zoo Wildl Med 2010;41:487–95.
81. Evans EE, Emery LC, Cox SK, et al. Pharmacokinetics of terbinafine after oral administration of a single dose to Hispaniolan Amazon parrots (Amazona ventralis). Am J Vet Res 2013;74:835–8.

Avian Vaccination
Current Options and Strategies

J. Jill Heatley, DVM, MS, DABVP (Avian, Reptilian, Amphibian), DACZM, Susan Payne, PhD,
Ian Tizard, BVMS, PhD, DACVM, DSc*

KEYWORDS

- Parrot • Immunization • Pet • Zoo • Vaccine • Disease prevention

KEY POINTS

- Most vaccines used in nonpoultry avian species are used in an off-label manner.
- The number of vaccines experimentally investigated and found efficacious in protecting birds from disease far outstrips the number of vaccines commercially available.
- There is a lack of commercially available, efficacious, and safe vaccines for the prevention of many threatening diseases in pet and nonpoultry avian species.
- Unless significant changes occur in the economics of vaccine production, including development, manufacture, and distribution, this trend is unlikely to change in the foreseeable future.
- Major differences in avian medicine and biology that contribute to the difficulty in creating and marketing of vaccines include the development of the avian immune system, continuing changes in popularity of pet bird species, and decreasing pet bird populations.

INTRODUCTION

Infectious viral diseases remain a constant threat to wild, exotic, and pet birds. Polyoma, herpes, and the Bornaviruses present a significant threat to some species and effective safe vaccines are urgently needed. Others, such as avian influenza and Newcastle disease, are potential threats to pet birds for which vaccines may be necessary in future. In general, these threats stem mainly from viral infections; however, clostridial and mycoplasmal infections are examples of bacterial diseases that are likely better prevented or avoided than treated.

The commercial production and applied use of avian viral vaccines has not kept pace with the research into the development of new and improved vaccines. Constraints on new vaccine production and marketing include not only the cost and

Disclosure: The authors have nothing to disclose.
Veterinary Pathobiology, Schubot Exotic Bird Health Center, College of Veterinary, Medicine & Biomedical Sciences, Texas A&M University, 668 Raymond Stotzer Parkway, VIDI Building 1813, College Station, TX 77843-4467, USA
* Corresponding author.
E-mail address: itizard@cvm.tamu.edu

complexity of production but also the small size of the market, especially for pet and exotic birds. Although veterinarians have been highly successful in promoting the routine vaccination of puppies and kittens, they have not yet been able to promote a similar coverage in pet birds. The relative complexity of many new vaccines, and their expensive and complex licensing requirements, are reflected in their cost. Thus a gap exists between clinicians' ability to make sophisticated vaccines in a laboratory setting and to manufacture and market these products at a reasonable price. As a result, companies are reluctant to make a large investment in new vaccine production. In contrast, chickens constitute the largest population of pet birds in the United States and waterfowl collections are widespread, which suggest that veterinarians must be prepared to use commercial poultry and duck vaccines in these species.

MODERN VACCINE TECHNOLOGY

Traditional vaccines were of 2 basic sorts: killed vaccines and modified live vaccines. Modern molecular techniques have greatly expanded the potential diversity, potency, and safety of vaccines. For example, cloning of viral antigens within bacteria and yeasts can create large quantities of very pure antigens. Irreversible attenuation of a virulent virus can be accomplished by deliberate, specific gene deletions. Incorporation of new or unusual antigens into such vaccines can also result in a DIVA (differentiate infected from vaccinated animals) vaccine. These vaccines have been used for avian influenza viruses (AIVs). Virus genes encoding their protein antigens can also be cloned into other viruses, which can then be used as recombinant vaccines. Recombinant vaccinia, fowlpox, and canarypox viruses have been most widely used as vectors because their large stable genomes are easy to manipulate. They express large amounts of antigen and their proteins undergo appropriate processing steps to facilitate antigen recognition. These live recombinant organisms are very safe. They are not secreted in body fluids or transmitted by arthropods and cannot revert to virulence. An additional benefit of canarypox-vectored vaccines is that they may overcome blocking by maternal antibodies and can thus prime very young animals. Examples of successful vaccines using this technology include Newcastle disease vaccine vectored by fowlpox virus, and the use of a yellow fever viral chimera to protect against West Nile virus (WNV).

Oral vaccination has long been considered a desirable route of vaccine administration but has been hindered by the digestion and destruction of oral antigens within the gastrointestinal tract. Cloning of vaccine antigen genes into tobacco, potato, soybean, rice, and corn has been achieved for viruses such as transmissible gastroenteritis, Norwalk virus, and Newcastle disease. A Newcastle disease vaccine produced in suspension-cultured tobacco cells has been licensed in the United States. As an alternative, vaccine antigens derived from recombinant yeasts seem to be very safe and effective.

DNA VACCINES

Instead of using protein antigens, DNA encoding specific vaccine antigens may also be inserted into a bacterial plasmid (a piece of circular DNA that acts as a vector) for use in vaccines. The plasmid, unlike viral vectors, cannot replicate but its encoded products are processed by the immune system so that they generate neutralizing antibodies as well as cytotoxic T cells. They have yet to reach commercial production but DNA vaccines are ideal for organisms that are difficult or dangerous to grow in the laboratory. DNA vaccines are often more effective than recombinant proteins and avoid the need for complex carrier organisms.

AVIAN DISEASES OF CONCERN AND VACCINE INFORMATION
Circoviruses

Psittacine beak and feather disease (PBFD) is caused by a DNA circovirus (PBFD virus [PBFDV]). Viral replication occurs first in the lymphoid organs, spreads to the liver and thymus, and leads to eventual viral invasion of the epithelium, resulting in beak and feather malformations. An acute form of the disease occurs in young birds in which death results from acute liver failure, despite normal feathering. Birds that recover from the acute disease may become chronic carriers. Secondary infections as a result of viral immunosuppression occur. Although no vaccine for PBFDV is currently available, multiple experimental vaccines have been assessed, including a subunit vaccine, a recombinant vaccine, and a live attenuated vaccine. A recombinant vaccine expressing the PBFDV capsid protein (CP), the major antigenic determinant, expressed in a plant, yeast, or bacterial system could be particularly useful and is promising based on recent research.[1,2]

The immunogenicity of a recombinant PBFDV-CP vaccine has been assessed in long-billed corellas (Cacatua tenuirostris). The birds were vaccinated, boosted on day 11, and challenged 16 days after boosting. Using polymerase chain reaction (PCR), 4 of 97 blood samples from vaccinated birds after virus challenge were positive, whereas 17 of 35 samples from nonvaccinated controls were positive. The vaccinated birds lacked feather lesions, had only transient viremia, and did not seem to develop persistent infections after challenge. In contrast, control birds developed transient feather lesions, had antibodies against PBFDV, and were PCR positive for up to 41 days postchallenge. Quantitative PCR showed reduced virus replication in vaccinated birds compared with controls.[3] In another PBFDV-CP study, adult and nestling galahs (Eolophus roseicapillus) vaccinated with an inactivated double-oil emulsion vaccine had comparable antibody responses to those induced by a primary-oil emulsion vaccine. Both vaccines protected nestlings. In this study, unvaccinated control chicks developed acute PBFD within 4 weeks of challenge.[4]

Adult umbrella cockatoos (Cacatua alba), Moluccan cockatoos (Cacatua moluccensis), African gray parrots (Psittacus erithracus), and a yellow-headed Amazon parrot (Amazona oratrix) have been vaccinated with a vaccine containing β-propiolactone (BPL)-inactivated PBFDV and all seroconverted. (BPL cross-links viral DNA, preventing viral growth but conserving its antigenicity.) Three African gray parrot chicks and 2 umbrella cockatoo chicks from vaccinated hens and 1 African gray parrot chick and 1 umbrella cockatoo chick from unvaccinated hens were exposed to PBFDV. The chicks from the vaccinated hens remained clinically normal. Chicks from the nonvaccinated hens developed PBFD. Thus, when administered to hens, this vaccine resulted in chicks that were, at least temporarily, resistant to virus challenge.[5] In conclusion, successful vaccination of psittacine birds against PBFDV is feasible should the economics of vaccine production permit.

Avian Polyoma Virus

Avian polyoma viruses (APVs) cause severe systemic disease in finches and psittacines. APVs cause acute mortality in fledgling budgerigars, nestling macaws, and finches. An inactivated vaccine is commercially available and is commonly used to vaccinate birds before shipment for commercial sales (**Table 1**). As a result, it has been possible to test the safety and immunogenicity of adjuvanted and nonadjuvanted inactivated APV vaccines administered either intramuscularly or subcutaneously in psittacines. In more than 200 vaccinated birds (macaws, cockatoos, conures, and other parrots), local reactions were limited to small scab formation at the injection

Table 1
Vaccines for consideration in ornamental avian species

Species Group	Disease	Vaccine Options[a]	Vaccine Strategy	References
Parrots, finches Adult birds seldom have disease	Polyomavirus	Polyomavirus (Psittimune APV, Creative Science), contains gentamicin and amphotericin B as preservatives. Inactive (killed) vaccine indicated for the prevention of avian polyomavirus	Birds > 200 g give 0.5 mL SQ. Birds < 200 g give 0.25 mL SQ. First dose at 35 d, repeat in 2–3 wk. Annual booster recommended. Repeat in 2–3 wk. Annual booster recommended	Creative Science http://www.creativesciencellc.com 455 Sovereign Court Ballwin, MO 63011 888-506-3039 Ritchie et al,[7] 1996
Parrots: macaws, Amazons, conures	Pacheco disease	PSITTIMUNE PDV: Ceva Biomune Pacheco Disease Vaccine, Inactivated Virus, Oil Emulsion	Vaccinate before exposure or disease outbreak	No longer commercially available
Cranes, pheasants, emu	EEE, WEE	Tissue culture propagated, inactivated bivalent eastern and western equine encephalomyelitis vaccine prepared and licensed for use in horses may contain equine tetanus antitoxin	Emu: give full equine dose IM at 6 wk, 10 wk, 5 mo and 6 mo, and annually thereafter before and after breeding season and if viral disease occurs within 16 km or before transfer to a known endemic area	Merck Veterinary Manual. Management of Ratites Tully,[69] TN
Raptors, corvids, penguins, flamingoes	WNV	WNV vaccinations (Fort Dodge killed equine product, or canarypox-vectored vaccine by Merial) annually at 1.0 mL IM using the pectoral muscle Duvaxyn WNV, Fort Dodge Laboratories, Zoetis Belgium SA, Louvain-la-Neuve, Belgium; United States: West Nile-Innovator, Zoetis Inc, Florham Park, NJ, and Recombitek Equine rWNV vaccine, Merial Limited, Duluth, GA. EU: Proteq West Nile, Merial, Lyon, France	Annually 1.0 mL IM pectoral muscle, preferred 1 mo before breeding season with 1 mo booster first year Condor example: 1.0 mL IM series of up to three, given 1 mo apart before mosquito season	Angenvoort et al,[28] 2014 AZA captive care manual for the Andean condor

Species susceptible	Disease	Vaccine	Strategy	References
Many different species susceptible	Avian influenza	EU accepts inactivated adjuvanted vaccines. Inactivated vaccines: monovalent, including either H5 or H7strains; bivalent, including H5 and H7 strains; combination vaccines (other antigens) should be considered if a prolonged vaccination program may be required Live recombinant vaccines (fowlpox H5) are efficacious only in 1-d-old chickens. Exposure in later life to wild-type fowlpox virus precludes use of this vectored vaccine	Emergency, preventive or prophylactic, and routine vaccination strategies may be used	European Commission Control Measures for Avian Influenza https://ec.europa.eu/food/animals/animal-diseases/control-measures/avian-influenza_en
Emu	Clostridium chauvoei	Ruminant vaccine ± tetanus antitoxin	2 mo, 3 mo, booster annually thereafter at end of breeding season in April	Merck Veterinary Manual. Management of Ratites. Tully,[69] TN
	Salmonella spp, Escherichia coli, clostridial diseases	Autogenous bacterins. These products may be difficult to obtain	Off-label use, uncommon use but may be indicated in specific flocks	
Chickens, turkeys, pheasants, pigeons, ostriches	Pox	Fowlpox vaccine for chickens, turkeys, pheasants, ostriches Pigeon pox vaccine for pigeons	Fowl: vaccine is missed and used within 24 h. Wing web stick or thigh skin stick method Pigeons: apply with small brush to feather follicle	Perelman et al,[68] 1988 Winterfield RW, Reed W. Avian pox: infection and immunity with quail, psittacine, fowl, and pigeon pox viruses. Poultry Science. 1985 Jan 1;64(1):65–70.
Kori bustard, pigeons	Newcastle disease	Inactivated Newcastle disease vaccine and live canarypox vaccine	Annual vaccination in the Middle East but typically not in zoos in the United States for bustards. Vaccinations best given during health-assessment catch-ups performed 1–2 mo before the start of the breeding season	Bailey & Hallager, 2003 AZA Care Manual Kori Bustard

Abbreviations: EEE, eastern equine encephalitis; EU, European Union; IM, intramuscular; rWNV, recombinant West Nile virus; SQ, subcutaneous; WEE, western equine encephalitis; WNV, West Nile virus.

[a] Vaccines used with either good serologic immunity demonstrated or challenge immunity demonstrated.

Table 2
Vaccines with experimental efficacy in ornamental avian species that are not commercially available

Disease of Concern	Vaccine Basis	Species with Demonstrated Protection
Psittacine beak and feather disease	Recombinant PBFDV	Long-billed corellas (C tenuirostris)
Psittacine beak and feather disease	Inactivated double-oil emulsion CP	Galahs (E roseicapillus)
Psittacine beak and feather disease	BPL-treated PBFDV	Umbrella cockatoos, Moluccan cockatoos, African gray parrots, and a yellow-headed Amazon parrot
Pacheco disease (PsHV1)	Multiple emulsion tissue culture vaccine	Budgerigars (Melopsittacus undulatus)
Pacheco disease (PsHV1)	Autogenous, formalin-inactivated vaccine, adjuvanted	Zoologic collection of parrots
PaBV-1–5	Adjuvanted recombinant N-protein	Cockatiels (Nymphicus hollandicus)

Abbreviations: CP, capsid protein; PaBV-1–5, psittacine Bornaviruses 1–5; PsHV1, psittacid herpesvirus 1; PBFDV, psittacine beak and feather disease virus.

site in 3 African gray parrots. Both vaccines stimulated a virus neutralizing antibody response in previously seronegative parrots. Two weeks after boosting, 93% of birds had seroconverted. Seroconversion did not significantly differ between the birds vaccinated with the adjuvanted or the nonadjuvanted vaccines.

The creation of an APV DIVA vaccine is technically possible by using a replication-competent deletion mutant virus where the CP VP4 (VP4Δ) is lost. Both wild-type and mutant viruses elicited neutralizing antibodies after infection of chickens. In addition, the reduced infectivity of VP4Δ compared with the wild-type virus suggests they could be considered for use as vaccines.[6] Thus inactivated or attenuated APV vaccines could both safely immunize psittacines.[7]

Herpesviruses

Herpesviruses are DNA viruses that characteristically cause acute disease. They also have the ability to cause latent infections and thus persist in surviving birds for a long time after clinical disease has resolved. Pacheco disease, caused by psittacid herpesvirus 1, is an acute fulminating hepatitis resulting in up to 100% mortality in New World parrots. Survivors may eventually develop cloacal papillomas or hepatomas. Several oil-adjuvanted, inactivated vaccines have been developed against this disease. However, none are commercially available at present. Although these vaccines are protective, immunity takes more than a week to develop after vaccination and does not prevent shedding of latent virus. Oil emulsion vaccines have been developed but these may cause serious injection site reactions, including swelling, muscle necrosis, or granuloma formation. Cockatoos seem to be most sensitive to these types of reactions. In addition, the vaccine may not protect against all forms of PDV.

In contrast, an autogenous vaccine has been used to control a Pacheco disease outbreak in a zoo. Thus an autogenous, formalin-inactivated vaccine, adjuvanted with aluminum hydroxide, was injected intramuscularly 14 days and 6 weeks after the onset of mortality in the zoo. The vaccine was well tolerated and seemed to stop virus spread, morbidity, and mortality. Serum obtained from vaccinated birds

9 months after the second vaccination contained neutralizing antibodies. Twenty-five months after vaccination 2 of 4 serum samples were still antibody positive. The autogenous vaccine seemed to play a major role in containing this outbreak.[8,9]

An experimental inactivated vaccine against Pacheco disease has also been shown to be effective in budgerigars (*Melopsittacus undulatus*). Infected chicken kidney cells were sonicated and adjuvanted to produce a multiple emulsion vaccine. Although this vaccine was protective against challenge exposure, it generated a negligible serologic response after vaccination, which suggests that cell-mediated responses may have been the prime reason for its efficacy.[10]

Pigeon Herpesvirus

Columbid herpesvirus 1 causes a generalized disease of doves and budgerigars as well as upper respiratory tract infections or encephalitis. Pigeon herpesvirus may also cause acute mortality in raptors that eat infected pigeons. Vaccination of domestic pigeons using an oil-adjuvanted inactivated vaccine does not prevent viral latency.[11] Although the feeding or hawking of pigeons may be avoided to prevent this disease, good sport and plentiful food is wasted. Further, falconers may be specifically called on to reduce pigeon numbers. A reliable, safe vaccine that prevents viral shedding is needed for the prevention of this disease.

Psittacine Bornaviruses

Proventricular dilatation disease (PDD) is caused by psittacine Bornaviruses (PaBV-1). Because the disease is T cell–mediated, PaBV vaccination should, theoretically, exacerbate the disease.[12] Nevertheless, 2 recent reports of the use of viral vector vaccines against parrot Bornaviruses used a prime boost strategy and showed that vaccinated cockatiels had a reduced viral load and shedding as well as a delayed course of infection. Nevertheless, this vaccine failed to prevent the vaccinated cockatiels from developing neurologic signs of PDD despite a low challenge dose.[13] In contrast, an adjuvanted recombinant PaBV N-protein vaccine protected cockatiels against PDD development but had minimal effect on viral load.[14] Overall, these vaccination results reflect the complex pathogenesis of PDD. The use of viral vectored vaccines would be expected to stimulate a type 1 immune response resulting in increased killing of viral infected cells (hence decreased viral load and shedding). However, they could exacerbate clinical disease as a result of this increased lymphocyte response. In contrast, use of the recombinant adjuvanted vaccine would be anticipated to stimulate a type 2 immune response but have little effect on viral load. These studies are ongoing and are especially important in view of the significance of PDD to the avicultural community.

Picornaviruses

Duck hepatitis virus

Duck hepatitis A viruses type 1 (DHAV-1) and type 3 (DHAV-3) are lethal for ducklings. Passive protection of ducklings can be provided by the vaccination of breeder birds. However, a licensed commercial vaccine to address both virus types is currently unavailable. Bacterial recombinants containing viral protein-1 (VP1) genes and expressing VP1 from both DHAV-1 and DHAV-3 have been generated. Ducks that received a single dose of this vaccine were protected against challenge with both viruses, as early as 3 days after vaccination. Viral replication was blocked in vaccinated ducks by 1 week postvaccination.[15] Tissue culture attenuated DHAV-1 also protected ducklings against challenge.[16] Immunization of ducklings with yeast-derived recombinant

VP1 induced a significant immune response and may also prove to be an effective vaccine.[17]

West Nile Virus

Since its introduction to North America in 1999, WNV has spread across both continents causing neurologic disease in humans, horses, and many avian species. Since then, outbreaks have occurred in Europe and, in 2012, the United States experienced a second severe outbreak that resulted in more than 200 human deaths. WNV is maintained in nature in an enzootic transmission cycle between birds and mosquitoes. Corvids seem to be highly susceptible to WNV infection. Other susceptible North American species include endangered or threatened species, such as the greater sage-grouse (*Centrocercus uropbasianuts*) and the eastern loggerhead shrike (*Lanius ludovicianus migrans*), the Florida scrub jay (*Aphelocoma coerulescens*), the California condor (*Gymnogyps californianus*), and the whooping crane (*Grus americana*) and sandhill cranes (*Grus canadensis*). As in humans, juvenile and aged birds may be more susceptible to disease. Although a clear threat, no avian-specific WNV vaccine is available. Therefore, at this time, susceptible species, especially captive cranes, raptors, penguins, flamingos, and corvids, in endemic areas are vaccinated using equine vaccines.

Commercially available equine vaccines

Several different vaccines have been developed for use in horses. There are 3 commercially available vaccines available for use in horses in the United States.[18]

Inactivated vaccines

A formalin-inactivated, adjuvanted whole virus vaccine, West Nile Innovator, is marketed by Zoetis. Innovator has been tested extensively in birds, especially in emergency zoo situations in which it is considered essential to protect large, valuable populations. For example, this vaccine has been evaluated in sandhill cranes (*Antigone canadensis*). Cranes inoculated with Innovator did not develop significant antibody titers, but no cranes inoculated with the vaccine and challenged died of WNV infection. It should be noted that no unvaccinated challenged sandhill cranes died. However, 2 days postchallenge, vaccinated cranes had significantly less viremia than unvaccinated cranes. Seven days postchallenge vaccinated cranes had significantly less cloacal shedding and significantly less weight loss compared with unvaccinated cranes. Vaccinated sandhill cranes developed significantly higher antibody titers postchallenge and were viremic for shorter periods of time after challenge than unvaccinated individuals. Unvaccinated challenged cranes had lesions in both the brain and brain stem that were not observed in vaccinated challenged cranes or in vaccinated unchallenged cranes.[19]

The serologic responses of adult thick-billed parrots (*Rhynchopsitta pachyrhyncha*) after 3 injections of Innovator and annual boosters over 6 years have also been evaluated. Most adult birds had seroconverted after 5 years of annual vaccination. None of their chicks seroconverted during the initial 3-vaccine series; 2 of 4 chicks seroconverted when tested at 1-year, and 3 of 4 chicks had seroconverted by 2 years. It is thus unclear whether this vaccine would be effective in thick-billed parrots.[20]

Five additional species have also been used to assess the antibody response to Innovator. These species are black-footed penguins (*Spheniscus demersus*), little blue penguins (*Eudyptula minor*), American flamingos (*Phoenicopterus ruber*), Chilean flamingos (*Phoenicopterus chilensis*), and Attwater's prairie chickens (*Tympanuchus cupido attwateri*). All birds were vaccinated intramuscularly at least twice. Significant differences in antibody titers over time were detected for black-footed penguins and both flamingo species.[21]

Greater flamingo chicks have also been vaccinated using Innovator. One group received two 1.0 mL intramuscular (IM) doses of vaccine 3 weeks apart, and another group received one 0.5 mL IM dose, followed by two 1.0 mL IM doses 3 weeks apart. A booster vaccination of 1.0 mL was administered to all birds 280 days after the initial vaccination series. Antibody titers were measured before and after the initial injection and 3 weeks after the booster vaccination. Serum neutralizing antibodies were detected in 60% of the samples after the booster. No adverse effects were observed. Passive transfer of maternal antibodies against WNV has been investigated in Chilean and greater flamingos. Transfer of WNV antibodies from hens to chicks was measured by the plaque-reduction test. Hen titers were significantly correlated to chick titers. The mean half-life of maternal WNV antibodies was 13.4 days in flamingo chicks.[22]

Sixteen Chilean flamingos and 10 red-tailed hawks (*Buteo jamacensis*) were vaccinated in the pectoral muscle with 0.2 mL of the Innovator vaccine. Half the birds of each species then received a booster vaccination 3 weeks after the first injection. Three weeks after the booster vaccination, none of 13 birds surveyed had detectable antibody to WNV.[23] Thus antibody responses are variable and may not correlate with protection.

Before the arrival of WNV to the western United States, prospective vaccination was conducted for the entire population of endangered California condors (*G californianus*), both in captivity and in the wild. The Innovator vaccine was safe and stimulated protective immunity in adults, nestlings, and newly hatched chicks. Most importantly, it provided protection to captive birds exposed to naturally circulating WNV during the 2004 transmission season. The prospective vaccination of the entire population of California condors before the arrival of WNV has thus potentially saved this species from subsequent lethal WNV encephalitis and possible extinction.[24]

Recombinant virus vaccines

A recombinant live canarypox-vectored WNV vaccine has also been licensed for use in horses (Merial, Recombitek). This vaccine expresses WNV prM and E genes.[25] It has been tested in comparative trials in birds (discussed later). A fowlpox virus vectored vaccine with inserts of WNV prM and E proteins (vFP2000) followed by a canarypox virus vectored vaccine can protect domestic geese.[26] American robins (*Turdus migratorius*) may be key WNV amplification hosts. However, a single dose of Recombitek injected intramuscularly into robins resulted in more than a 400-fold decrease in average viremia. Although sample sizes were small, these results suggest that vaccinated robins would likely develop viremias that were insufficient to infect *Culex* mosquitoes, the disease vector.[27]

Chimeric virus vaccines

A third equine WNV vaccine is a live chimera vaccine expressing prM and E antigens in a yellow fever 17D vector (Prevnile, Intervet).[18] It has not yet seem to have been tested in birds.

Comparative testing

The relative immunogenicities of both Recombitek and Innovator have been evaluated in gyrfalcons (*Falco rusticolus*) and other falcons.[28] Recombitek gave slightly better protection than innovator, but mild reactions were observed at the injection sites. Using the recommended 2-dose regimen, both vaccines gave only partial protection following WNV challenge. Better results were obtained for both vaccines after a third dose.[30]

Scrub jays (*Aphelocoma californica*) have been used to test 3 WNV equine vaccines: Innovator, an experimental DNA plasmid vaccine called pCBWN, and Recombitek. Overall, vaccination lowered peak viremia compared with nonvaccinated positive controls, but this viremia was probably sufficient to infect susceptible vector mosquitoes. The Innovator vaccine and the experimental pCBWN vaccine stimulated antibody formation and had limited side effects. Five of the 6 birds vaccinated with the Recombitek vaccine, including a vaccinated, non–WNV-challenged control, developed inoculation site lesions.[29]

Responses of 4 species of penguins to WNV vaccines were also evaluated: Humboldt (*Spheniscus humboldti*), Magellanic (*Spheniscus magellanicus*), Gentoo (*Pygoscelis papua*), and rockhopper (*Eudyptes chrysoscome*) penguins. Birds were inoculated with either killed Innovator or the DNA Innovator vaccine. Both vaccines induced seroconversion in all 4 species, and no adverse reactions were noted. In all species, the killed vaccine resulted in greater and faster seroconversion than the DNA vaccine. In addition, the duration of the antibody response was significantly longer in birds vaccinated with the killed vaccine compared with those vaccinated with the DNA vaccine.[30]

Non–commercially available vaccines
Experimental WNV vaccines have been evaluated in American crows (*Corvus brachyrhynchos*), including an intramuscular DNA vaccine, a DNA vaccine with adjuvant, an orally administered microencapsulated DNA vaccine, and the killed Innovator vaccine. Neutralizing antibodies developed in 80% of crows that received the DNA vaccine (with or without adjuvant), and in 44% that received the killed vaccine. However, crows that received the oral microencapsulated DNA vaccine or the placebo failed to produce antibodies. All crows were challenged 10 weeks after initial vaccination. No unvaccinated crows survived challenge, and survival rates were 44% (DNA vaccine), 60% (DNA vaccine with adjuvant), 0% (oral microencapsulated DNA vaccine), and 11% (killed vaccine). Thus administration of some DNA vaccines was associated with reduced mortality but did not result in sterile immunity.[31]

Two experimental DNA vaccines encoding the ectodomains of the envelope protein of WNV lineages 1 and 2 have been evaluated in falcons. Four different vaccination protocols were used, including electroporation and booster injections of recombinant WNV domain III protein, before challenge with the live WNV. Antibody responses following vaccination were low and only lasted for 3 weeks. Viremia, mortality and levels, but not duration, of oral virus shedding were reduced in all the vaccinated birds following challenge compared with nonvaccinated controls. Likewise, clinical scoring, cloacal virus shedding, and viral load in organs were significantly reduced in the vaccinated birds, but full protection was not achieved.[31] WNV NS3 "genes" have also been constructed and assessed for immunogenicity. Both the level of WNV specific antibodies and the number of T cells in vaccinated birds were increased compared with unvaccinated controls.[32]

Captive, nonbreeding Nēnē (*Branta hawaiiansis*) were immunized with 2 doses of the WN-80E recombinant protein adjuvanted with Montanide ISA720. Two birds received a sham vaccine as controls. This vaccine seemed to be safe and immunogenic in this species.[33]

The use of WNV envelope recombinant (rE) protein has also been examined in red-legged partridges (*Alectoris rufa*). Birds were immunized 3 times at 2-week intervals. All vaccinated partridges elicited anti-WNV antibodies before challenge and survived the infection, whereas a third of the sham-immunized birds died. Most unvaccinated birds developed viremia, but this was only detected in 14% of the vaccinated birds. WNV-RNA was detected in feathers and swabs from sham-immunized but not in vaccinated birds. Thus, rE vaccination may not only protect partridges against WNV but may also reduce the risk of virus spread.[34]

A recombinant avirulent Newcastle disease virus (NDV) LaSota strain expressing WNV premembrane/envelope proteins has been assessed in chickens, ducks, and geese.[35] It induced significant levels of neutralizing antibodies and specific CD4+ and CD8+ T-cell responses. Moreover, it also elicited significant levels of specific immunoglobulin (Ig)G in these birds following intramuscular, oral, or intranasal immunization. It too is a promising WNV vaccine candidate.

An experimental adjuvanted DNA vaccine against WNV has been tested in red-tailed hawks (*Buteo jamaicensis*). Hawks were injected with the vaccine in an aluminum phosphate adjuvant or adjuvant only. All birds received 2 injections at a 3-week interval. Four weeks after the second injection the hawks were challenged. Three vaccinated birds seroconverted after the second vaccine injection; all other birds seroconverted following challenge. Vaccinated birds had significantly lower viremia and less shedding compared with the control birds.[36]

Tembusu virus

In 2010 a disease outbreak occurred in egg-laying and breeder ducks in China. It was caused by a flavivirus with 90% homology to Tembusu virus. Its major effect was a decrease in egg production. This virus has also been isolated from house sparrows (*Passer domesticus*). Tembusu virus was grown in duck embryos and inactivated with formaldehyde. The inactivated viral antigen was emulsified with mineral oil. More than 80% of vaccinated ducks were protected against virus challenge after 2 intramuscular or subcutaneous injections.[37]

Viral encephalitides

The equine encephalitis viruses (eastern equine encephalitis [EEE]; western equine encephalitis [WEE]; and Venezuelan equine encephalitis [VEE]), are pathogenic for many birds and, as a result, vaccination may be desirable. A trivalent EEE/WEE/VEE equine vaccine seems to be protective in cranes, pheasants, and emus. EEE virus (EEEV) and WEE virus (WEEV) cause fatal disease in ostriches and other ratites, with mortality ranging from 20% to 80%. Equine and human vaccines are apparently safe and efficacious in ratites.[38] The antibody response against EEEV is short lived. It peaks and disappears within 30 days. The secondary response is dominated by IgM and is relatively long lasting. These results are contrary to classic expectations.[39]

The responses of whooping cranes (*G americana*) and sandhill cranes to a formalin-inactivated EEE vaccine have also been examined. Neutralizing antibodies were elicited in both species after intramuscular vaccination. Subcutaneous and intravenous vaccination failed to elicit detectable antibody in sandhill cranes. Booster doses consistently elicited detectable antibodies in the whooping cranes. Even though EEEV vaccine induced neutralizing antibodies and produced no adverse side effects, its protective efficacy is unclear.[39] Based on seroconversion of sandhill cranes, and a previous 35% case fatality rate in whooping cranes, 37% of susceptible whooping cranes should have been exposed to virus and 6 should have died. Because there were no deaths in these birds, the EEE vaccination program seemed to be efficacious.[40]

Humoral immune responses have been evaluated in emus (*Dromaius novaehollandiae*) vaccinated with commercially available equine polyvalent or experimental monovalent EEEV and WEEV vaccines. Birds were vaccinated with 1 of 2 commercially available polyvalent equine vaccines, a monovalent EEEV vaccine, or a monovalent WEEV vaccine. All 4 vaccines induced neutralizing antibodies, and all birds that received the vaccines were fully protected against an otherwise lethal dose of EEEV. Unvaccinated challenged birds developed viremia and shed virus. Thus commercially available polyvalent equine vaccines protect emus against EEEV infection.[41]

Avian influenza

The recent emergence of pandemic influenza A strains such as H1N1, H7N9, and H5N1 reveals the tremendous challenges to the current influenza vaccine strategies. Better vaccines that provide protection against a wide spectrum of influenza viruses and long-lasting immunity are urgently needed.[42] Although influenza viruses may be acutely lethal for domestic poultry, until recently, vaccination was not permitted in the United States and slaughter was the accepted control policy. However recent outbreaks have made mass slaughter prohibitively expensive. As a result, vaccination is now practiced, but with strict government control. Vaccination is used in control programs for both highly pathogenic (HP) and low pathogenicity (LP) AIV. More than 95% of all AIV vaccines used in poultry are inactivated, adjuvanted products. Challenge studies have found that adjuvants based on mineral and vegetable oils generally induced the highest antibody titers. Formalin-inactivated vaccines induced similar antibody titers and protection against challenge compared with BPL-inactivated vaccines.[43] Inactivated adjuvanted vaccines made from LP field strains have been used for vaccination, but advances in molecular biology have allowed viral vectored vaccines, expressing the AIV hemagglutinin (HA) gene, to be sold commercially. As a group, these vectored vaccines can stimulate both cellular and humoral immunity and are effective at preventing clinical disease and reducing virus shedding. All the licensed recombinant vaccines, because they only express the HA gene, may be used to differentiate vaccinated from vaccinated and infected birds (a DIVA strategy). The vectored vaccines also work well with a prime boost strategy in which the vectored vaccine is given first and a killed adjuvanted vaccine is given 2 or 3 weeks later.[44]

These vaccines have been tested and used in species other than poultry. For example, in 3 zoos, 543 birds were vaccinated twice against AIV using an inactivated H5N9 vaccine. Serologic responses were evaluated by hemagglutination inhibition tests. Eighty-four percent of the birds seroconverted after the second vaccine dose. Significant species variation in response was noted; penguins, pelicans, ducks, geese, herons, guinea fowl, cranes, cockatiels, lovebirds, and barbets showed very poor response to vaccination, whereas very good responses were seen in flamingos, ibis, rheas, Congo peafowl, blackwinged stilts, amazon parrots, and kookaburras.[45] Similar vaccines have been tested in pelicans.[46]

In another study, the efficacy of H5 vaccination was evaluated in flamingos. Antibody titers were maintained at high levels for more than 7 years, against both H5N9 and H5N3, as well as H5N3 and H5N1 reference strains. Thus vaccination may provide long-term protection from HP AIV outbreaks in zoos.[47] Cross-reactive neutralizing antibodies against pandemic influenza virus A/H1N1 have been generated in ostrich eggs produced by females immunized with seasonal influenza viral vaccine.[48]

Because waterfowl, especially ducks, play an important role in the maintenance of H9 AIV in nature, successful control of the spread of AIVs in ducks is desirable. Duck enteritis virus (DEV) is a promising candidate viral vector for duck vaccination. A recombinant DEV vaccine has been made by inserting the HA gene from duck-origin H9N2 AIV into DEV. A single dose of this recombinant vaccine induced solid protection against both DEV and H9N2 AIV challenge.[49]

HP avian influenza H5N1 virus infections cause morbidity and mortality in a wide range of bird species. Vaccination with a commercial H5N2 vaccine using doses adapted to mean body weight per species is safe. After boosting, the mean antibody titer in 334 birds was 190, and 80.5% of vaccinated birds developed a titer of greater than or equal to 40. Titers to the HP H5N1 virus followed a similar trend but were lower. The breadth of the immune response was shown by measuring antibody titers against 4 antigenic clades of currently circulating H5N1 viruses. Vaccination should be regarded as a beneficial component of the preventive measures (in addition to increased biosecurity and monitoring).[50]

Prevaccination and postvaccination AIV antibody titers in 211 birds of several different orders have been determined. After booster vaccination, 81.5% of vaccinated birds developed a titer of greater than or equal to 40, whereas the overall mean titer was 190. Birds of the orders Anseriformes, Galliformes, and Phoenicopteriformes showed higher mean titers, and larger percentages developed titers greater than or equal to 40 than those of the other orders. AIV antibody responses decreased with increasing mean body weight in birds weighing1.5 kg or heavier.[51] The long-term efficacy of AIV H5 vaccination has been evaluated in flamingoes in the Barcelona Zoo. Specific antibody titers were maintained at high levels for more than 7 years against both the H5N9 and H5N3 vaccine strains, as well as the H5N3 and H5N1 reference strains.[47]

Newcastle Disease Virus

Newcastle disease virus (NDV; avian avulavirus-1) affects all avian species. Newcastle disease severity depends on the virus strain and the species involved. Viscerotropic velogenic Newcastle disease is most severe, resulting the development of diphtheritic and necrotic or hemorrhagic lesions along the gastrointestinal tract. Live or inactivated/adjuvanted vaccines are widely used in the domestic poultry industry. NDV vaccines can be applied by eye-nose drops or by a coarse spray. Reactions in spray-vaccinated birds are significantly more severe than in those receiving eye-nose drops, whereas their antibody responses are slightly but significantly stronger.[52]

Bivalent NDV-vectored vaccines against several important pathogens have been developed. These bivalent vaccines confer solid protective immunity against NDV. In most cases, they also induce strong local and systemic immune responses against the targeted pathogen.[53] Although NDV vaccines can prevent clinical disease and mortality in chickens, a major impediment to preventing outbreaks is uneven vaccine application when using mass administration techniques. Another cause of decreased vaccine efficacy is the presence of maternal antibodies that can neutralize the vaccine virus.[54]

NDV vaccines are used in ostriches but NDV may be transmitted from vaccinated to unvaccinated ostriches within a flock.[55] The ability to transmit NDV can be reduced by effective vaccination. Ostriches respond to vaccination with LaSota strain NDV vaccines. In contrast, immunization by eye drops with a live LaSota vaccine of 5-week-old ostrich chicks failed to elicit detectable antibodies.[56]

NDV causes neurologic disease and diarrhea in pigeons. Clinical signs include watery droppings, polydipsia, and neurologic signs. The chronic enteritis may persist for many months. Morbidity may reach 100% but mortality is low. Good immunity can be induced by subcutaneous vaccination with an inactivated oil-adjuvant poultry NDV vaccine. Vaccination is mandatory for racing pigeons in many countries.[57]

In the United States, sampling for NDV is generally conducted when disease occurs in families of wild birds known to be affected by the virus, such as cormorants, pigeons, doves, or pelicans.[58] Three strains have been tested as monovalent oil emulsion vaccines. For example, a pigeon paramyxovirus type 1 (PPMV-1) isolate and the NDV strains LaSota and Ulster were used to prepare BPL-inactivated vaccines. Chickens and pigeons were vaccinated subcutaneously with one of the vaccines and their antibody responses determined. Pigeons were challenged after 10 weeks with a virulent PPMV-1. All these vaccines protected the pigeons against morbidity and death but not against infection with the challenge virus. However, the shedding of the challenge virus from PPMV-1 vaccinates was greatly reduced 6 days after challenge.[59]

Pigeon chicks may be vaccinated, subcutaneously, with an inactivated aqueous suspension of NDV LaSota vaccine. Irrespective of the level of maternally derived antibodies, a single vaccination gave protection lasting 1 year.[60] The vaccine occasionally causes the development of granulomas or abscesses at the injection site. Although protective, some vaccinated pigeons do not react with the formation of detectable antibodies.[61]

Paramyxovirus type 3 (PMV-3) can cause severe illness in small psittacines (*Neophema* spp and other parakeets) and passerines (finches). This disease is characterized by acute or chronic pancreatitis and central nervous symptoms resulting in high mortality in affected flocks. An experimental inactivated adjuvanted PMV-3 vaccine is well tolerated and has been used in a PMV-3 vaccine for parakeets.[62]

Pox Viruses

Avipoxvirus (APV) infections are have been reported in more than 200 bird species. However, passerines, galliformes, and raptors do not commonly show morbidity or mortality as a result of poxvirus infection. Several vaccines have been used to control APV infections. Live virus homologous vaccines are currently in use for fowlpox and effectively elicit long-lasting immunity. Attenuated strains of poxviruses (fowlpox and canarypox) have been exploited as vaccine vectors to deliver heterologous immunogens. These vaccines are thermostable and stimulate both cellular and humoral immune responses.[63] A multivalent vaccine consisting of quail, psittacine, and fowlpox viruses induced excellent protection in chickens against challenge with the 3 respective viruses. However, wing web reactions following vaccination do not necessarily correlate with immunity development.[64] A live pigeon pox vaccine has been tested in hunting falcons.[65] A fowlpox vaccine provided safe and appropriate protection for zebra finches and may be used where APV threatens endangered passerines.[66] Birds were vaccinated using fowlpox virus vaccine and subsequently challenged with either a silvereye or a blackbird APV isolate. Both APV strains caused either swelling or hyperplasia at the inoculation site of nonvaccinated birds. The swelling was less severe and no foot lesions were observed in vaccinated birds.

APV regularly affects captive houbara bustards (*Chlamydotis undulata*), despite a strict implementation of both vaccination and biosecurity. Molecular typing revealed that these infections were mostly caused by canarypoxlike viruses in Morocco, whereas fowlpoxlike viruses predominated in the United Arab Emirates. APVs remain a major threat in bird conservation initiatives and priority should be given to developing a vaccine for these birds.[67]

CONSIDERATIONS FOR VACCINATION STRATEGIES IN NONPOULTRY AVIAN SPECIES

Three major considerations must be reviewed when vaccination is considered for use in avian species (**Table 2**): should vaccination occur, what vaccination protocol to use, and whether or how to assess vaccination efficacy.

1. Should clinicians vaccinate? Consider the following questions:
   a. What is the risk of disease to the population?
   b. Is the population in decline or at risk of actual or functional extinction or extirpation?
   c. Has the population already been exposed
   d. Is the vaccine safe?
   e. Is the vaccination process safe?
   f. Has the vaccine been proved (immunogenic and protective) efficacious?
   g. Is the vaccine available?
   h. What is the cost of vaccination?
2. What vaccination protocol should be adopted? Consider the following questions:
   a. What vaccine is available?
   b. Is the vaccine licensed for use in the species?
   c. Has a vaccine protocol for the available vaccine been used safely in this species or another avian species?
   d. Has the vaccine protocol for the available vaccine been proved efficacious in this species or another species?
   e. Is the vaccination protocol process safe?
   f. What is the cost of the vaccination protocol?
3. Should clinicians assess vaccination efficacy, and if so how? Consider the following questions:
   a. Has the at-risk population already been exposed?
   b. Does the vaccine create measurable antibody levels?
   c. Can the antibody levels from vaccine and natural exposure be differentiated?
   d. How long are vaccine or natural antibody levels maintained?
   e. What is the cost of antibody level measurement?

SUMMARY

Recent advances in virus technology and immunology have the potential to revolutionize the use of antiviral vaccine in exotic avian species. Numerous investigators have used ingenious methods to develop safe and effective vaccines. However, few have proceeded to commercial development. Vaccine complexity, the cost of vaccine production, and the small size of potential markets relative to the mammalian populations all contribute to this problem. The question of vaccination based on vaccine safety and efficacy for many exotic bird species remains unexplored or at least unsatisfactorily answered. Nevertheless, exotic animal veterinarians must continue to push for the production and commercial sale of such products. Vaccination remains an especially important, and critically needed, tool to protect critically endangered bird species.

REFERENCES

1. Duvenage L, Hitzeroth II, Meyers AE, et al. Expression in tobacco and purification of beak and feather disease virus capsid protein fused to elastin-like polypeptides. J Virol Methods 2013;191(1):55–62.

2. Patterson EI, Swarbrick CM, Roman N, et al. Differential expression of two isolates of beak and feather disease virus capsid protein in *Escherichia coli*. J Virol Methods 2013;189(1):118–24.

3. Bonne N, Shearer P, Sharp M, et al. Assessment of recombinant beak and feather disease virus capsid protein as a vaccine for psittacine beak and feather disease. J Gen Virol 2009;90(Pt 3):640–7.

4. Raidal SR, Firth GA, Cross GM. Vaccination and challenge studies with psittacine beak and feather disease virus. Aust Vet J 1993;70(12):437–41.

5. Ritchie BW, Niagro FD, Latimer KS, et al. Antibody response to and maternal immunity from an experimental psittacine beak and feather disease vaccine. Am J Vet Res 1992;53(9):1512–8.

6. Johne R, Paul G, Enderlein D, et al. Avian polyomavirus mutants with deletions in the VP4-encoding region show deficiencies in capsid assembly and virus release, and have reduced infectivity in chicken. J Gen Virol 2007;88(Pt 3): 823–30.

7. Ritchie BW, Niagro FD, Latimer KS, et al. An inactivated avian polyomavirus vaccine is safe and immunogenic in various Psittaciformes. Vaccine 1996;14(12): 1103–7.

8. Barao Da Cunha M, Correia JJ, Fagulha T, et al. Pacheco's parrot disease in macaws of the Lisbon's Zoological Garden. Description of an outbreak, diagnosis and management, including vaccination. Dtsch Tierarztl Wochenschr 2007; 114(11):423–8.

9. Fudge AM. Psittacine vaccines. Vet Clin North Am Small Anim Pract 1991;21(6): 1273–9.

10. Hitchner SB, Calnek BW. Inactivated vaccine for parrot herpesvirus infections (Pacheco's disease). Am J Vet Res 1980;41(8):1280–2.

11. Vindevogel H, Pastoret PP, Leroy P. Vaccination trials against pigeon herpesvirus infection (Pigeon herpesvirus 1). J Comp Pathol 1982;92(4):483–94.

12. Briese T, Hornig M, Lipkin WI. Bornavirus immunopathogenesis in rodents: models for human neurological diseases. J Neurovirol 1999;5(6):604–12.

13. Runge S, Olbert M, Herden C, et al. Viral vector vaccines protect cockatiels from inflammatory lesions after heterologous parrot Bornavirus 2 challenge infection. Vaccine 2017;35(4):557–63.

14. Hameed SS, Guo J, Tizard I, et al. Studies on immunity and immunopathogenesis of parrot bornaviral disease in cockatiels. Virology 2018;515:81–91.

15. Song C, Liao Y, Gao W, et al. Virulent and attenuated strains of duck hepatitis A virus elicit discordant innate immune responses in vivo. J Gen Virol 2014;95(Pt 12):2716–26.

16. Wang C, Li XK, Wu TC, et al. Recombinant VP1 protein of duck hepatitis virus 1 expressed in *Pichia pastoris* and its immunogenicity in ducks. Acta Virol 2014; 58(4):333–9.

17. Wang W, Said A, Wang Y, et al. Establishment and characterization of duck embryo epithelial (DEE) cell line and its use as a new approach toward DHAV-1 propagation and vaccine development. Virus Res 2016;213:260–8.

18. Seino KK, Long MT, Gibbs EP, et al. Comparative efficacies of three commercially available vaccines against West Nile virus (WNV) in a short-duration challenge trial involving an equine WNV encephalitis model. Clin Vaccin Immunol 2007; 14(11):1465–71.

19. Olsen GH, Miller KJ, Docherty DE, et al. Pathogenicity of West Nile virus and response to vaccination in sandhill cranes (*Grus canadensis*) using a killed vaccine. J Zoo Wildl Med 2009;40(2):263–71.

20. Glavis J, Larsen RS, Lamberski N, et al. Evaluation of antibody response to vaccination against West Nile virus in thick billed parrots (*Rhynchopsitta pachyrhyncha*). J Zoo Wildl Med 2011;42(3):495–8.

21. Okeson DM, Llizo SY, Miller CL, et al. Antibody response of five bird species after vaccination with a killed West Nile virus vaccine. J Zoo Wildl Med 2007;38(2): 240–4.

22. Baitchman EJ, Tlusty MF, Murphy HW. Passive transfer of maternal antibodies to West Nile virus in flamingo chicks (*Phoenicopterus chilensis* and *Phoenicopterus ruber ruber*). J Zoo Wildl Med 2007;38(2):337–40.

23. Nusbaum KE, Wright JC, Johnston WB, et al. Absence of humoral response in flamingos and red-tailed hawks to experimental vaccination with a killed West Nile virus vaccine. Avian Dis 2003;47(3):750–2.

24. Chang GJ, Davis BS, Stringfield C, et al. Prospective immunization of the endangered California condors (*Gymnogyps californianus*) protects this species from lethal West Nile virus infection. Vaccine 2007;25(12):2325–30.

25. Minke JM, Toulemonde CE, Dinic S, et al. Effective priming of foals born to immune dams against influenza by a canarypox-vectored recombinant influenza H3N8 vaccine. J Comp Pathol 2007;137(Suppl 1):S76–80.

26. Sá E Silva M, Ellis A, Karaca K, et al. Domestic goose as a model for West Nile virus vaccine efficacy. Vaccine 2013;31(7):1045–50.

27. Kilpatrick AM, Dupuis AP, Chang GJ, et al. DNA vaccination of American robins (*Turdus migratorius*) against West Nile virus. Vector Borne Zoonotic Dis 2010; 10(4):377–80.

28. Angenvoort J, Fischer D, Fast C, et al. Limited efficacy of West Nile virus vaccines in large falcons (*Falco* spp.). Vet Res 2014;45:41.

29. Wheeler SS, Langevin S, Woods L, et al. Efficacy of three vaccines in protecting Western Scrub-Jays (*Aphelocoma californica*) from experimental infection with West Nile virus: implications for vaccination of island scrub-jays (*Aphelocoma insularis*). Vector Borne Zoonotic Dis 2011;11(8):1069–80.

30. Davis MR, Langan JN, Johnson YJ, et al. West Nile virus seroconversion in penguins after vaccination with a killed virus vaccine or a DNA vaccine. J Zoo Wildl Med 2008;39(4):582–9.

31. Bunning ML, Fox PE, Bowen RA, et al. DNA vaccination of the American crow (*Corvus brachyrhynchos*) provides partial protection against lethal challenge with West Nile virus. Avian Dis 2007;51(2):573–7.

32. Young JA, Jefferies W. Towards the conservation of endangered avian species: a recombinant West Nile Virus vaccine results in increased humoral and cellular immune responses in Japanese quail (*Coturnix japonica*). PLoS One 2013;8(6): e67137.

33. Jarvi SI, Hu D, Misajon K, et al. Vaccination of captive nene (*Branta sandvicensis*) against West Nile virus using a protein-based vaccine (WN-80E). J Wildl Dis 2013;49(1):152–6.

34. Escribano-Romero E, Gamino V, Merino-Ramos T, et al. Protection of red-legged partridges (*Alectoris rufa*) against West Nile virus (WNV) infection after immunization with WNV recombinant envelope protein E (rE). Vaccine 2013;31(41):4523–7.

35. Wang J, Yang J, Ge J, et al. Newcastle disease virus-vectored West Nile fever vaccine is immunogenic in mammals and poultry. Virol J 2016;13:109.

36. Redig PT, Tully TN, Ritchie BW, et al. Effect of West Nile virus DNA-plasmid vaccination on response to live virus challenge in red-tailed hawks (*Buteo jamaicensis*). Am J Vet Res 2011;72(8):1065–70.

37. Lin J, Liu Y, Wang X, et al. Efficacy evaluation of an inactivated duck tembusu virus vaccine. Avian Dis 2015;59(2):244–8.

38. Verwoerd DJ. Ostrich diseases. Rev Sci Tech 2000;19(2):638–61.

39. Griffiths BB, McClain O. Immunological response of chickens to eastern equine encephalomyelitis virus. Res Vet Sci 1985;38(1):65–8.

40. Olsen GH, Turell MJ, Pagac BB. Efficacy of eastern equine encephalitis immunization in whooping cranes. J Wildl Dis 1997;33(2):312–5.

41. Tengelsen LA, Bowen RA, Royals MA, et al. Response to and efficacy of vaccination against eastern equine encephalomyelitis virus in emus. J Am Vet Med Assoc 2001;218(9):1469–73.

42. Zhu W, Wang C, Wang BZ. From variation of influenza viral proteins to vaccine development. Int J Mol Sci 2017;18(7). pii: E1554.

43. Lone NA, Spackman E, Kapczynski D. Immunologic evaluation of 10 different adjuvants for use in vaccines for chickens against highly pathogenic avian influenza virus. Vaccine 2017;35(26):3401–8.

44. Suarez DL, Pantin-Jackwood MJ. Recombinant viral-vectored vaccines for the control of avian influenza in poultry. Vet Microbiol 2017;206:144–51.

45. Bertelsen MF, Klausen J, Holm E, et al. Serological response to vaccination against avian influenza in zoo-birds using an inactivated H5N9 vaccine. Vaccine 2007;25(22):4345–9.

46. Oh S, Martelli P, Hock OS, et al. Field study on the use of inactivated H5N2 vaccine in avian species. Vet Rec 2005;157(10):299–300.

47. Fernandez-Bellon H, Vergara-Alert J, Almagro V, et al. Vaccination against H5 avian influenza virus induces long-term humoral immune responses in flamingoes (Phoenicopterus spp.). Vaccine 2016;34(27):3082–6.

48. Adachi K, Takama K, Tsukamoto M, et al. Ostrich produce cross-reactive neutralization antibodies against pandemic influenza virus A/H1N1 following immunization with a seasonal influenza vaccine. Exp Ther Med 2011;2(1):41–5.

49. Sun Y, Yang C, Li J, et al. Construction of a recombinant duck enteritis virus vaccine expressing hemagglutinin of H9N2 avian influenza virus and evaluation of its efficacy in ducks. Arch Virol 2017;162(1):171–9.

50. Philippa J, Baas C, Beyer W, et al. Vaccination against highly pathogenic avian influenza H5N1 virus in zoos using an adjuvanted inactivated H5N2 vaccine. Vaccine 2007;25(19):3800–8.

51. Philippa JD, Munster VJ, Bolhuis HV, et al. Highly pathogenic avian influenza (H7N7): vaccination of zoo birds and transmission to non-poultry species. Vaccine 2005;23(50):5743–50.

52. Landman WJM, Vervaet C, Remon JP, et al. Primary Newcastle disease vaccination of broilers: comparison of the antibody seroresponse and adverse vaccinal reaction after eye-nose drop or coarse spray application, and implication of the results for a previously developed coarse dry powder vaccine. Avian Pathol 2017;46(4):451–61.

53. Choi KS. Newcastle disease virus vectored vaccines as bivalent or antigen delivery vaccines. Clin Exp Vaccine Res 2017;6(2):72–82.

54. Dimitrov KM, Afonso CL, Yu Q, et al. Newcastle disease vaccines–A solved problem or a continuous challenge? Vet Microbiol 2017;206:126–36.

55. Ruenphet S, Satoh K, Tsujimura M, et al. Strategies of Newcastle disease vaccination for commercial ostrich farms in Japan. J Vet Med Sci 2012;74(7):905–8.

56. Blignaut A, Burger WP, Morley AJ, et al. Antibody responses to La Sota strain vaccines of Newcastle disease virus in ostriches (Struthio camelus) as detected by enzyme-linked immunosorbent assay. Avian Dis 2000;44(2):390–8.

57. Lumeij JT, Stam JW. Paramyxovirus disease in racing pigeons. Clinical aspects and immunization. A report from the Netherlands. Vet Q 1985;7(1):60–5.

58. Pedersen K, Marks DR, Afonso CL, et al. Identification of avian paramyxovirus serotype-1 in wild birds in the USA. J Wildl Dis 2016;52(3):657–62.

59. Stone HD. Efficacy of oil-emulsion vaccines prepared with pigeon paramyxovirus-1, Ulster, and La Sota Newcastle disease viruses. Avian Dis 1989;33(1):157–62.

60. Duchatel JP, Flore PH, Hermann W, et al. Efficacy of an inactivated aqueous-suspension Newcastle disease virus vaccine against paramyxovirus type 1 infection in young pigeons with varying amounts of maternal antibody. Avian Pathol 1992;21(2):321–5.

61. Bonner BM, Koehler K, Reichel U, et al. Undesirable reactions of domestic pigeons to vaccination against paramyxovirus type 1. Dtsch Tierarztl Wochenschr 2003;110(10):403–6.

62. Beck I, Gerlach H, Burkhardt E, et al. Investigation of several selected adjuvants regarding their efficacy and side effects for the production of a vaccine for parakeets to prevent a disease caused by a paramyxovirus type 3. Vaccine 2003;21(9–10):1006–22.

63. Bhanuprakash V, Hosamani M, Venkatesan G, et al. Animal poxvirus vaccines: a comprehensive review. Expert Rev Vaccines 2012;11(11):1355–74.

64. Winterfield RW, Reed W. Avian pox: infection and immunity with quail, psittacine, fowl, and pigeon pox viruses. Poult Sci 1985;64(1):65–70.

65. Samour JH, Cooper JE. Avian pox in birds of prey (order Falconiformes) in Bahrain. Vet Rec 1993;132(14):343–5.

66. Ha HJ, Alley M, Howe L, et al. Evaluation of the pathogenicity of avipoxvirus strains isolated from wild birds in New Zealand and the efficacy of a fowlpox vaccine in passerines. Vet Microbiol 2013;165(3–4):268–74.

67. Le Loc'h G, Paul MC, Camus-Bouclainville C, et al. Outbreaks of pox disease due to canarypox-like and fowlpox-like viruses in large-scale houbara bustard captive-breeding programmes, in Morocco and the United Arab Emirates. Transbound Emerg Dis 2016;63(6):e187–96.

68. Perelman B, Gur-Lavie A, Samberg Y. Pox in ostriches. Avian Pathol 1988;17(3):735–9.

69. Tully TN. Ratites. In: Tully TN, Dorrestein G, Jones A, editors. Handbook of Avian Medicine. 2nd edition. Saunders; 2009. p. 258–74.

Cardiovascular Drugs in Avian, Small Mammal, and Reptile Medicine

Brenna Colleen Fitzgerald, DVM, DABVP (Avian Practice)[a],*,
Sara Dias, DVM, MSc[b],
Jaume Martorell, DVM, PhD, DECZM (Small Mammal)[c]

KEYWORDS

- Cardiovascular • Avian • Exotic mammal • Reptile • Heart failure
- Pericardial effusion • Atherosclerosis • Treatment

KEY POINTS

- Cardiovascular disease, including congestive heart failure (CHF), pericardial disease and effusion, and atherosclerosis, is becoming increasingly better recognized in companion birds, small mammals, and reptiles.
- Animals with cardiac disease often present with signs of CHF. The mainstays for treatment of CHF in small animal medicine, namely diuretics, vasodilators, and positive inotropes, can also be applied to treatment of the condition in birds, reptiles, and small mammals. Negative inotropic drugs and lifestyle changes can also have merit.
- CHF may be accompanied by disease processes, such as hypertrophic cardiomyopathy, systemic and/or pulmonary hypertension, and arrhythmias, which need to be addressed accordingly.
- Treatment of pericardial effusion and cardiac tamponade should initially focus on fluid removal, followed by treatment of the underlying cause.
- Atherosclerosis is a disease that predominantly affects psittacine birds; treatment of this condition involves both controlling risk factors and managing sequelae, including peripheral hypoperfusion, ischemic stroke, and CHF.

INTRODUCTION

Cardiovascular disease has traditionally been thought to be a rare occurrence in companion birds, but a growing body of evidence collected over the last few decades indicates otherwise. It is frequently encountered in practice, predominantly in psittacine

Disclosure Statement: The authors have nothing to disclose.
[a] Medical Center for Birds, 3805 Main Street, Oakley, CA 94561, USA; [b] Exotic Animals Department, Hospital Clínic Veterinari, Universitat Autònoma de Barcelona, Carrer de l'Hospital, Campus UAB, Bellaterra (Cerdanyola del Vallés), Barcelona 08193, Spain; [c] Facultat de Veterinaria, Universitat Autònoma de Barcelona, Hospital Clinic Veterinari, Bellaterra, Barcelona 08193, Spain
* Corresponding author.
E-mail address: fitzgeraldvm@gmail.com

Vet Clin Exot Anim 21 (2018) 399–442
https://doi.org/10.1016/j.cvex.2018.01.015
1094-9194/18/© 2018 Elsevier Inc. All rights reserved.

birds, and poses a serious threat to the quality of life and longevity of these and many other avian species. Similarly, in small mammals, cardiac diseases seem to be seen with increasing frequency and are no longer limited to the "predisposed" species, such as the ferret and hedgehog. In reptiles, cardiovascular disease still appears a relatively uncommon condition, predominantly occurring secondary to other abnormalities. Nevertheless, several case reports on reptiles with cardiac disease can be found in the literature. Improved acuity of available diagnostic methods, along with growing owner interest in more sophisticated veterinary care, enables the clinician to better recognize and pursue treatment of cardiovascular disease. Successful intervention requires a foundational understanding of relevant anatomy and physiology, heightened awareness of risk factors and clinical disease states, accurate and timely diagnosis, and innovative treatment approaches.

At the present time, therapeutic interventions for cardiovascular disease in birds and other exotic animals are largely empirical and extrapolated, where possible, from small animal and human medicine. Case reports of cardiovascular disease in which treatment was attempted are relatively few, but include cases of endocardial (eg, endocarditis), myocardial (eg, myocarditis), pericardial (eg, pericardial effusion), and vascular disease (eg, atherosclerosis and associated abnormalities, such as stroke and intermittent claudication syndrome in birds; heartworm disease in ferrets), cardiac arrhythmias (eg, second-degree atrioventricular [AV] block), and end-stage cardiac disease (ie, congestive heart failure [CHF]).[1–20] There is a paucity of pharmacokinetic and pharmacodynamic data and no clinical trials in exotic species for cardiovascular therapeutic agents. At present, the wide array of causative conditions, affected species, therapeutic interventions proposed or attempted, and outcomes precludes any conclusive association between therapeutic protocols and survival time.

Regardless of the species, long-term prognosis for most cardiovascular diseases is considered guarded to poor, given that treatment is limited to management, rather than resolution of disease in most cases. In addition, prognosis is partly contingent on timely diagnosis, which proves challenging given the absence or subtlety of clinical signs and the limited sensitivity of available diagnostic modalities before disease has become advanced. Primary goals are to identify and control risk factors, where possible, and following diagnosis of cardiovascular disease, to maintain quality of life and extend survival time. The following sections review treatment options that show promise for management of recognized disease states, including CHF and related conditions, pericardial disease/effusion, and clinical atherosclerotic disease in birds, reptiles, and small mammals. Medications that have been used empirically, and those for which pharmacokinetic and pharmacodynamic data are available, are presented in **Table 1**.

CONGESTIVE HEART FAILURE AND RELATED CONDITIONS

CHF occurs when the heart is unable to empty the venous reservoirs, manifested by vascular congestion and transudation of fluid within tissues and body cavities (congestive signs).[21,88–91] In the case of right-sided CHF, peripheral venous congestion, hepatic congestion, ascites, and pericardial (or pleural, in case of small mammals) effusion are often present. Pulmonary edema and congestion of the pulmonary veins occur with left-sided CHF, and a combination of signs may be seen with biventricular failure.[17,18,21,22,29,88,91,92] Heart failure can further be characterized as systolic (inadequate ventricular ejection), diastolic (inadequate ventricular filling), or a combination of the 2. In either scenario, stroke volume and cardiac output decrease.[89,90]

Table 1
Selected agents for treatment of cardiovascular disease in birds, small mammals, and reptiles

Drug	Species	Dose/Frequency	Basis	Ref
Diuretics				
Furosemide	Parrots, raptors, mynah birds, African penguins (Spheniscus demersus)	0.1–2.2 mg/kg IM, PO q6–24h	EU	4,5,21–27
	Parrots	1–5 mg/kg IM q2–12h (acute treatment)	EU	Author (B.C.F.)
	Parrots	1–13 mg/kg PO q8–12h (maintenance)	EU	Author (B.C.F.)
	Chickens (G gallus domesticus)	2.5 mg/kg IM	PD	28
		5 mg/kg PO	PD	28
	Small mammals (all)	1–5 mg/kg IV, IM, SC, PO q8–12h	EU	29–32
	Ferrets	2–3 mg/kg IV, IM (initially for fulminant CHF)	EU	33
	Ferrets	1–2 mg/kg PO q12h (long-term maintenance therapy)	.EU	33
	Ferrets	1–4 mg/kg IV, IM, SC, PO q8–12h	EU	14,34
	Rabbits	1–4 mg/kg IV, IM q4–6h (pulmonary edema)	EU	35
		2–5 mg/kg IV, IM, SC, PO q12h (CHF)	EU	35
	Rodents	5–10 mg/kg IM, SC, PO q12h	EU	29,36
	Hedgehogs	2.5–5 mg/kg IM, SC, PO q8h	EU	37
	Hedgehogs	1–4 mg/kg IM, SC, PO q8–12h	EU	38
	Reptiles	2–5 mg/kg IV, IM, PO q12–24h	EU	39,40
Spironolactone	Chickens	1 mg/kg PO	PD	28
	Gray parrot (Psittacus erithacus)	1 mg/kg PO q12h	EU	4 , author (B.C.F.)
	Yellow-naped Amazon parrot (A auropalliata)	2 mg/kg PO q12h	EU	Author (B.C.F.)
	Small mammals (all)	1–2 mg/kg PO q12h	EU	14,29,30
Hydrochlorothiazide	Reptiles	1 mg/kg PO q24–72h	EU	40
Vasodilators				
Isoxsuprine	Yellow-naped Amazon parrot	10 mg/kg PO q24h	EU	41
	Parrots	10 mg/kg PO q12–24h	EU	Author (B.C.F.)

(continued on next page)

Table 1
(continued)

Drug	Species	Dose/Frequency	Basis	Ref
Enalapril	Pigeons (Columba livia)	1.25 mg/kg PO q8–12h	PK	42
	Amazon parrots	1.25 mg/kg PO q8–12h	PK	42
	Parrots	1.25–5 mg/kg PO q12h	EU	7,8, author (B.C.F.)
	African penguin	0.8 mg/kg PO q12h	EU	26
	African penguin	0.25 mg/kg PO q24h	EU	27
	Small mammals (all)	0.25–0.5 mg/kg PO q24–48h	EU	14,29,30,32–34
	Rabbits	0.1–0.5 mg/kg PO q24–48h	EU	43
	Rats	10 mg/kg PO q24h	PD	44
	Rats	17–25 mg/L drinking water	PD	45
	Hedgehogs	0.5 mg/kg PO q24h	EU	38
Benazepril	Gray parrot	0.5 mg/kg PO q24h	EU	4
	Ferrets, rabbits	0.25–0.5 mg/kg PO q24h	EU	14,29
	Rats	0.3–10 mg/kg PO q24h	PD	46
Sildenafil	Parrots	1–5 mg/kg PO q8–12h	EU	47, Author (B.C.F.)
	African penguin	1 mg/kg PO q12h	EU	26
Nitroglycerin 2% ointment	Ferrets	1/16–1/8 inch/animal (applied to shaved skin) q12–24h	EU	14,34
Positive inotropes				
Digoxin	Budgerigars (M undulatus)	0.02 mg/kg PO q24h	PK	48
	Quaker parrots (Myiopsitta monachus)	0.05 mg/kg PO q24h	PK	49
	Sparrows	0.02 mg/kg PO q24h	PK	48
	Indian ringneck parakeet (Psittacula krameri)	0.025 mg/kg PO q24h	EU	5
	Indian hill mynah (G religiosa)	0.01 mg/kg PO q24h	EU	23
	Chickens	0.01 mg/kg PO q24h	EU	50
	Small mammals (all)[a]	0.005–0.01 mg/kg PO q12–24h	EU	30,32
	Ferrets	0.01 mg/kg PO q12h (start at 75% lean body weight)	EU	33,51
	Ferrets	0.005–0.01 mg/kg PO q12–24h	EU	14,34
	Rabbits	0.07 mg/kg PO	PK	52
		0.02 mg/kg PO	PK	52
	Guinea pigs	0.125 mg/kg IV	PK	53
	Rats	1 mg/kg IV	PK	54
	Hamsters	0.05–0.1 mg/kg PO q12h	EU	36
	Hedgehogs	0.01–0.05 mg/kg PO	EU	38

Drug	Species	Dose		
Pimobendan	Hispaniolan Amazon parrots (*A ventralis*)	10 mg/kg PO q12h	PK	55
	Parrots	6–10 mg/kg PO q12h	EU	Author (B.C.F.)
	Parrots	0.25 mg/kg PO q12h	EU	4,56
	Harris hawk (*P unicinctus*)	0.25 mg/kg PO q12h	PK, EU	24
	African penguin	6 mg/kg PO q12h	EU	26
	African penguin	0.25 mg/kg PO q12h	EU	27
	Small mammals (all)	0.2–0.5 mg/kg PO q12h	EU	29,57
	Ferrets	0.5–1.25 mg/kg PO q12h	EU	14,29
	Rabbits	0.1–0.3 mg/kg PO	PD	58
	Hamsters	2.8 mg/kg PO q24h	PD	59
	Mice[b]	100 mg/kg PO q24h, 30 d	PD	60
	Lizards	0.2 mg/kg PO q24h	EU	39
Dobutamine	Hispaniolan Amazon parrots	5–15 µg/kg/min (CRI)	PD	61
	Small mammals (all)	5–15 µg/kg/min (CRI)	EU	62
	Ferrets	5–10 µg/kg/min (CRI)	EU	14
Dopamine	Hispaniolan Amazon parrots	5–10 µg/kg/min (CRI)	PD	61
	Small mammals (all)	5–15 µg/kg/min (CRI)	EU	62
	Ferrets	1–3 µg/kg/min (CRI)	EU	14
	Guinea pigs	0.08 mg/kg IV	EU	63
Negative inotropes				
Carvedilol	Turkeys (*Meleagris gallopavo*)[c]	1–20[d] mg/kg PO q24h	PD	64
	Parrots	1–9 mg/kg PO q12–24h	EU	Author (B.C.F.)
Propranolol	Turkeys[c]	10 mg/kg PO q8h	PD	65
	Turkeys[c]	10–30 mg/kg PO q8h	PD	66
	Ferrets	0.5–2 mg/kg SC, PO q12–24h	EU	34
	Ferrets	0.2 mg/kg PO q8–12h	EU	14
Atenolol	Most species	0.2 mg/kg IM, 0.04 mg/kg IV	EU	22
	Turkeys[c]	10–30 mg/kg PO q24h	PD	66
	Small mammals (all)	3–6.25 mg/kg PO q24h	EU	30
	Ferrets	6.25 mg/ferret PO q24h	EU	34
	Ferrets	3.125–6.25 mg/kg PO q24h	EU	14
	Rodents	0.2–2 mg/kg PO q24h	EU	43

(continued on next page)

Table 1
(continued)

Drug	Species	Dose/Frequency	Basis	Ref
Carteolol	Turkeys[c]	0.01–10 mg/kg PO q12h	PD	67
Nifedipine	Turkeys[c]	10–50 mg/kg PO q8h	PD	66
Diltiazem	Most species	1–2 mg/kg PO q8–12h	EU	68
	Chickens	15 mg/kg PO q12h	PD	69
	Small mammals (all)	1.5–7.5 mg/kg PO q12h	EU	14,30,34
	Rabbits, rodents	0.5–1 mg/kg PO q12–24h	EU	29,43,70
Verapamil	Chickens	5 mg/kg PO q12h	PD	71
Parasympatholytics				
Atropine	Most species	0.01–0.1 mg/kg IM, IV	EU	21
	Moluccan cockatoo (*C moluccensis*)	0.05 mg/kg IM	EU	56
	Small mammals (all)	0.02–0.05 mg/kg IM, SC	EU	14,30,34
	Rabbits	0.1–0.5 mg/kg IV	EU	35
	Rabbits	0.05–3 mg/kg IM	EU	72,73
	Guinea pigs, chinchillas	0.1–0.2 mg/kg IM, SC	EU	74
	Rats, mice, hamsters, gerbils	0.1–0.4 mg/kg IM, SC	EU	74
	Hedgehogs	0.05–0.2 mg/kg SC	EU	75
	Reptiles	0.01–0.04 mg/kg IV, IM, SC	EU	40

Drug	Species	Dosage	Type	Ref
Glycopyrrolate	Most species	0.01–0.02 mg/kg IM	EU	76
	Small mammals (all)	0.01–0.02 mg/kg IM, SC	EU	30,34
	Rabbits	0.01–0.1 mg/kg IM, SC	EU	35,72
	Rodents	0.01–0.1 mg/kg IV, IM, SC	EU	77
	Reptiles	0.01 mg/kg IV, IM, SC	EU	40
Other Antiarrhythmics				
Lidocaine (preservative-free)	Hispaniolan Amazon parrots	2.5 mg/kg IV	PK, PD	78
	Chickens	6 mg/kg IV	PD	79
	Chickens	2.5 mg/kg IV	PK, PD	80
	Small mammals (all)	1–2 mg/kg IV	EU	30,43
Propantheline	Moluccan cockatoo	0.3 mg/kg PO q8h	EU	56
Filaricides				
Ivermectin	Ferrets	0.05–0.2 mg/kg SC, PO q30d (larvicide)	PD	81–83
	Ferrets	0.05 mg/kg SC, PO q30d (adulticide)	EU	14,29
Selamectin	Ferrets	6–18 mg/kg spot-on q30d (larvicide)	PD	84
Moxidectin	Ferrets	0.17–2 mg/ferret SC once (adulticide)	EU	85,86
Moxidectin/imidacloprid	Ferrets	1%/10% 0.4 mL spot-on q30d (larvicide)	PD	87

Abbreviations: CRI, continuous rate infusion; EU, empirical use; PD, pharmacodynamic study; PK, pharmacokinetic study; q8/12/24h, every 8/12/24 hours.
[a] Therapeutic levels: 0.8 to 1.2 ng/mL.
[b] Troponin knockout mice.
[c] Broad-breasted white turkey poults.
[d] Some birds receiving carvedilol at 20 mg/kg had significantly decreased heart rate and blood pressure for up to 8 h.

CHF is not a primary disease in itself, but an ultimate consequence of structural or functional abnormalities of the cardiovascular or pulmonary systems, compounded by the chronic effects of compensatory mechanisms (**Table 2**). Not all cardiovascular disease necessarily leads to CHF, but it is a frequent clinical endpoint encountered in exotic species. Heart failure can result from primary myocardial failure (eg, dilated cardiomyopathy [DCM]), ventricular pressure overload (eg, outflow obstruction, systemic or pulmonary hypertension [PH]), or volume overload (eg, valvular insufficiency), conduction disturbances, or diastolic dysfunction (eg, myocardial hypertrophy, cardiac tamponade). For more details, please see Refs.[89,90,93]

To diagnose CHF, radiographic imaging and ultrasonography often have the greatest value.[17,21,95,96] In addition, electrocardiography (ECG),[21,22,96,97] blood pressure measurement,[98,99] angiography, complete blood count and serum biochemistry, computed tomography (CT), magnetic resonance imaging (MRI),[100–102] and other ancillary tests (fluid analysis, culture, cytology, histopathology, pathogen-specific tests) can be used to characterize the nature, extent, and underlying causes of cardiovascular disease.

Successful medical management is partly contingent on the earliest possible detection of disease. Timely detection can be enabled by teaching the exotic pet owner to identify clinical signs, even if subtle, by regular physical examinations on an annual or semiannual basis, by considering the option of baseline diagnostic imaging for at-risk individuals, and by heightened awareness in the clinical setting. By doing so, one of the authors (B.C.F.) has identified right-sided cardiac insufficiency in birds wherein the first premonitory sign was delayed absorption of subcutaneous fluids administered for a noncardiovascular indication.

In a patient presenting with acute or decompensated heart failure, initial treatment aims to stabilize the patient, followed by design of a longer-term management strategy. In the experience of one of the authors (B.C.F.), stabilization and long term management have met with highly variable success in avian species, but some have been maintained in stable condition for up to 5 years. A review of 17 published clinical cases of CHF in birds, using a variety of treatments, shows a median survival time of 35 days

Table 2
Documented causes of congestive heart failure in birds, small mammals, and reptiles

Domestic and Companion Birds[93]	Small Mammals[94]	Reptiles[94]
DCM	DCM	Restrictive cardiomyopathy
HCM	HCM	Cardiac infection
Atherosclerosis	Restrictive cardiomyopathy	Myocardial fibrosis
Systemic hypertension	Hyperthyroidism	Atherosclerosis
PH	Stress-induced	Valvular insufficiency
Pulmonary fibrosis/mycosis	Anesthesia-induced	Valvular stenosis
Arrhythmias	Cardiac infection	Pericardial effusion
Cardiac infection	Heartworm disease	
Nutritional causes	Autoimmune disease	
Iron storage disease	Drug-induced (chemotherapy, doxorubicin)	
Toxic causes	Neoplasia	
Valvular insufficiency	Genetic defects	
Valvular stenosis	Valvular insufficiency	
Septal defects	Valvular stenosis	
Pericardial effusion	Septal defects	
	Pericardial effusion	

(**Table 3**). Overall, CHF in exotic mammals carries a poor long-term prognosis. A review of 19 published clinical cases of CHF in companion exotic mammals with various conditions and under various treatments showed a median survival time of 88 days, with a maximum survival of 1.5 years (see **Table 3**). Reports on treatment of CHF in reptiles are scarce, with 135 days being the longest survival time reported in the literature thus far (see **Table 3**).

The mainstays of treatment of CHF in small animal medicine, namely diuretics, vasodilators (including angiotensin-converting enzyme inhibitors [ACEI]), and positive inotropes, can be applied to treatment of the condition in birds, reptiles, and small mammals (see later discussion).[4,14,18,19,21,93,119,120] β-Blockers (BBs), considered part of standard treatment in humans, may also have potential application.[64,121,122] In addition, known or hypothesized underlying causes should be addressed, if possible. Some causes, including bacterial and fungal infections, parasitic disease, and certain toxic insults, carry a better prognosis for recovery.

Diuretics

Marked reduction of excessive circulating plasma volume (hypervolemia), edema, and effusion is an immediate treatment priority in any exotic patient with CHF. Alleviation of this relative fluid overload can be accomplished through the use of diuretics, principally furosemide. Diuretics should not be used alone long term because they further activate the renin-angiotensin-aldosterone system (RAAS).[123] Of the various diuretics available, furosemide is most commonly used in exotic pets.

Furosemide

Furosemide is a potent loop diuretic that inhibits the sodium, potassium, and chloride cotransporter in the ascending limb of the loop of Henle, thereby promoting diuresis and excretion of sodium and chloride.[123,124] Parenteral administration of furosemide is an essential step in management of the acute crisis in most species because this route allows for a fast onset of action. A relatively high initial dose is often required, especially in patients in which renal blood flow is impaired because of severe CHF, plasma volume concentration, or the administration of a nonsteroidal anti-inflammatory drug, which can impair effective delivery of the drug to the proximal nephron. In such cases, a constant rate intravenous (IV) infusion of furosemide can be considered. Following stabilization of the patient, a maintenance dose of furosemide can be used to enable the long-term management of chronic CHF.[123–125]

Despite the fact that only 10% to 30% of the nephrons in the avian kidney are looped, furosemide has been found efficacious with a rapid onset of action in birds,[126] and as such, has been used successfully for treatment of pericardial effusion, CHF, pulmonary edema, and ascites.[8,21,22,104] Route of administration may significantly influence bioavailability, as suggested by the results of a study examining the diuretic effects of furosemide in chickens (adult laying hens). In this study, it was found that urine output significantly increased following parenteral administration (2.5 mg/kg), but did not in birds receiving the drug orally, even at twice the parenteral dose (5 mg/kg).[28]

In reptiles, the use of furosemide has been suggested for the management of cardiogenic pulmonary edema, but because reptiles do not have a loop of Henle, its efficacy is questionable. In a study in freshwater turtles, furosemide (2 and 5 mg/kg) failed to alter plasma renin activity, suggesting turtles lack a tubular mechanism for altering renin release. Nevertheless, tubular reabsorption was inhibited, as indicated by a doubling of the urine volume and presence of a net potassium secretion.[127] Similarly, the drug appeared to exert clinical effect in 2 iguanas with CHF that were treated with a dose of 2 mg/kg subcutaneously (SC) every 12 hours.[39] However, in a carpet

Table 3
Survival time after diagnosis and treatment of selected cases of congestive heart failure in birds, small mammals, and reptiles

Species	Ultimate Diagnosis	CHF	Treatment	Survival Time	Ref
Gray parrot (Psittacus erithacus)	Atherosclerosis Right AV valve insufficiency Cor pulmonale Myocardial fibrosis	Right	Coelomocentesis Furosemide Spironolactone Benazepril Pimobendan	35 d	4
Gray parrot (P erithacus)	Valve regurgitations, hyperechoic aorta	Biventricular	Furosemide Imidapril Pimobendan	30 d	103
Indian ringneck parakeet (P krameri)	Left and right AV valve insufficiency (myxomatous degeneration of left AV valve and hypertrophy of right AV valve) Myocardial degeneration and necrosis	Biventricular	Furosemide Digoxin	10 mo	5
Blue-fronted Amazon parrot (A aestiva)	Right AV valve insufficiency (congenital defect)	Right	Supportive Furosemide Digoxin	8 d	104
Yellow-crowned Amazon parrot (A ochrocephala)	Cause undetermined	Right	Supportive Furosemide Enalapril	27 mo	8
Severe macaw (Ara severa)	Atherosclerosis Diffuse fatty infiltration of the right ventricular myocardium	Biventricular	Furosemide	70 d	3
Gray-cheeked parakeet (Brotogeris pyrrhopterus)	Atherosclerosis Left and right AV valve insufficiency Myocardial degeneration and fibrosis	Biventricular	Supportive	3 d	105
Umbrella cockatoo (Cacatua alba)	Atherosclerosis Aneurysm of right coronary artery Myocardial fibrosis	Right	Supportive Furosemide	Euthanized at diagnosis	106

Species	Cardiac lesions/diagnosis	Location	Treatment	Outcome	Reference
Umbrella cockatoo (C alba)	Atherosclerosis Left AV valve insufficiency (myxomatous degeneration and mineralization)	Left		Euthanized within 1 d of diagnosis	107
Pukeko (Porphyrio melanotus)	Atherosclerosis Left AV valve insufficiency (endocardiosis) Left atrial thrombus Atrial fibrillation Myocardial degeneration	Biventricular	Supportive Digoxin	49 d	108
Red-tailed hawk (Buteo jamaicensis)	DCM	Right	Supportive Furosemide	Euthanized 2 d after presentation	1
Indian hill mynah (G religiosa)	Left AV valve insufficiency	Biventricular	Supportive Coelomocentesis Furosemide Digoxin	10 mo	23
Greater hill mynah (Gracula religiosa intermidia)	Coronary mineralization	Right	Coelomocentesis	12 d	2
Mallard hybrid duck (Anas spp)	Congenital left AV valve stenosis and subvalvular aortic stenosis	Biventricular	Supportive Coelomocentesis Furosemide	29 d	6
African penguin (S demersus)	Right AV valve insufficiency (endocardiosis)	Right	Supportive Coelomocentesis Furosemide Enalapril Pimobendan Sildenafil	124 d	26
African penguin	Right AV valve insufficiency (congenital valvular dysplasia and myxomatous degeneration) Myocardial fibrosis	Right	Supportive Furosemide Enalapril Pimobendan	10 d	27
Harris hawk (P unicinctus)	Cardiomyopathy	Biventricular	Furosemide Pimobendan	6 mo	24

(continued on next page)

Table 3
(continued)

Species	Ultimate Diagnosis	CHF	Treatment	Survival Time	Ref
Yellow-naped Amazon parrot (*A auropalliata*)	Atherosclerosis	Biventricular	Supportive Coelomocentesis Furosemide Spironolactone Enalapril Sildenafil Pimobendan Carvedilol	8 mo	Author (B.C.F.)
Gray parrot (*P erithacus*)	DCM Atherosclerosis	Right	Supportive Furosemide Spironolactone Enalapril	30 d	Author (B.C.F.)
Gray parrot (*P erithacus*)	Atherosclerosis	Biventricular	Supportive Furosemide Spironolactone Enalapril Pimobendan	14 mo	Author (B.C.F.)
Gray parrot (*P erithacus*)	Open	Right	Supportive Furosemide Enalapril Sildenafil Pimobendan Omega-3 fatty acid supplementation	65 months to present	Author (B.C.F.)
Gray parrot (*P erithacus*)	Left AV valve insufficiency Atherosclerosis	Left	Supportive Furosemide Spironolactone Enalapril Sildenafil Pimobendan	17 mo	Author (B.C.F.)

	Open		Supportive		Author (B.C.F.)
Gray parrot (P erithacus)		Left	Furosemide, Enalapril, Pimobendan	30 months to present	
Ferret	DCM	Biventricular	Furosemide, Digoxin	7 mo	[109]
Ferret	DCM	Biventricular	Furosemide, Digoxin	21 d	[110]
Ferret	DCM, Cryptococcosis	Biventricular	Furosemide, Digoxin	1 d	[111]
Ferret	DCM	Biventricular	Furosemide, Digoxin, Taurine	12 mo	[112]
Ferret	Ventricular septal defect, Valvular disease	Biventricular	Furosemide, Benazepril, Pimobendan, Thoracocentesis	5 mo	[113]
Ferret	Atrial septal defect	Right	Furosemide	12 d	[114]
Ferret	Tetralogy of Fallot	Biventricular	Furosemide, Benazepril	4 d	[115]
Rabbit	DCM	Left	Furosemide, Spironolactone, Enalapril, Pimobendan	42 d	[57]
Rabbit	Valvular disease	Biventricular	Furosemide, Enalapril, Pimobendan	7 mo	[57]
Rabbit	HCM	Biventricular	Thoracocentesis	1 d	[16]
Rabbit	DCM, Valvular disease	Right	Furosemide	Few days	[16]

(continued on next page)

Table 3
(continued)

Species	Ultimate Diagnosis	CHF	Treatment	Survival Time	Ref
Rabbit	Cardiomyopathy	Right	Furosemide	3 d	116
Guinea pig	DCM	Biventricular	Furosemide Enalapril	56 d	15
Guinea pig	HCM	Left	Furosemide Benazepril	18 mo	117
Rat	DCM	Biventricular	Furosemide Benazepril Pimobendan Digoxin	5 d	118
Rat	DCM	Biventricular	Furosemide Benazepril Pimobendan Digoxin	27 d	118
Syrian hamster	DCM Atrial thrombosis	Biventricular	Furosemide Pimobendan	21 d	57
Syrian hamster	DCM	Left	Furosemide Pimobendan	17 d	57
Carpet python (*Morelia spilota variegata*)	Right AV valve insufficiency	Bilateral	Furosemide	63 d (euthanized)	20
Bearded dragon (*Pogona vitticeps*)	Ventricular hypertrophy	Right	Supportive Furosemide Pimobendan (only one dose)	35 d	39
Green iguana (*Iguana iguana*)	Ventricular hypertrophy	Bilateral	Supportive Furosemide Pimobendan	130 d	39

python, furosemide administered in a dose of 5 mg/kg SC every 48 hours failed to result in a clinical response.[20] These ambiguous results emphasize the need of further studies regarding the efficacy of furosemide in these species.

Doses that have been used vary widely within and across taxa (see **Table 1**). Similar to dogs and cats, the dose and administration interval are best determined by clinical response (namely normalization of respiratory rate and effort), the degree of which can be of diagnostic and prognostic value. In the experience of one of the authors (B.C.F.), a dose range of 1 to 5 mg/kg intramuscularly (IM) has been most efficacious when stabilizing psittacine patients with severely decompensated disease. An initial frequency of 2 hours is usually followed by a shift to 6- to 12-hour intervals. Once the patient has been stabilized, furosemide can be administered orally, with the dose increased at least 2-fold (presuming oral bioavailability is 60%–75% as in humans[128]) given every 8 to 12 hours. Ultimately, the goal for long-term management is to identify the lowest dose that controls congestive signs.

Adverse effects of loop diuretics include polydipsia, polyuria, reduction in blood pressure, plasma volume depletion, (prerenal) azotemia, and depletion of electrolytes, especially chloride, potassium, and magnesium.[14,120,123] With chronic use, renal functional status (blood uric acid in birds) and electrolytes should therefore be monitored carefully.[21] In addition, caution is warranted when using this drug in patients with renal disease as well as in lories and lorikeets (subfamily Loriinae), which have been reported to be extremely susceptible to adverse effects of furosemide. As a result, lower doses are recommended for these species.[22]

Other diuretics
Spironolactone, an aldosterone antagonist that is classified as a potassium-sparing diuretic, may have merit as part of the treatment regimen in cases where congestive signs cannot be controlled with furosemide and an ACEI alone.[129] Its combined use with furosemide may also be considered to offset potassium loss.[4,124,129] Aside from its diuretic effects, spironolactone is thought to prevent or decrease myocardial fibrosis in humans[123] and counteract the myriad deleterious effects of aldosterone in CHF.[130] However, thus far, reports on its use or efficacy in exotics are scarce.

Hydrochlorothiazide, a thiazide diuretic with calcium-sparing properties that is, used in humans to treat hypertension and fluid retention, has been used to promote diuresis in reptiles.[40]

Vasodilators

Angiotensin-converting enzyme inhibitors
ACEI are typically combined with diuretics and positive or negative inotropes and comprise an essential component of long-term medical management of CHF by blunting the effects of the RAAS. By interfering with AII formation and limiting aldosterone production, ACEI promote vasodilation and reduce sodium and water retention, thereby decreasing total peripheral resistance and pulmonary vascular resistance (afterload) and circulating volume (preload), allowing an increase in cardiac output.[21,42,131,132] Enalapril is thought to attenuate myocardial remodeling in humans and dogs.[133] In both species,[134,135] ACEI have been found beneficial to increase survival times. Similar effects were observed during a placebo-controlled study using an experimental CHF model in rats, which demonstrated that animals treated with enalapril had a 95% higher median survival time than controls.[45]

Because of their longer half-life, enalapril and benazepril are the most commonly used ACEI in small mammals. Of the different ACEI that are available, enalapril has been the most commonly used in birds, with empirical evidence suggesting it is both safe and efficacious.[42] Enalapril has been used, both alone and in combination with furosemide, to treat CHF with reduction in pericardial effusion, ascites, and hepatic congestion documented by echocardiography, and reportedly increased quality of life and longevity in birds with severe cardiac abnormality.[8,42] Pharmacokinetic data support a dose of at least 1.25 mg/kg orally (PO) every 8 to 12 hours in pigeons and Amazon parrots, although the half-life was shorter and lower maximum plasma concentrations were reached in the latter species.[42] As a result, one of the authors (B.C.F.) has used higher doses (1.25–5 mg/kg PO every 12 hours) in psittacine birds with appreciable symptomatic benefit.

No information is available on the use of these drugs in pet reptiles.[136] ACEI have experimentally been used in alligators. However, in comparison to α-adrenergic receptor antagonists (phentolamine and phenoxybenzamine), ACEI (captopril and enalapril) seemed less capable of controlling arterial blood pressure. As a result, their efficacy in reptiles remains uncertain.

Potential adverse effects of using ACEI include hypotension, renal dysfunction, and hyperkalemia. Dehydration has been reported with long-term, higher-dose therapy (5 mg/kg daily) in birds, although the drug generally appears well tolerated.[42] To prevent side effects, some investigators have recommended to carefully titrate the dose to effect, especially in patients with renal compromise, severe CHF, or dehydration. The risk of hyperkalemia is likely diminished by concurrent use of furosemide, but may be relatively greater if spironolactone is used as well.[131] When using ACEI, it is reasonable to consider similar biochemical and hematologic monitoring as for furosemide, but no significant changes in these parameters were found in pigeons receiving 10 mg/kg enalapril once daily for 3 weeks.[42]

Other vasodilators

Other vasodilators/venodilators used in small animal cardiology are the nitrates (including nitroglycerin), amlodipine, and hydralazine. These drugs are typically used in patients with acute heart failure.[131] To the authors' knowledge, their use has not been reported in birds and reptiles. In small mammals (eg, ferrets, rabbits), the use of nitroglycerine 2% cream applied on the inside of the pinna has been reported for the initial (ie, first 24 hours) treatment of life-threatening pulmonary edema because the drug is considered to dilate mainly systemic veins and venules, causing blood to pool away from the lungs.[14,120] Because of the risk for hypotension, careful monitoring is recommended.

Positive Inotropes

Positive inotropes such as digoxin and pimobendan have been used or proposed for treatment of heart failure in exotic species, but pharmacodynamic data are lacking and pharmacokinetic data and information as to their efficacy and margin of safety are extremely limited.[7,21,42,55] Both drugs are used to enhance myocardial contractility and are appropriate for treatment of heart failure due to systolic dysfunction. They are contraindicated in cases of hypertrophic cardiomyopathy (HCM; where diastolic dysfunction is the primary problem), and of outflow obstruction (eg, aortic stenosis).[21,124,137] Likewise, it should be questioned whether their use is appropriate in birds with heart failure secondary to atherosclerotic disease and luminal stenosis of major arteries. In those cases with severe systolic dysfunction, however, it is fair to consider their inclusion in the treatment regimen in an effort to stabilize the patient. Once the patient has been stabilized, the clinician should consider either alternative or concurrent use of a BB (discussed in the next section).

Digoxin
Digoxin is a digitalis glycoside that increases myocardial contractility by directly inhibiting the Na^+/K^+ ATPase pump, resulting in intracellular calcium accumulation through the activation of the Na^+/Ca^{2+} exchanger. Other effects include mild diuresis, increased parasympathetic tone, and decreases in sympathetic tone and renin release. Digoxin acts as both a weak positive inotrope and a negative chronotrope, slowing the sinus rate and decreasing AV nodal conduction. In mammals, including ferrets, digoxin has been beneficial for treatment of heart failure that is complicated by supraventricular tachycardia (including atrial fibrillation).[14,138] Similarly, in birds, digoxin may have value in certain heart failure cases when used in combination with diuretics and ACEI, particularly when supraventricular tachyarrhythmia is a feature.[22] Nevertheless, its narrow therapeutic index is a concern, and chronic, maintenance administration may prove problematic because of the high risk for proarrhythmic and gastrointestinal side effects.[21,55] In addition, studies have failed to demonstrate its efficacy in reducing overall mortality. As a result, its use is becoming more controversial in small animal and human cardiology.[138]

Pharmacokinetics of digoxin has been investigated in several bird and mammalian species.[48,49,52–54,139,140] In sparrows and budgerigars, a plasma concentration of 1.6 ng/mL was achieved by administration of 0.02 mg/kg PO every 24 hours for 5 days.[48] In Quaker parrots, a single oral dose of 0.05 mg/kg produced a maximum plasma concentration of 1.8 ± 0.36 ng/mL.[49] In experimental studies with rabbits, single oral doses of 0.02 mg/kg and 0.07 mg/kg resulted in plasma concentrations between 2.02 to 2.26 and 5.6 to 6.0 ng/mL, respectively. Reported half-times varied from 9.4 to 20 hours.[52,54] However, repeated administration resulted in lower plasma concentrations due to increased clearance.[141] Therefore, pharmacokinetic parameters derived from single-dose studies should be interpreted with caution because these may not necessarily reflect plasma levels following prolonged administration.

Because of the risk of side effects, any patient receiving digoxin should be carefully monitored. Aside from a clinical examination and evaluation of biochemical and hematologic parameters, risks posed by digoxin toxicity necessitate therapeutic drug monitoring and follow-up ECG.[21,142] Recommended therapeutic levels for digoxin in the dog are 0.8 to 1.2 ng/mL.[138] In ferrets, slightly higher therapeutic plasma concentrations of 1 to 2 ng/mL should occur 10 to 12 hours after oral administration.[14] For other species, therapeutic plasma concentrations have not been properly established, but anecdotal evidence from individual case reports suggests that the levels may also range higher for (some) birds.[5,23] In an Indian hill mynah bird (*Gracula religiosa*) with biventricular CHF, marked clinical improvement was seen with digoxin (0.01 mg/kg PO every 24 hours) and furosemide (2.2 mg/kg PO every 12 hours), with trough serum digoxin concentration maintained at 1.6 ng/mL.[23] Administration of the drug to chickens with right-sided CHF (ascites syndrome) at a dose of 0.01 mg/kg PO every 24 hours over a 6-week period resulted in decreased ventricular size and ascites.[50] To the authors' knowledge, no information is available on the clinical use, efficacy, or therapeutic plasma concentrations for digoxin in reptiles.

Digoxin toxicity can produce any type of arrhythmia, which may be further potentiated by hypokalemia due to diuretic use.[22] As a result, its use is contraindicated in patients with sinoatrial nodal dysfunction or AV blocks and in those with ventricular arrhythmias given the risk of inducing ventricular fibrillation.[22,143] In the case of the Indian hill mynah mentioned above, second-degree AV block developed when digoxin was used at 0.02 mg/kg PO every 24 hours and trough serum digoxin concentration was 2.4 ng/mL.[23] Similarly, digoxin administered at a dose of 0.22 mg/kg PO every 24 hours produced arrhythmias in pigeons.[144] Digoxin is furthermore contraindicated in patients with moderate to severe renal dysfunction because the drug is eliminated by the kidneys.[120,138]

Pimobendan

Pimobendan, a calcium sensitizer and phosphodiesterase inhibitor, is a positive inotrope and vasodilator (inodilator), as well as a positive lusitrope. It enhances myocardial contractility, primarily through calcium sensitization of cardiac myofibrils and by phosphodiesterases III inhibition, without increasing myocardial oxygen consumption.[55,138] Inhibition of phosphodiesterase III and V promotes systemic and pulmonary arterial and venous dilation, thereby reducing afterload and preload, respectively.[55] Pimobendan is commonly used in small animal cardiology and has been shown to increase both survival time and quality of life in dogs with DCM and heart failure secondary to mitral valve disease.[145]

In small mammals, pimobendan has been used with mixed results.[57] In experimental studies in hamsters and mice with DCM, survival times of animals treated with pimobendan were significantly increased in comparison to the control group.[59,60] However, in 2 hamster patients with DCM, survival times were poor. The difference in results may in part be due to differences in dosing regimen (0.3 mg/kg PO every 12 hours vs 2.8 mg/kg PO every 24 hours) or severity of condition at the start of therapy. In a rabbit diagnosed with DCM, clinical improvement was seen following addition of pimobendan to the treatment protocol. This rabbit ended up living for 7 months following diagnosis. In another rabbit, outcome was less favorable, with the animal only surviving for 42 days after diagnosis.[57] In ferrets with DCM, pimobendan has also been used anecdotally, often in combination with other drugs.[113,146]

In psittacine birds, there are 2 reported cases whereby pimobendan (0.25–0.6 mg/kg every 12 hours) was used in conjunction with a diuretic and an ACEI to treat CHF. Similar to small mammals, results have been variable.[4,103] The apparent limited clinical effect may be explained by underdosing. A pharmacokinetic study in Hispaniolan Amazon parrots (*Amazona ventralis*) demonstrated that a single oral dose of 10 mg/kg is required to achieve a peak plasma concentration of 8.26 ng/mL, comparable to levels considered therapeutic in dogs and humans.[55] Extrapolation of the dose used in this study to other species groups should be done with caution. Plasma concentrations in a Harris hawk (*Parabuteo unicinctus*) with CHF receiving 10 mg/kg pimobendan PO peaked at 25,196 ng/mL. However, there was no indication of toxicosis.[24]

Bioavailability of pimobendan can be affected by pharmacologic composition. An oral suspension formulated from commercially available tablets (crushed and combined with a suspending vehicle) produced 6 times greater plasma concentrations than a suspension made from the bulk chemical (powder). The investigators proposed that the difference might be attributed to the citric acid excipient present in the commercially available tablets, which facilitated oral absorption.[55]

In lizards, pimobendan has been recommended at dose of 0.2 mg/kg PO every 24 hours.[40] However, in a bearded dragon with CHF, this dose resulted in lethargy and weakness that disappeared 1 day after cessation of the drug.[39]

In birds and other exotics, adverse effects have thus far not been recognized, but because of lack of information regarding safety and efficacy of this drug, care is warranted when using this drug in these species.

Other positive inotropes

The sympathomimetics dopamine and dobutamine are used in small animal medicine for short-term, life-saving intervention in cases of acute, profound myocardial failure. Both drugs act via β_1-adrenoreceptors to increase myocardial contractility and relaxation and induce peripheral vasodilation. They can also promote vasoconstriction through their action at α-adrenoceptors.[124,147] Because their action is short lived, they must be administered by constant rate infusion (CRI). In exotics, their use thus far has been limited to experimental studies (eg, in rats, rabbits, Hispaniolan Amazon parrots),[61,148,149] or as part of cardiopulmonary-cerebral resuscitation.[150]

In Hispaniolan Amazon parrots anesthetized with isoflurane, dopamine (5, 7, and 10 μg/kg/min) and dobutamine (5, 10, and 15 μg/kg/min) CRIs significantly increased heart rate and arterial blood pressure (as determined by direct method) in a dose-dependent manner (dopamine > dobutamine). Four of the birds included in the study developed second-degree AV block and hypotension while receiving dobutamine at 15 μg/kg/min, emphasizing the need for ECG monitoring to detect changes in heart rate and rhythm in an early phase.[61] The effects of these drugs on systolic function and cardiac output have thus far not been established.

Negative Inotropes

Negative inotropes, including BBs and calcium channel blockers (CCBs), may have merit as adjunctive treatment of CHF, particularly when ventricular hypertrophy and tachyarrhythmia are contributing factors. These 2 drug classes are discussed in detail later.

β-Blockers

BBs are sympatholytic agents that block the binding of endogenous catecholamines to β-adrenoreceptors. They are negative inotropes, chronotropes, and lusitropes that also slow AV nodal conduction:

- First-generation, nonselective BBs (eg, propanolol, carteolol) block both β_1-adrenoreceptors and β_2-adrenoreceptors.
- Second-generation BBs (eg, atenolol, metoprolol) are relatively β_1-selective.
- Carvedilol, a third-generation BB, is both a nonselective β-adrenoreceptor antagonist and selective α_1-adrenoreceptor antagonist, such that it also has vasodilatory action to reduce afterload.[122,151–154]

BBs are part of core therapy for heart failure in humans, in both early and advanced stages.[121,155,156] They counter the increased sympathetic tone and RAAS activation characteristic of the neuroendocrine system that is central to the pathogenesis and progression of CHF.[124,157] By retarding its deleterious effects, β-blockade is beneficial in treatment of heart failure, ultimately improving systolic function despite the attendant negative inotropic effect. Longer-term actions of BBs include regression of myocardial hypertrophy, reversal of remodeling, and normalization of ventricular geometry. In addition, the antioxidant properties of some BBs, including carvedilol, may also contribute to their beneficial effects. In human cardiovascular medicine, second- and third-generation BBs are used in combination with diuretics and ACEI for treatment of chronic, stable CHF related to left ventricular systolic dysfunction (including DCM).[121,124,155,157] In dogs, these drugs have also garnered interest as adjunctive treatment of CHF, although their efficacy has not yet been established.[122,124,153]

BBs and ACEI are also used to prevent heart failure in cases with structural cardiac abnormalities (eg, left ventricular hypertrophy, valvular disease) and systolic dysfunction that are as yet asymptomatic.[121] Similarly, BBs have been suggested as part of treatment for preclinical chronic degenerative AV valve disease (chronic valve disease [CVD]) and preclinical DCM in dogs, because they might delay progression to heart failure.[122] Although similar considerations may apply to small mammals, recommendations regarding the use of BBs have thus far been limited to cases of HCM. One case report in a ferret noted favorable results following the use of atenolol in a 17-month-old ferret diagnosed with tetralogy of Fallot.[158]

The beneficial effects of BBs have been documented in avian models of heart failure. Propranolol, carteolol, atenolol, metoprolol, and carvedilol have been investigated in the furazolidone-induced model of DCM in turkey poults as well as in spontaneously occurring, idiopathic DCM in these birds. Cardioprotective effects of these agents, both grossly and at the microscopic level, have been repeatedly demonstrated in birds concurrently receiving furazolidone:

- Propranolol has been found to prevent the gross morphologic changes (chamber dilatation, wall thinning) and microscopic changes (including cardiomyocyte hypertrophy) characteristic of the disease, benefits not seen with digoxin.
- Atenolol has similar, although lesser, cardioprotective effects, and both drugs have been shown to normalize myocardial contractility.
- Cardioprotective efficacy of BBs is dose dependent and greatest with nonselective BBs; efficacy is ranked in descending order as carteolol > propranolol > atenolol ≥ metoprolol.[64–67]

Other studies have focused on treatment of established, advanced furazolidone-induced heart failure in turkeys, in which cardiac chamber dilatation and decreased systolic function were documented by echocardiography. All BBs examined were found to improve systolic performance and decrease mortality:

- Treatment with carteolol, at both low dose (0.01 mg/kg PO every 12 hours) and high dose (10 mg/kg PO every 12 hours, uptitrated from 2.5 mg/kg over a period of 4 days) resulted in significant decreases in cardiac chamber sizes and wall thinning, improvement in systolic performance, reduction in myocardial fibrosis, and reversal of cardiomyocyte hypertrophy.[67]
- Birds receiving carvedilol for 4 weeks, at 1 mg/kg or 20 mg/kg PO every 24 hours, showed significant improvements in left ventricular volume and fractional shortening (by 80% in some individuals) and had reduced apoptosis of cardiomyocytes (possibly because of the drug's antioxidant properties).[64]

Adverse effects of BBs are typically dose dependent and include bradycardia, hypotension, and precipitation or worsening of heart failure.[122,151–154] However, most human heart failure patients will stabilize with reduction in the BB dose and appropriate adjustments to their conventional therapy.[121] In dogs, concurrent administration of pimobendan may enable patients to tolerate initiation and uptitration of β-blockade. In normal dogs receiving both carvedilol and pimobendan, there are synergistic vasodilatory effects and conserved positive inotropic effects.[122,124]

If BB administration is abruptly stopped, tachyarrhythmia and sudden death may occur.[122] BBs are contraindicated in patients with decompensated heart failure, bradycardia, or greater than first-degree AV block.[151–154] They should not be combined with other BBs or CCBs.[122]

In turkey poults with furazolidone-induced DCM, studies have evaluated maximum tolerated doses of several BBs:

- One study indicated a maximum dose of 30 mg/kg propranolol PO every 8 hours and 30 mg/kg atenolol PO every 24 hours, each defined by an absence of adverse effects (sedation, persistent bradycardia, hypotension).[66]
- In the carteolol study, neither the low nor high dose reduced blood pressure (as determined by indirect method), but heart rate acutely decreased (by <10%) for up to 4 hours in birds receiving the high dose.[67]

- Some individual birds receiving high-dose carvedilol (20 mg/kg) became moribund with significantly decreased heart rate and blood pressure for up to 8 hours. However, results of that study demonstrated that the beneficial effects of the drug do not require high enough doses to produce bradycardia and hypotension.[64]

One of the authors (B.C.F.) suggests that BBs may have application in avian cardiology as adjunctive treatment of CHF, provided the condition is first stabilized using conventional management strategies. This author has used carvedilol, in conjunction with diuretics and an ACEI, as part of treatment of CHF in psittacines, specifically when concentric ventricular hypertrophy, tachycardia, and diastolic dysfunction were features. Goals and guidelines for BB use should realistically mirror those set forth for canine and feline patients with heart disease or failure (**Box 1**).[122] Concurrent administration of a positive inotrope, such as pimobendan, during the period of BB uptitration may allow patients to tolerate initiation of treatment. Close monitoring during initiation of treatment as well as regular follow-up over the long term are essential.

Calcium channel blockers

CCBs, including nifedipine, verapamil, diltiazem, and amlodipine, inhibit influx of extracellular calcium ions across cardiomyocyte and vascular smooth muscle cell membranes, thereby inhibiting contraction. Effects are negative inotropy and chronotropy, slowing of the sinus rate and AV nodal conduction, and vasodilation. CCBs are classified by their relative selectivity for the vasculature or for the myocardium; those that predominately promote peripheral vasodilation and reduce total peripheral resistance (eg, nifedipine and amlodipine) are indicated primarily for treatment of hypertension, and those that influence conduction (eg, verapamil and diltiazem) are indicated for treatment of supraventricular tachyarrhythmias.[68,159–161] Similar indications for use of CCBs have been mentioned in small mammals.[14,29,30,34,43,70,162]

In human heart failure patients with systolic dysfunction, CCBs confer no survival benefit and may exacerbate the condition.[121] Nevertheless, CCBs warrant mention because their cardioprotective effects have been investigated in furazolidone-induced DCM of turkey poults and found to rival those of BBs. Both nifedipine and

---

Box 1
Goals and guidelines for β-blocker therapy in small animal heart disease and failure

- Begin with a low initial dose (*especially* in patients with systolic dysfunction or HF).
- Uptitrate the dose gradually.
  - Increase dose by 25% to 100% at weekly-biweekly intervals.
  - If a dose increase precipitates clinical signs of HF, reduce dose to the last tolerated dose and institute/adjust HF therapy.
    - If HF is severe, reduce the dose by 50%. Once the patient is stabilized, gradual uptitration can recommence if tolerated.
- Aim for the highest tolerated dose (dose that achieves adequate clinical effect).
  - Benefits of β-blockade may take months to achieve.
- Never stop treatment abruptly; instead reduce dose gradually if treatment must be discontinued.

Abbreviation: HF, heart failure.
Modified from Gordon SG. Beta blocking agents. In: Ettinger SJ, Feldman EC, editors. Textbook of veterinary internal medicine. 7th edition. St Louis (MO): Elsevier Saunders; 2010. p. 1207–11.

verapamil are cardioprotective (nifedipine > verapamil), but the mechanisms by which these drugs confer their benefits are unknown.[66,163] In addition, CCBs have been evaluated as preventative agents in experimentally induced PH and right-sided CHF (ascites syndrome) of broiler chickens[69,71] (see the following section). Given an absence of systemic effects, the investigators concluded that diltiazem is more selective for the pulmonary vasculature than for the systemic vasculature in these birds.[69] To the authors' knowledge, no reports are available on the clinical use of CCBs in birds, nor in small mammals or reptiles.

Adverse effects of CCBs include bradycardia, hypotension and reflex tachycardia, and AV block.[68,159–161] Contraindications include SA nodal dysfunction, second- or third-degree AV block, and decompensated heart failure.[68,160,161]

Treatment of Related Conditions

CHF may be accompanied by disease processes such as HCM, systemic and/or PH, and arrhythmias. These conditions thus deserve special consideration and are discussed below.

Hypertrophic cardiomyopathy

HCM comprises hyperplasia or thickening of individual muscle fibers of the heart. Although the disease has been reported to occur in ferrets, rabbits, rats, and hamsters, actual cases have been poorly documented, with little to no information available on its treatment. In birds, HCM is more common, but is usually secondary to pressure overload states (cardiomyopathy of overload), including arterial luminal stenosis due to advanced atherosclerosis, and PH.[3,21,91,143,164,165] As in mammals, the affected ventricle or ventricles ultimately undergo concentric hypertrophy, in which the ventricular wall thickens with a corresponding decrease in chamber volume. Eventual ischemia of the hypertrophied myocardium results in fibrosis and increased collagen content, impairing both systolic and diastolic function.[89,90] Analogous conditions in human and small animal medicine are ventricular outflow obstructions such as subvalvular aortic stenosis and primary HCM to include the obstructive type characterized by systolic anterior motion of the mitral valve. BBs are used in treatment of these conditions; their potential benefit is based on reduction of heart rate and myocardial oxygen consumption as well as improved diastolic filling and coronary artery flow.[122,166] However, in cats, evidence of their efficacy is scarce, with little to no indication that they improve survival in patients with CHF.[122,167]

Anecdotally, BBs can have merit for treatment of HCM in birds. One of the authors (B.C.F.) has used carvedilol, with or without an ACEI, in a small number of psittacines with suspected atherosclerotic disease and concentric ventricular hypertrophy that had not yet progressed to failure. In each of these cases, there has been symptomatic improvement in the form of increased energy and activity level, appetite, and body weight. One of these cases included a 34-year-old, female yellow-naped Amazon parrot (Amazona auropalliata) that was treated for biventricular CHF secondary to advanced atherosclerotic disease. There was marked concentric hypertrophy of both ventricles, diastolic dysfunction, and sinus tachycardia. Following initial management with standard therapy (furosemide, spironolactone, enalapril, sildenafil, and pimobendan), clinical status deteriorated and carvedilol was added to the treatment regimen; pimobendan was discontinued. Following these changes in the treatment protocol, rapid and marked clinical improvement was seen, after which the patient remained stable for an additional 7 months.

Systemic hypertension

Systemic hypertension can be encountered in several small mammal species and can lead to CHF. It is particularly common in aged male rats, wherein it appears to occur in association with other age-related diseases (eg, renal failure). Systemic hypertension has also been suspected to occur in conjunction with pheochromocytomas (eg, in ferrets[162]) or hyperthyroidism (eg, in guinea pigs[168]). Systemic hypertension occurs in poultry species and can result in severe ventricular hypertrophy and CHF.[169] Although not defined in psittacines,[170] systemic hypertension probably is a disease entity in this group as well.[171] In human and small animal medicine, BBs are often used in conjunction with ACEI, CCBs, and/or diuretics to reduce arterial blood pressure.[121,122,172] In humans, such treatment markedly reduces the risk of developing heart failure, and combined therapy with a BB and ACEI is recommended in cases of diastolic heart failure with concurrent hypertension.[121] In cats, CCB amlodipine is the treatment of choice for systemic hypertension; it has been shown to significantly reduce blood pressure, and in one study, resolved secondary ventricular hypertrophy in 50% of subjects.[172] In birds and other exotics, application of BBs, CCBs, or other antihypertensive drugs for treatment of systemic hypertension is largely precluded by the fact that there is no practical means to obtain accurate and repeatable arterial blood pressure measurements in the clinical setting, and, in birds, no established definition of hypertension exists.[98,173,174] However, if in select cases, direct blood pressure measurements are obtained and support a diagnosis of hypertension (systolic blood pressure >240 mm Hg in birds; >180 mm Hg in small mammals),[99,170] combined treatment of an ACEI with a BB or a CCB may be considered. Because indirect blood pressure measurements thus far do not seem to correlate well with direct arterial blood pressures in either birds or mammals, monitoring of the actual effects of these treatments is complicated because it would require the use of invasive techniques.

Pulmonary hypertension

Compared with mammals, birds are thought to have a greater propensity for developing PH and right-sided, rather than left-sided CHF owing to the morphology of the right AV valve, less deformable nucleated erythrocytes, and the rigid, nondistensible lungs that limit the ability of the blood capillaries to expand and accommodate greater blood flow.[91,175] PH can result from pulmonary vascular disease (to include atherosclerosis), chronic pulmonary disease and/or hypoxia, congenital left-to-right shunts, or left-sided heart disease and failure.[3,21,47,91,143,164,165,176,177] Secondary polycythemia, which develops as a consequence of chronic hypoxemia, can be a complicating factor in several disease conditions, including PH. Increased blood viscosity and larger and less deformable erythrocytes result in increased resistance to blood flow in the lung and other tissues.[47,69,71,164,165,178–180]

Certainly the known or hypothesized underlying cause or causes of PH should be addressed, if possible, but pulmonary vasodilators (sildenafil), CCBs, pentoxifylline, and periodic phlebotomy may have symptomatic benefit in birds with a presumptive or definitive diagnosis of PH.[47] Similarly, the inclusion of these drugs should be considered in treatment of CHF patients with cor pulmonale.

Pulmonary Vasodilators

Sildenafil is a selective pulmonary vasodilator that acts by specifically inhibiting phosphodiesterase V, an enzyme that degrades cyclic guanosine monophosphate (cGMP) in pulmonary vascular smooth muscle cells. The resulting increase in cGMP enhances nitric oxide–mediated pulmonary vasodilation, thereby reducing pulmonary vascular resistance and right ventricular afterload. The drug does not typically lower systemic arterial blood pressure or alter heart rate.[176,177,181–183] Its hypotensive effects may be increased upon concurrent use of α-adrenoceptor blockers, amlodipine, or other hypotensive drugs. In addition, its metabolism may be reduced by administration of azole antifungals.[181] In humans and dogs, sildenafil is an effective treatment of PH[176,177,181–183] and has been shown to improve quality of life and mitigate secondary polycythemia in dogs.[176,181,182]

In birds, prolonged (>15 months) use of sildenafil (2.5–3 mg/kg PO every 8 hours) has been described in a 25-year-old male mealy Amazon parrot (Amazona farinosa) with suspected PH (based on clinical signs, secondary, absolute polycythemia, and consistent echocardiographic findings), in addition to therapeutic phlebotomy, and supplemental oxygen. In this bird, resolution and reappearance of the clinical signs (lethargy, anorexia, ataxia, tachypnea/dyspnea, and oxygen dependence) were found to coincide with changes to the dosing frequency (from every 8 to every 12 hours).[47] In addition, one of the authors (B.C.F.) has treated an unknown-age, female rose-breasted cockatoo (Eolophus roseicapilla) with suspected PH, in which the clinical signs (lethargy and exercise intolerance) rapidly resolved with administration of sildenafil (2 mg/kg PO every 12 hours) and enalapril (3 mg/kg PO every 12 hours). Over a period of 1 year, doses of both drugs have been gradually increased to 5 mg/kg PO every 12 hours. Right ventricular hypertrophy had decreased 6 months into treatment.

Other Treatment Options

Patients with suspected PH may also benefit from the following therapies:

- ACEI, which reduce pulmonary vascular resistance as well as total peripheral resistance.[132] In growing broiler chickens exposed to low temperatures to induce PH and right-sided CHF (ascites syndrome), enalapril administration (in the drinking water, 42 days) reduced right ventricular hypertrophy and mortality.[184] Similarly, imidapril (3 mg/kg PO every 24 hours for 30 days) prevented low temperature–induced PH and right ventricular hypertrophy in broilers.[185,186]
- Pimobendan, which has both systemic and pulmonary vasodilatory effects.[55,138,177]
- CCBs, including diltiazem (15 mg/kg PO every 12 hours, 27 days) and low-dose verapamil (5 mg/kg PO every 12 hours, 27 days), which were both capable of preventing low temperature–induced PH, right ventricular hypertrophy, and polycythemia in growing broilers. Nifedipine, in contrast, was comparably ineffective and had systemic side effects.[69,71]
- Pentoxifylline, which is a methylxanthine derivative with hemorrheologic and immunomodulatory effects. In mammals, pentoxifylline increases flexibility and deformability of erythrocytes and leukocytes (thereby promoting their passage through damaged or occluded microvasculature) and decreases blood viscosity by reducing plasma fibrinogen and increasing fibrinolytic activity.[187,188] Because of these effects, pentoxifylline may have merit in patients with PH and secondary polycythemia and hyperviscosity syndrome.
- Therapeutic phlebotomy, which is indicated in humans with secondary polycythemia when hematocrit exceeds 56% or when there are hyperviscosity symptoms.[178] In small animals, hyperviscosity syndrome develops when hematocrit exceeds 65% to 68%, and periodic phlebotomy (with crystalloid volume replacement) is performed to maintain hematocrit between 62% and 68%.[166] Phlebotomy was also used as part of the treatment regimen in the previously mentioned Amazon parrot diagnosed with PH. In this bird, intermittent epistaxis

was seen and attributed to hyperviscosity syndrome resulting from secondary, absolute polycythemia (hematocrit 71%; reference interval 40%–55%). Following phlebotomy, during which 10 mL/kg blood was removed (while 60 mL/kg crystalloid fluids were administered concurrently), hematocrit decreased to 58%. Ongoing treatment, consisting of regular phlebotomy (5–10 mL/kg every 4–6 weeks) and oral sildenafil, resulted in long-term resolution of the clinical signs.[47]

Arrhythmias

Cardiac arrhythmias range from clinically insignificant to life-threatening and/or terminal events. Clinical signs may be absent or include weakness, syncope, or sudden death. Arrhythmias rarely constitute a primary disease process; they can develop secondary to cardiac chamber dilatation, myocarditis, or cardiomyopathy of any cause as well as toxicoses, nutritional deficiencies, electrolyte imbalances, and various anesthetic agents.[22,159,189–192] They can be potentiated by catecholamine release as occurs with handling stress and painful conditions.[22,193,194] Clinically significant cardiac arrhythmias likely represent the minority, but those that are symptomatic, causing hemodynamic instability, and complicating or precipitating heart failure warrant characterization and appropriate treatment.[121,159] To date, reports of antiarrhythmic therapy in birds, small mammals, and reptiles are extremely few.

Reported arrhythmias in birds and small mammals can be categorized by relative clinical significance[22,29,56,61,97,159,189–196]:

- Physiologic basis and/or clinically benign:
  - Respiratory sinus arrhythmia (Note: *not* seen in rabbits), wandering pacemaker, and occasional sinus arrest and SA block can occur with increased vagal tone.
  - Supraventricular premature complexes (SPCs) and ventricular premature complexes (VPCs) have been reported in apparently healthy, unanesthetized chickens, Amazon and gray parrots, ferrets, and rabbits.
  - First-degree AV block and second-degree AV block (Mobitz type 1) may be found in healthy individuals of some species, including chickens, racing pigeons, and Amazon and gray parrots, ferrets, and rabbits. These arrhythmias may occur with some frequency during anesthetic events.
- Greater likelihood of pathologic basis and clinical disease:
  - Sinus bradycardia
  - Sinus tachycardia
  - SPC and supraventricular tachycardia
  - Atrial fibrillation
  - VPC
  - Sinus arrest and SA block
  - Mobitz type 2 second-degree AV block; has the potential to progress to third-degree AV block
- Pathologic basis and high probability of severe clinical disease:
  - Ventricular tachycardia
  - Ventricular fibrillation
  - Third-degree AV block
  - Bundle branch block

In reptiles, diagnosis of rate or rhythm disturbances is complicated because of the limited amount of reference material available to assist in interpretation as well as the limited degree of sensitivity associated with the available equipment. In addition, results can vary greatly between and within species, and even within the individual based on the environmental temperature and physiologic status of the animal.[17,19]

Treatment of Tachyarrhythmias

Aside from digoxin, BBs and CCBs are used in small animal cardiology for treatment of supraventricular tachyarrhythmias, including atrial fibrillation, in order to slow the ventricular response rate.[159] Their use is generally contraindicated in patients with acute or decompensated CHF unless the arrhythmia is contributing to the condition such that conventional treatment alone has failed to stabilize the patient.[68,159–161] However, even in this scenario, these drugs must be used with great caution, beginning at low dosages, with the aim of decreasing ventricular rate only marginally.[159]

Lidocaine is a parenteral antiarrhythmic agent used to control life-threatening ventricular tachyarrhythmias.[159] It reduces automaticity by blocking fast sodium channels, particularly in damaged or ischemic portions of the myocardium. At usual doses, there is minimal effect on the cardiac conduction system or on myocardial contractility. Adverse effects, including central nervous system signs (reduced mentation, ataxia, or seizures), may be seen at higher doses.[159,197] To the authors' knowledge, there are no reports describing its use for treatment of tachyarrhythmias in exotic animals. Nevertheless, its pharmacokinetics and cardiovascular effects have been evaluated during experimental studies. Two recent studies in isoflurane-anesthetized broiler chickens (*Gallus gallus domesticus*) and Hispaniolan Amazon parrots identified mild, transient bradycardia and, in Amazon parrots, mild increases in arterial blood pressure following IV administration of lidocaine (2.5 mg/kg).[78,80] Similarly, infusion of 6 mg/kg lidocaine over 2 minutes was well tolerated in chickens, with only mild decreases in heart rate and mean arterial blood pressure. ED_{50} (ie, the dose at which 50% of test subjects would have mild cardiovascular depression) was determined to be 6.3 mg/kg.[79]

Treatment of Bradyarrhythmias

Bradyarrhythmias, and in particular, second- and third-degree AV blocks, have been noted in both birds and small mammals (ferrets, rabbits) with cardiac disease.[56,159,191,192,198,199] Escape beats and escape rhythms may be seen with severe bradyarrhythmias; they are of ectopic origin and perform an essential salvage function by preventing asystole at low heart rates. QRS morphology of ventricular escape beats may be abnormal (wide and bizarre), but these should not be confused with premature beats (additional beats added to already normal or rapid heart rate), because in the case of escape beats, antiarrhythmic therapy is contraindicated.[159,192]

Antimuscarinic agents, including atropine and glycopyrrolate, competitively inhibit binding of acetylcholine (and other cholinergic stimulants) to muscarinic receptors and can be used for both the diagnosis and the treatment of bradycardias related to increased vagal tone, including SA arrest and first- and second-degree AV block.[21,76,143,200] In rabbits, the effects of atropine may be lowered because of the presence of atropinase. In comparison with birds and mammals, reptiles have low heart rates so use of atropine or glycopyrrolate is rarely indicated. Nevertheless, when real bradycardia is encountered, the use of both drugs can be considered because reptile catecholamines share similarities with those of mammals, such as the presence of β-adrenergic receptors that mediate the chronotropic and ionotropic effect of catecholamines.[18,201] However, in iguanas, both drugs were found ineffective in blocking the negative chronotropic effects of vagal stimulation of the heart.[202]

Because the activity of atropine and glycopyrrolate is short-lived, these drugs are mainly used during treatment of bradycardia during anesthesia. For long-term use, propantheline, an oral antimuscarinic agent, has been used at a dose of 0.3 mg/kg

PO every 8 hours to normalize heart rate and rhythm in a 30-year-old Moluccan cockatoo (*Cacatua moluccensis*) with second-degree AV block (Mobitz type 2). Clinical signs of periodic dyspnea and syncopal episodes improved, and the bird remained stable for at least 2 years.[56]

Other drugs that can be used in an attempt to increase the ventricular rate with second- or third-degree AV block include theophylline, metaproterenol, pseudoephedrine, or isoproterenol. Metaproterenol is considered more convenient than isoproterenol because of the longer duration of action but is not as effective at maintaining heart rates of greater than 80 bpm.[14,119,120] However, in many patients, these aforementioned drugs will have insufficient effect, necessitating placement of a pacemaker. For most species, this may not be a feasible option because of their size or heart rate, but in ferrets and a rabbit, such pacemakers have been successfully implanted using transvenous or transabdominal techniques.[191,198,199]

Supportive Care and Husbandry Considerations

Along with medical management of CHF, it is often necessary to address concurrent problems and meet specific supportive needs. Patients may be presented in a severely debilitated state, with cachexia, dehydration, secondary renal dysfunction, and injuries.

In-patient supportive care measures may include oxygen supplementation, nutritional support, and fluid therapy (although parenteral fluid administration must be carefully questioned). Once the patient has been stabilized and discharged, longer-term management strategies should also incorporate exercise restriction, housing modifications, and dietary and lifestyle changes.

Supportive care

General supportive principles apply to the exotic heart failure patient, namely rest, minimizing stress with judicious, limited handling and restraint, and provision of supplemental oxygen when appropriate. Patients are typically dyspneic because of pulmonary edema, intracoelomic air sac compression by ascitic fluid, and/or pleural (in the case of mammals) or pericardial effusion. Oxygen supplementation is indicated for patients with pulmonary edema, whereas physical fluid removal is more efficacious to stabilize those with air sac or pulmonary compression and cardiac tamponade (for pericardiocentesis, see the next section).

When providing supplemental oxygen, care must be taken to avoid oxygen toxicity by excessive supplementation. For example, repeated acute exposures (95% concentration for 3 hours on 3 consecutive days) and chronic exposure (95% concentration for 72 hours) resulted in pulmonary congestion, edema, inflammatory infiltrates, and thickening of the blood-gas barrier in budgerigars (*Melopsittacus undulatus*).[203] Thoracocentesis or abdominocentesis/coelomocentesis will rapidly relieve air sac or pulmonary compression in case of ascites or pleural effusion, respectively. Although the procedure can be performed periodically over the longer term, it should not be substituted for pharmacologic management.

Fluid therapy challenges

Maintaining the delicate balance between management of hypervolemia and concurrent dehydration and renal dysfunction is a profound clinical challenge, requiring close monitoring for changes in clinical status and adjustment of the treatment plan accordingly. In-patient treatment is necessary until the patient has been stabilized to the extent that appetite and water intake are acceptable, hypervolemia is adequately controlled and hydration adequate, oxygen supplementation no longer needed, and parenteral medications withdrawn. Fluid therapy is generally not indicated in the treatment of CHF wherein a primary, immediate goal is reduction of fluid overload. Initial treatment of acute and decompensated CHF frequently results in some degree of dehydration and prerenal azotemia, but these abnormalities can resolve over a few days once food and water intake have normalized.

In cases with persistent, severe azotemia, it may be necessary to administer small volumes of parenteral fluids, but patients for which hemodynamic stability cannot be achieved without severe renal compromise have a poor prognosis. Subcutaneous fluid absorption may fail in cases of right-sided CHF.

Exercise restriction and housing

Weakness and ataxia may limit patient mobility and access to food and water and predispose to falls (in the case of birds). Impaired mobility necessitates housing modifications designed to limit exertion and allow easy, immediate access to food and water. As even debilitated bird, ferret, and rodent patients will often persist in trying to climb or perch, enclosures that prevent or limit this activity are ideal. Incubators, aquarium setups, or plastic or acrylic bins with a soft substrate serve this purpose well and permit visual monitoring. Depending on patient strength and stability, a low, secure, and stable perch can be provided for birds (eg, rope perch or rolled towel situated on the bottom of the enclosure). Once the patient regains strength and exercise tolerance, housing can be adjusted to allow greater activity (eg, small cage or crate, furnished with low perches and readily accessible dishes in case of birds); some patients will ultimately be able to return to a traditional cage with no specific exercise restrictions.

Diet and lifestyle

For birds, longer-term husbandry considerations, including dietary changes (which should also entail sodium restriction) and lifestyle changes, mirror those discussed for atherosclerosis. However, dietary changes should not be made until the patient is well stabilized. Given that CHF often arises secondary to atherosclerotic disease in psittacine birds, preventative considerations may be applicable to both conditions (see following section).

Dietary management in small mammals likely follows similar guidelines, such as those described for dogs and cats, that is, ensuring adequate caloric intake to prevent obesity or cachexia; ensuring adequate protein intake (including intake of essential amino acids such as L-carnitine and taurine, because taurine deficiency has been proposed as a cause for DCM in carnivorous species such as the ferret),[112,162] and ensuring adequate mineral intake (ie, restricting sodium intake, and supplementing chloride, potassium, and/or magnesium, if needed). In addition, increased intake of omega-3 fatty acids (present in fish oil supplements) has been considered beneficial because of their anti-inflammatory properties and propensity to exert antihypertensive effects and reduce mortality from coronary heart disease in humans.[204–206]

Other

Considering that most patients will require long-term (if not life-long) medical management, operant learning methods and food vehicles should be used to facilitate low-stress medication administration (please see Brian L. Speer and colleagues' article, "Low Stress Medication Techniques in Birds and Small Mammals," in this issue).

Effective long-term management furthermore requires regular follow-up (to include physical examination, repeat imaging, and biochemical monitoring) to reevaluate patient status and make necessary adjustments to the treatment regimen. Success is dependent in large part on owner compliance, so thorough client education and communication are essential.

PERICARDIAL EFFUSION/CARDIAC TAMPONADE

Pericardial effusion is characterized by an inappropriate accumulation of fluid within the pericardial sac. Possible causes are listed in **Table 4**, although in some cases an underlying cause cannot be identified and the condition is ruled idiopathic. Severe pericardial effusion or restrictive pericarditis can compress the heart, resulting in impaired ventricular filling (diastolic dysfunction), and subsequent decreases in stroke volume and cardiac output. This condition, which can become life threatening, is referred to as cardiac tamponade. Because the intramural pressure of the thinner-walled right ventricle is overcome more rapidly than that of the left, cardiac tamponade results more quickly in right-sided CHF than in left-sided failure.[22,208]

Echocardiography is undoubtedly the most efficient, highest-yield method for diagnosis of pericardial effusion.[21,22,143,209] The elements of a comprehensive diagnostic workup for CHF apply also to differentiating between possible causes of pericardial disease and effusion.

Regardless of the species involved, treatment of pericardial effusion and cardiac tamponade is based first on removal of the fluid, and second on treatment of the underlying cause of fluid accumulation.[21,22,94,208,210] Fluid removal can be accomplished either by ultrasound-guided[7,21,42,207] or, in birds, endoscopic pericardiocentesis, or by endoscopic or surgical fenestration of the pericardium.[22,94,143,210,211] Although diuretics are generally contraindicated in cardiac tamponade because they decrease the preload necessary to maintain ventricular filling pressure and cardiac output, furosemide with or without an ACEI may be useful to reduce pericardial fluid of low volume related to CHF in birds.[8,21,22,42,104] For example, furosemide has been used as part of combination medical management of CHF in a yellow-crowned Amazon parrot (*Amazona ochrocephala*) and in a blue-fronted Amazon parrot (*Amazona aestiva*) in which low-grade pericardial effusion was also a feature.[8,104] In the first case, furosemide was administered at a dose of 0.15 mg/kg IM every 24 hours in combination with enalapril, resulting in resolution of pericardial effusion.[8] In the second case, furosemide was administered at a dose of 0.2 mg/kg IM every 12 hours in combination with a cardiac glycoside (digoxin), resulting in reduction, although not resolution, of pericardial effusion.[104]

Endoscopic partial pericardiectomy was used by one of the authors (B.C.F.) to relieve cardiac tamponade in a 14-year-old, female jenday conure (*Aratinga jandaya*) with pericardial effusion and fibrinous pericarditis of undetermined primary cause. The bird remained clinically healthy for 6 years afterward.

Table 4
Causes of pericardial effusion in birds, small mammals, and reptiles

Birds[93,207]	Small Mammals[94]	Reptiles[94]
Infectious pericarditis	Infectious pericarditis	Infectious pericarditis
Noninfectious pericarditis (visceral gout)	Primary myocardial disease or CHF	Noninfectious pericarditis (visceral gout)
Right-sided CHF	Hemopericardium (trauma, aneurismal rupture, coagulopathy)	CHF
Hemopericardium (trauma, aneurismal rupture, coagulopathy)	Neoplasia (lymphoma)	Hemopericardium (trauma, aneurismal rupture, coagulopathy)
Cardiac or pericardial neoplasia	Hypoproteinemia	Neoplasia
Metabolic derangements (eg, hypoproteinemia)		
Toxic causes		

ATHEROSCLEROTIC DISEASE

Atherosclerosis is a chronic inflammatory and degenerative disease of the arterial wall wherein the lumen narrows by progressive accumulation of fibrofatty atheromatous plaques within the intima. Advanced lesions are characterized by severe arterial stenosis and occlusion, and by calcification and osseous metaplasia. Although atherosclerosis has been reported to occur in small mammals and reptiles,[94] the disease rarely causes clinical disease. However, in companion psittacine birds, atherosclerosis is likely an underlying factor in most noninfectious cardiovascular diseases. Lesions are most frequently recognized in the ascending aorta, brachiocephalic trunks, and pulmonary arteries, but occur in the peripheral vasculature as well (eg, coronary and carotid arteries, descending aorta, subclavian arteries, celiac artery, and ischiatic arteries). Prevalence is highest in gray parrots (*Psittacus* spp), Amazon parrots (*Amazona* spp), and cockatiels (*Nymphicus hollandicus*). Other risk factors include increasing age, female sex, high-calorie, -fat, and -cholesterol diets, dyslipidemia (eg, hypercholesterolemia), and limited physical activity.[171,212–215]

Clinical signs are attributed to advanced lesions, whereas early and intermediate lesions are generally silent and subclinical. Unlike humans, recognizable clinical disease is primarily the product of progressive, flow-limiting arterial stenosis rather than thrombosis and hemorrhage of disrupted plaques that results in thromboembolism and acute arterial obstruction.[171,212,213,215] Clinical signs vary depending on the vessels affected, severity of atherosclerotic lesions, and presence of concurrent disease, including cardiac disease and CHF.[171,214] Patients often present for falling or collapse, frequently accompanied by transient or persistent weakness and dysfunction of one or more limbs. There may be persistent neurologic abnormalities identified on physical examination, including reduced mentation, blindness, anisocoria, seizures, vestibular signs, paresis of one or both pelvic limbs, and ataxia. These signs are considered most consistent with stroke, but rarely is this confirmed diagnostically.[9,171] Diagnostic options include radiography, angiography, CT, and MRI.[9,102,105,171,216,217]

Treatment of atherosclerosis involves both controlling risk factors and managing sequelae, including peripheral hypoperfusion, ischemic stroke, and CHF.[171] Atherosclerotic lesions cannot be resolved, but diet, husbandry, and lifestyle changes may help to prevent, slow progression, or decrease the size of lesions. Medical management focuses primarily on improving peripheral perfusion. Peripheral vasodilators, used either singly or in combination, may have symptomatic benefit by decreasing vascular resistance and reducing afterload.

Vasodilation

Isoxsuprine

Isoxsuprine is a peripheral vasodilator that causes vascular smooth muscle relaxation predominately through α-adrenoceptor blockade.[218,219] It furthermore is a β-adrenoreceptor agonist and as such may have positive chronotropic and inotropic effects.[220] In addition, it is known to increase erythrocyte deformability in humans.[221] In veterinary medicine, isoxsuprine is used to increase peripheral blood flow in horses with vascular disorders of the lower limb and to address trauma-induced wingtip edema in raptors.[41,222] In a published report, a 35-year-old yellow-naped Amazon (*A auropalliata*) with presumptive atherosclerosis (based on clinical signs and suggestive radiographic findings) was treated with isoxsuprine (10 mg/kg PO every 24 hours). Clinical signs of lethargy, weakness, hyporexia, weak grip, and ataxia resolved with treatment and repeatedly recurred when the drug was discontinued, again resolving once it was reinstituted.[41] One of the authors (B.C.F.) has observed similar, apparent symptomatic improvement when using isoxsuprine (beginning at 10 mg/kg PO every 12–24 hours) in numerous cases of presumed atherosclerosis (some of which were later confirmed at necropsy and by histopathology). Many of these patients have been treated and followed for several months to several years, over which time frequency and severity of strokelike events and other clinical signs appeared to decrease.

Angiotensin-converting enzyme inhibitors
ACEI, including enalapril and benazepril, result in vasodilation by blocking the formation of angiotensin II (AII).[131] AII promotes vasoconstriction and venoconstriction by mediating release of catecholamines, which act on vascular smooth muscle via α-adrenergic receptors.[223] As a result, they reduce both total peripheral resistance and pulmonary vascular resistance.[132] Although the relative vasodilatory effect of an ACEI compared with isoxsuprine in birds is not known, it is conceivable that the 2 used in combination would have synergistic effects: an ACEI by limiting α-adrenoreceptor stimulation and isoxsuprine by α-adrenoreceptor antagonism.

Sildenafil
Sildenafil has predominantly been used for treatment of PH in humans and dogs.[176,177,181–183] In birds, the drug may have merit in cases with suspected atherosclerosis of the pulmonary arteries, potentially in combination with other vasodilators.

Other Medical Managements

Pentoxifylline
In human medicine, pentoxifylline has been used for the treatment of peripheral vascular and cerebrovascular disease.[187,188,224] In studies using small mammal models, the drug was found to increase tissue perfusion and mitigate inflammation, thereby significantly improving tissue survival after frostbite.[187,224] In addition, pentoxifylline was found to attenuate plaque formation in New Zealand white rabbits with experimentally induced (by cholesterol feeding) atherosclerosis, possibly through anti-inflammatory effects.[187] Based on these findings, pentoxifylline has been suggested as an adjunct therapy for frostbite in birds and used empirically at a dose of 15 mg/kg PO every 8 to 12 hours for 2 to 6 weeks (numerous species) and 25 mg/kg PO every 12 hours for 2 weeks (gray-headed parrot, *Poicephalus fuscicollis suahelicus*) with no apparent adverse effects.[224,225] The drug may furthermore have value in improving peripheral perfusion in birds with atherosclerotic disease and has been recommended as part of treatment of burns in reptiles, but not reported for treatment of cardiovascular disease.[187,226]

Statins
Statins are a group of lipid-lowering drugs used extensively in human medicine for their antiatherosclerotic effects through inhibition of cholesterol synthesis and other mechanisms. Statins reduce both plasma total cholesterol and low-density lipoprotein (LDL) cholesterol concentrations, whereas to a lesser extent increasing high-density lipoprotein cholesterol concentration.

Several products are commercially available for human use, including lovastatin, simvastatin, pravastatin, fluvastatin, atorvastatin, and rosuvastatin. Of these, only atorvastatin (Lipitor) and rosuvastatin (Crestor) have a long half-life in humans and are most commonly used.[227]

In chickens (*G gallus domesticus*), statins have been used experimentally to establish their cholesterol-lowering effect. One study demonstrated significantly lower plasma total cholesterol concentrations in white leghorn hens fed either a 0.03% or a 0.06% atorvastatin or simvastatin diet.[228] Statins have furthermore been used empirically in psittacine birds, but their use is controversial because no pharmacodynamic information is available for these species. In addition, target levels of plasma total cholesterol and LDL that would reduce atherosclerosis risk are unknown. A recent study investigated the pharmacokinetics of orally administered rosuvastatin (Crestor) in Hispaniolan Amazon parrots (*A ventralis*). This study found that a dose of 10 mg/kg or 25 mg/kg (approximately 30 and 100 times the human dose, respectively) resulted in plasma concentrations below the limits of quantitation.[229] Consequently, the authors do not recommend use of statins in psittacines considered either to have or to be at risk for atherosclerotic disease. Instead, vasodilatory therapy (for symptomatic patients) and dietary and lifestyle changes are more appropriate.

Supportive Care and Husbandry Considerations

In addition to medical treatment, patients with clinical atherosclerosis and associated disease can benefit greatly from the following measures:

Supportive care
Patients with signs of stroke may have marked neurologic deficits to include reduced mentation, limb paresis, and ataxia that prevent normal eating and drinking and impair mobility. They may experience seizures or suffer injuries from falls. Supportive care measures to consider for these patients include fluid and nutritional support, analgesia, anticonvulsant therapy when needed, and management of secondary conditions, such as trauma and aspiration pneumonia.

Exercise restriction versus promotion of exercise
For patients with advanced, clinical atherosclerotic disease, exercise restriction should be part of the longer-term treatment plan as well as appropriate housing modifications to accommodate and protect birds with persistent deficits. In contrast, increasing opportunities for exercise (especially flight) from early in life may have preventative value.[171] Physical activity can be promoted through training and by designing captive environments to facilitate locomotion and foraging behaviors.

Dietary management
Dietary management may have both therapeutic and preventative value, particularly for at-risk species. Such measures include[171,215]

- Moderation of dietary calories and fat to prevent and resolve obesity
- Avoidance of dietary sources of cholesterol
- Supplementation with omega-3 fatty acids, particularly α-linolenic acid (found in flaxseed oil), has been shown to improve lipid metabolism, reduce inflammation, and minimize development of atherosclerosis in several avian species.[230–232]

Other
Along with dietary changes, control of female reproductive activity may help prevent atherosclerotic disease. For patients receiving medications long term, training to allow low-stress administration is indicated.

SUMMARY

Cardiovascular disease, including CHF, pericardial disease and effusion, and atherosclerosis, is becoming increasingly better recognized in companion birds, small mammals, and reptiles. Accurate and timely diagnosis, requiring comprehensive clinical assessment and essential diagnostic imaging (radiographs and ultrasound), provides an opportunity for successful intervention. Given limited pharmacologic data in exotic species, treatment approaches remain largely empirical and extrapolated from small animal and human medicine. Long-term prognosis for most cardiovascular diseases is guarded to poor, but the management strategies presented here have the potential to maintain quality of life and extend survival time for these patients.

REFERENCES

1. Knafo SE, Rapoport G, Williams J, et al. Cardiomyopathy and right-sided congestive heart failure in a red-tailed hawk (Buteo jamaicensis). J Avian Med Surg 2011;25(1):32–9.
2. Ensley PK, Hatkin J, Silverman S. Congestive heart failure in a greater hill mynah. J Am Vet Med Assoc 1979;175(9):1010–3.
3. Phalen DN, Hays HB, Filippich LJ, et al. Heart failure in a macaw with atherosclerosis of the aorta and brachiocephalic arteries. J Am Vet Med Assoc 1996;209:1435–40.
4. Sedacca CD, Campbell TW, Bright JM, et al. Chronic cor pulmonale secondary to pulmonary atherosclerosis in an African grey parrot. J Am Vet Med Assoc 2009;234(8):1055–9.
5. Oglesbee BL, Lehmkuhl L. Congestive heart failure associated with myxomatous degeneration of the left atrioventricular valve in a parakeet. J Am Vet Med Assoc 2001;218(3):376–80, 360.
6. Mitchell EB, Hawkins MG, Orvalho JS, et al. Congenital mitral stenosis, subvalvular aortic stenosis, and congestive heart failure in a duck. J Vet Cardiol 2008; 10(1):67–73.
7. Straub J, Pees M, Enders F, et al. Pericardiocentesis and the use of enalapril in a Fischer's lovebird (Agapornis fischeri). Vet Rec 2003;152:24–6.
8. Pees M, Schmidt V, Coles B, et al. Diagnosis and long-term therapy of right-sided heart failure in a yellow-crowned amazon (Amazona ochrocephala). Vet Rec 2006;158(13):445–7.
9. Beaufrere H, Nevarez J, Gaschen L, et al. Diagnosis of presumed acute ischemic stroke and associated seizure management in a Congo African grey parrot. J Am Vet Med Assoc 2011;239(1):122–8.
10. Beaufrere H, Holder KA, Bauer R, et al. Intermittent claudication-like syndrome secondary to atherosclerosis in a yellow-naped Amazon parrot (Amazona ochrocephala auropalliata). J Avian Med Surg 2011;25(4):266–76.
11. Raymond JT, Garner MM. Cardiomyopathy in captive African hedgehogs (Atelerix albiventris). J Vet Diagn Invest 2000;12(5):468–72.
12. Cox I, Haworth P. Cardiac disease in guinea pigs. Vet Rec 2000;146(21):620.
13. Schmidt R, Reavill D. Cardiovascular disease in hamsters: review and retrospective study. J Exot Pet Med 2007;16(1):49–51.
14. Wagner R. Diseases of the cardiovascular system. In: Fox J, Marini R, editors. Biology and diseases of the ferret. 3rd edition. Ames (IA): Wiley Blackwell; 2014. p. 401–19.
15. Franklin J, Guzman D. Dilated cardiomyopathy and congestive heart failure in a guinea pig. Exotic DVM 2006;7(6):9–12.
16. Lord B, Devine C, Smith S. Congestive heart failure in two pet rabbits. J Small Anim Pract 2010;52(1):46–50.
17. Kik MJL, Mitchell MA. Reptile cardiology: a review of anatomy and physiology, diagnostic approaches, and clinical disease. Semin Avian Exot Pet Med 2005; 14:52–60.

18. Murray MJ. Cardiology. In: Mader DR, editor. Reptile medicine and surgery. 2nd edition. Philadelphia: Elsevier; 2006. p. 181–95.

19. Mitchell MA. Reptile cardiology. Vet Clin North Am Exot Anim Pract 2009;12(1): 65–79.

20. Rishniw M, Carmel BP. Atrioventricular valvular insufficiency and congestive heart failure in a carpet python. Aust Vet J 1999;77:580–3.

21. Pees M, Krautwald-Junghanns ME, Straub J. Evaluating and treating the cardio-vascular system. In: Harrison GJ, Lightfoot TL, editors. Clinical avian medicine, vol. 1. Palm Beach (FL): Spix Publishing; 2006. p. 379–94.

22. Lumeij J, Ritchie B. Cardiology. In: Ritchie BW, Harrison GJ, Harrison LR, edi-tors. Avian medicine: principles and applications. Lake Worth (FL): Wingers Publishing; 1994. p. 695–722.

23. Rosenthal K, Stamoulis M. Diagnosis of congestive heart failure in an Indian hill mynah bird (Gracula religiosa). J Assoc Avian Vet 1993;7(1):27–30.

24. Brandao J, Reynolds CA, Beaufrere H, et al. Cardiomyopathy in a Harris hawk (Parabuteo unicinctus). J Am Vet Med Assoc 2016;249:221–7.

25. Ritchie BW, Harrison GJ. Formulary. In: Ritchie BW, Harrison GJ, Harrison LR, editors. Avian medicine: principles and application. Lake Worth (FL): Wingers Publishing, Inc; 1994. p. 457–78.

26. Cusack L, Field C, McDermott A, et al. Right heart failure in an African penguin (Spheniscus demersus). J Avian Med Surg 2016;30:243–9.

27. McNaughton A, Frasa S Jr, Mishra N, et al. Valvular dysplasia and congestive heart failure in a juvenile African penguin (Spheniscus demersus). J Zoo Wildl Med 2014;45:987–90.

28. Esfandiary A, Rajaian H, Asasi K, et al. Diuretic effects of several chemical and herbal compounds in adult laying hens. Int J Poult Sci 2010;9(3):247–53.

29. Morrisey J, Kraus M. Cardiovascular and other diseases. In: Quesenberry K, Carpenter J, editors. Ferrets, rabbits, and rodents: clinical medicine and sur-gery. 3rd edition. St Louis (MO): Elsevier Saunders; 2012. p. 62–77.

30. Carpenter J, Marion C. Exotic animal formulary. 4th edition. St Louis (MO): Sa-unders; 2012.

31. Huston S, Lee P, Quesenberry K, et al. Cardiovascular disease, lymphoprolifer-ative disorders, and thymomas. In: Quesenberry K, Carpenter J, editors. Fer-rets, rabbits, and rodents: clinical medicine and surgery. 3rd edition. St Louis (MO): Elsevier Saunders; 2012. p. 257–68.

32. Pariaut R. Cardiovascular physiology and diseases of the rabbit. Vet Clin North Am Exot Anim Pract 2009;12(1):135–44.

33. Hoeffer H. Heart disease in ferrets. In: Boragure J, editor. Kirk's current veteri-nary therapy: XIII small animal practice. Philadelphia: WB Sounders; 2000. p. 1144–8.

34. Williams B. Therapeutics in ferrets. Vet Clin North Am Exot Anim Pract 2000;3(1): 131–53.

35. Ivey E, Monkisey J. Therapeutics for rabbits. Vet Clin North Am Exot Anim Pract 2000;3(1):183–213.

36. Adamcak A, Otten B. Rodent therapeutics. Vet Clin North Am Exot Anim Pract 2000;3(1):221–40.

37. Stocker L. Medication for use in the treatment of hedgehogs. Aylesbury (United Kingdom): Marshcliff, The Wildlife Hospital Trust; 1992.

38. Lightfoot TL. Therapeutics of African pygmy hedgehogs and prairie dogs. Vet Clin North Am Exot Anim Pract 2000;3(1):155–72.

39. Simone-Freilicher E, Sullivan P, Quinn R, et al. Two cases of congestive heart failure in lizards. In: Baer CK, editor. Proc 1st Exot Conf. Weatherford (TX): Association of Avian Veterinarians (AAV); 2015. p. 505–9.
40. Carpenter J, Klaphake E, Gibbons P. Reptile formulary and laboratory normals. In: Mader D, Divers S, editors. Current therapy in reptile medicine and surgery. St Louis (MO): Elsevier Saunders; 2014. p. 382–410.
41. Simone-Freilicher E. Use of isoxsuprine for treatment of clinical signs associated with presumptive atherosclerosis in a yellow-naped Amazon parrot (Amazona ochrocephala auropalliata). J Avian Med Surg 2007;21(3):215–9.
42. Pees M, Kuhring K, Demiraij F, et al. Bioavailability and compatibility of enalapril in birds. In: Bergman E, editor. Proc Annu Assoc Avian Med. Weatherford (TX): Association of Avian Veterinarians (AAV); 2006. p. 7–11.
43. Jepson L. Exotic animal medicine: a quick reference guide. Philadelphia: Elsevier Saunders; 2009.
44. Pahor M, Bernabei R, Sgadari A, et al. Enalapril prevents cardiac fibrosis and arrhythmias in hypertensive rats. Hypertension 1991;18(2):148–57.
45. Sweet C, Emmert S, Inez I, et al. Increased survival in rats with congestive heart failure treated with enalapril. J Cardiovasc Pharmacol 1987;10:636–42.
46. Webb RL, Miller D, Traina V, et al. Benazepril. Cardiovasc Drug Rev 1990;8(2): 89–104.
47. Brady SM, Burgdorf-Moisuk A, Silverman S, et al. Successful treatment of suspected pulmonary arterial hypertension in a mealy Amazon parrot (Amazona farinosa). J Avian Med Surg 2016;30:368–73.
48. Hamlin R, Stalnaker P. Basis for use of digoxin in small birds. J Vet Pharmacol Ther 1987;10(4):354–6.
49. Wilson R, Zenoble R, Horton C, et al. Single dose digoxin pharmacokinetics in the Quaker conure (Myiopsitta monachus). J Zoo Wildl Med 1989;20(4):432–4.
50. Alvarez Maldonado MVZ. Reporte preeliminar: digitalizacion en pollos de engorda como metodo preventivo en el syndrome ascitico. In: Proc 35th Western Poult Dis Conf. 1986.
51. Hillyer EV, Brown SA. Ferrets. In: Birchard SJ, Sherding RG, editors. Saunders manual of small animal practice. Philadelphia: WB Saunders Co; 1994. p. 1317–44.
52. He ZG, Li YS, Zhang TH, et al. Effects of 2-hydroxypropyl-β-cyclodextrin on pharmacokinetics of digoxin in rabbits and humans. Pharmazie 2004;59(3): 200–2.
53. Nishihara K, Hibino J, Kotaki H, et al. Effect of itraconazole on the pharmacokinetics of digoxin in guinea pigs. Biopharm Drug Dispos 1999;20(3):145–9.
54. Wojcicki M, Drozdzik M, Sulikowski T, et al. Pharmacokinetics of intragastrically administered digoxin in rabbits with experimental bile duct obstruction. J Pharm Pharmacol 1997;49(11):1082–5.
55. Guzman DS, Beaufrere H, KuKanich B, et al. Pharmacokinetics of single oral dose of pimobendan in Hispaniolan Amazon parrots (Amazona ventralis). J Avian Med Surg 2014;28(2):95–101.
56. Van Zeeland Y, Schoemaker N, Lumeij J. Syncopes associated with second degree atrioventricular block in a cockatoo. In: Bergman E, editor. Proc Annu Conf Assoc Avian Vet. Weatherford (TX): Association of Avian Veterinarians (AAV); 2010. p. 345–6.
57. Mitchell E, Zehnder A, Hsu A, et al. Pimobendan: treatment of heart failure in small mammals. In: Bergman E, editor. Proc of the Annu Conf Assoc Exotic Mammal Vet. Bedford (TX): Association of Avian Veterinarians (AAV); 2008. p. 71–9.

58. Van Meel JC, Diederen W. Hemodynamic profile of the cardiotonic agent pimobendan. J Cardiovasc Pharmacol 1989;14(S2):s1–6.

59. van Meel JC, Mauz AB, Wienen W, et al. Pimobendan increases survival of cardiomyopathic hamsters. J Cardiovasc Pharmacol 1989;13:508–9.

60. Du CK, Morimoto S, Nishii K, et al. Knock-in mouse model of dilated cardiomyopathy caused by troponin mutation. Circ Res 2007;101:185–94.

61. Schnellbacher RW, da Cunha AF, Beaufrère H, et al. Effects of dopamine and dobutamine on isoflurane-induced hypotension in Hispaniolan Amazon parrots (Amazona ventralis). Am J Vet Res 2012;73(7):952–8.

62. Haskins S. Monitoring anesthetized patients. In: Tranquilli W, Thurmon J, Grimm K, editors. Veterinary anesthesia and analgesia. 4th edition. Ames (IA): Blackwell Publishing; 2007. p. 533–58.

63. Laird KL, Swindle MM, Flecknell PA. Handbook of rodent and rabbit medicine. New York: Pergamon; 1996.

64. Okafor CC, Perreault-Micale C, Hajjar RJ, et al. Chronic treatment with carvedilol improves ventricular function and reduces myocyte apoptosis in an animal model of heart failure. BMC Physiol 2003;3:6.

65. Gwathmey JK. Morphological changes associated with furazolidone-induced cardiomyopathy: effects of digoxin and propranolol. J Comp Pathol 1991;104: 33–45.

66. Glass MG, Fuleihan F, Liao R, et al. Differences in cardioprotective efficacy of adrenergic receptor antagonists and Ca^{2+} channel antagonists in an animal model of dilated cardiomyopathy. Circ Res 1993;73(6):1077–89.

67. Gwathmey JK, Kim CS, Hajjar RJ, et al. Cellular and molecular remodeling in a heart failure model treated with the β-blocker carteolol. Am J Physiol 1999;276: H1678–90.

68. Plumb DC. Diltiazem. In: Plumb's veterinary drug handbook. 6th edition. Ames (IA): Blackwell Publishing; 2008. p. 396–8.

69. Yang Y, Gao M, Guo Y, et al. Calcium antagonists, diltiazem and nifedipine, protect broilers against low temperature-induced pulmonary hypertension and pulmonary vascular remodeling. Anim Sci J 2010;81:494–500.

70. Orcutt C. Cardiovascular disease. In: Meredith A, Lord B, editors. BSAVA manual of rabbit medicine. Gloucester (United Kingdom): British Small Animal Veterinary Association; 2014. p. 205–13.

71. Yang Y, Qiao J, Wang H, et al. Calcium antagonist verapamil prevented pulmonary arterial hypertension in broilers with ascites by arresting pulmonary vascular remodeling. Eur J Pharmacol 2007;561:137–43.

72. Harcourt-Brown FM. Therapeutics. In: Textbook of rabbit medicine. Oxford (United Kingdom): Butterworth Heineman; 2002. p. 94–120.

73. Heard DJ. Principles and techniques of anesthesia and analgesia for exotic practice. Vet Clin North Am Small Anim Pract 1993;23:1301–27.

74. Bauck L, Boyer TH, Brown SA, et al. Exotic animal formulary. Lakewood (CO): American Animal Hospital Association; 1995.

75. Heatley JJ. Hedgehogs. In: Mitchell MA, Tully TN Jr, editors. Manual of exotic pet practice. St Louis (MO): Elsevier Saunders; 2009. p. 433–55.

76. Plumb DC. Glycopyrrolate. In: Plumb's veterinary drug handbook. 6th edition. Ames (IA): Blackwell Publishing; 2008. p. 582–5.

77. Huerkamp MJ. Anesthesia and postoperative management of rabbits and pocket pets. In: Bonagura JD, editor. Kirk's current veterinary therapy XII: small animal practice. Philadelphia: WB Saunders Co; 1995. p. 1322–7.

78. da Cunha AF, et al. Pharmacokinetics and pharmacodynamics of lidocaine in Hispaniolan Amazon parrots (Amazona ventralis). In: Bergman E, editor. Proc Annu Conf Assoc Avian Vet. Denver (CO): Association of Avian Veterinarians (AAV); 2012. p. 313.

79. Brandao J, da Cunha AF, Pypendop B, et al. Cardiovascular tolerance of intravenous lidocaine in broiler chickens (Gallus gallus domesticus) anesthetized with isoflurane. Vet Anaesth Analg 2014;42(4):442–8.

80. da Cunha AF, et al. Pharmacokinetics/pharmacodynamics of bupivacaine and lidocaine in chickens. In: Bergman E, editor. Proc Annu Conf Assoc Avian Vet. Denver (CO): Association of Avian Veterinarians (AAV); 2011. p. 313.

81. Blair LS, Williams E, Ewanciw DV. Efficacy of ivermectin against third-stage Dirofilaria immitis larvae in ferrets and dogs. Res Vet Sci 1982;33(3):386–7.

82. Blair LS, Campbell WC. Trial of avermectin B1a, mebendazole and melarsoprol against pre-cardiac Dirofilaria immitis in the ferret (Mustela putorius furo). J Parasitol 1978;64(6):1032–4.

83. Blair LS, Campbell WC. Suppression of maturation of Dirofilaria immitis in Mustela putorius furo by single dose of ivermectin. J Parasitol 1980;66(4):691–2.

84. Fisher M, Beck W, Hutchinson M. Efficacy and safety of selamectin (Stronghold/Revolution) used off-label in exotic pets. Int J Appl Res Vet Med 2007;5(3):87–96.

85. Powers LV. Bacterial and parasitic disease of ferrets. Vet Clin North Am Exot Anim Pract 2009;12:531–61.

86. Cottrell D. Use of moxidectin as a heartworm adulticide in four ferrets. Exotic DVM 2004;6:9–12.

87. Schaper R, Heine J, Arther R, et al. Imidacloprid plus moxidectin to prevent heartworm infection (Dirofilaria immitis) in ferrets. Parasitol Res 2007;101(1):6.

88. Krautwald-Junghanns ME, Braun S, Pees M, et al. Research on the anatomy and pathology of the psittacine heart. J Avian Med Surg 2004;18:2–11.

89. de Morais HA, Schwartz DS. Pathophysiology of heart failure. In: Ettinger SJ, Feldman EC, editors. Textbook of veterinary internal medicine. 6th edition. St Louis (MO): Elsevier Saunders; 2005. p. 914–40.

90. Sisson DD. Pathophysiology of heart failure. In: Ettinger SJ, Feldman EC, editors. Textbook of veterinary internal medicine. 7th edition. St Louis (MO): Elsevier Saunders; 2010. p. 1143–58.

91. Oglesbee BL, Oglesbee MJ. Results of postmortem examination of psittacine birds with cardiac disease: 26 cases (1991-1995). J Am Vet Med Assoc 1998; 212:1737–42.

92. Heatley J. Cardiovascular anatomy, physiology, and disease of rodents and small exotic mammals. Vet Clin North Am Exot Anim Pract 2009;12:99–113.

93. Fitzgerald BC, Beaufrere H. Cardiology. In: Speer BL, editor. Current therapy in avian medicine and surgery. St Louis (MO): Elsevier; 2016. p. 252–328.

94. Beaufrere H, Schilliger L, Pariaut R. Cardiovascular system. In: Mitchell MA, Tully TN, editors. Current therapy in exotic pet practice. St Louis (MO): Elsevier; 2016. p. 151–220.

95. Ono S, Onuma M, Ueki M, et al. Radiographic measurement of cardiac size in ferrets with heart disease. Adv Anim Cardiol 2008;4(2):37–43.

96. Malakoff RL, Laste NJ, Orcutt CJ. Echocardiographic and electrocardiographic findings in client-owned ferrets: 95 cases (1994-2009). J Am Vet Med Assoc 2012;241(11):1484–9.

97. Martinez L, Jeffrey J, Odom T. Electrocardiographic diagnosis of cardiomyopathies in Aves. Poult Avian Biol Rev 1997;8(1):9–20.

98. Acierno MJ, de Cunha A, Smith J, et al. Agreement between direct and indirect blood pressure measurements obtained from anesthetized Hispaniolan Amazon parrots. J Am Vet Med Assoc 2008;233:1587–90.

99. Schnellbacher R, da Cunha A, Olson EE, et al. Arterial catheterization, interpretation, and treatment of arterial blood pressures and blood gases in birds. J Exot Pet Med 2014;23:129–41.

100. Helmer P. Advances in diagnostic imaging. In: Harrison GJ, Lightfoot TL, editors. Clinical avian medicine, vol. 2. Palm Beach (FL): Spix Publishing; 2006. p. 653–9.

101. Silverman S, Tell LA. Radiology equipment and positioning techniques. In: Silverman S, Tell LA, editors. Radiology of birds: an atlas of normal anatomy and positioning. St Louis (MO): Saunders Elsevier; 2010. p. 1–15.

102. Beaufrère H, Pariaut R, Rodriguez D, et al. Avian vascular imaging: a review. J Avian Med Surg 2010;24(3):174–84.

103. Beaufrere H, Aertsens A, Fouquet J. Un cas d'insuffisance cardiaque congestive chez un perroquet gris. L'Hebdo Veterinaire 2007;200:8–10.

104. Pees M, Straub J, Krautwald-Junghanns ME. Insufficiency of the muscular atrioventricular valve in the heart of a blue-fronted Amazon (Amazona aestiva aestiva). Vet Rec 2001;148:540–3.

105. Mans C, Brown CJ. Radiographic evidence of atherosclerosis of the descending aorta in a grey-cheeked parakeet (Brotogeris pyrrhopterus). J Avian Med Surg 2007;21(1):56–62.

106. Vink-Nooteboom M, Schoemaker N, Kik M, et al. Clinical diagnosis of aneurysm of the right coronary artery in a white cockatoo (Cacatua alba). J Small Anim Pract 1998;39(11):533–7.

107. Baine K. Atypical heart disease in an umbrella cockatoo. In: Bergman E, editor. Proc Annu Conf Assoc Avian Vet. Denver (CO): Association of Avian Veterinarians (AAV); 2012. p. 285.

108. Beehler B, Montali R, Bush M. Mitral valve insufficiency with congestive heart failure in a pukeko. J Am Vet Med Assoc 1980;177:934–7.

109. Ensley P, Van Winkle T. Treatment of congestive heart failure in a ferret (Mustela putorius furo). J Zoo Wildl Med 1982;12:23–5.

110. Lipman N, Murphy J, Fox J. Clinical, functional and pathological changes associated with a case of dilatative cardiomyopathy in a ferret. Lab Anim Sci 1987; 37(2):210–2.

111. Greenlee P, Stephens E. Meningeal cryptococcosis and congestive cardiomyopathy in a ferret. J Am Vet Med Assoc 1984;184(7):840–1.

112. Moneva-Jordan A, Moneva-Jordon A. What is your diagnosis? J Small Anim Pract 1998;39(6):263–303.

113. Girolamo N, Critelli M, Zeyen U, et al. Ventricular septal defect in a ferret (Mustela putorius furo). J Small Anim Pract 2012;53(9):549–53.

114. Schaik-Gerritsen KM, Schoemaker NJ, Kik MJL, et al. Atrial septal defect in a ferret (Mustela putorius furo). J Exot Pet Med 2013;22:70–5.

115. Dias S, Planellas M, Canturri A, et al. Extreme tetralogy of Fallot with polycythemia in a ferret (Mustela putorius furo). Top Companion Anim Med 2017;32: 80–5.

116. Martin M, Darke P, Else R. Congestive heart failure with atrial fibrillation in a rabbit. Vet Rec 1987;121:570–1.

117. Dias S, Todó M, Planellas M, et al. Unusual presentation of cardiac disease in two guinea pigs (Cavia porcellus). In: Proc X Southern Europ Vet Conf. 2016.

118. Dias S, Anselmi C, Casanova M, et al. Clinical and pathological findings in 2 rats (Rattus norvegicus) with dilated cardiomyopathy. J Exot Pet Med 2017;26: 205–12.
119. Varga M. Cardiorespiratory disease. In: Varga M, editor. Textbook of rabbit medicine. 2nd edition. Butterworth-Heinemann Elsevier; 2014. p. 390–404.
120. Bonagura JD, Keene BW. Drugs for treatment of heart failure in dogs. In: Bonagura JD, Twedt DC, editors. Kirk's current veterinary therapy XV. St Louis (MO): Elsevier Saunders; 2014. p. 762–72.
121. Yancy CW, Jessup M, Bozkurt B, et al. 2013 ACCF/AHA guideline for the management of heart failure: a report of the American College of Cardiology Foundation/American Heart Association Task Force on practice guidelines. Circulation 2013;128:e240–327.
122. Gordon SG. Beta blocking agents. In: Ettinger SJ, Feldman EC, editors. Textbook of veterinary internal medicine. 7th edition. St Louis (MO): Elsevier Saunders; 2010. p. 1207–11.
123. Schroeder N. Diuretics. In: Ettinger SJ, Feldman EC, editors. Textbook of veterinary internal medicine. 7th edition. St Louis (MO): Elsevier Saunders; 2010. p. 1212–4.
124. Bulmer BJ, Sisson DD. Therapy of heart failure. In: Ettinger SJ, Feldman EC, editors. Textbook of veterinary internal medicine. 6th edition. St Louis (MO): Elsevier Saunders; 2005. p. 948–72.
125. Cote E. Clinical veterinary advisor: dogs and cats. St Louis (MO): Mosby Inc; 2007.
126. Goldstein D, Skadhauge E. Renal and extrarenal regulation of body fluid composition. In: Whittow G, editor. Sturkie's avian physiology. 5th edition. San Diego (CA): Academic Press; 2000. p. 265–97.
127. Stephens GA, Robertson FM. Renal responses to diuretics in the turtle. J Comp Physiol B 1985;155:387–93.
128. Plumb DC. Furosemide. In: Plumb's veterinary drug handbook. 6th edition. Ames (IA): Blackwell Publishing; 2008. p. 553–6.
129. Plumb DC. Spironolactone. In: Plumb's veterinary drug handbook. 8th edition. Ames (IA): Wiley-Blackwell; 2015. p. 974–6.
130. Swift S. Aldosterone inhibitors. In: Ettinger SJ, Feldman EC, editors. Textbook of veterinary internal medicine. 7th edition. St Louis (MO): Elsevier Saunders; 2010. p. 1223–5.
131. Bulmer B. Angiotensin converting enzyme inhibitors and vasodilators. In: Ettinger SJ, Feldman EC, editors. Textbook of veterinary internal medicine. 7th edition. St Louis (MO): Elsevier Saunders; 2010. p. 1216–23.
132. Plumb DC. Enalapril maleate. In: Plumb's veterinary drug handbook. 6th edition. Ames (IA): Blackwell Publishing; 2008. p. 453–5.
133. Cohn JN. Structural basis for heart failure. Circulation 1995;91:2504–7.
134. BENCH (BENazepril in Canine Heart disease) Study Group. The effect of benazepril on survival times and clinical signs of dogs with congestive heart failure: results of a multicenter, prospective, randomized, double-blinded, placebo-controlled, long-term clinical trial. J Vet Cardiol 1999;1(1):7–18.
135. SOLVD Investigators. Effect of enalapril on survival in patients with reduced left ventricular ejection fractions and congestive heart failure. N Engl J Med 1991; 325:293–302.
136. Silldorff E, Stephens G. Effects of converting enzyme inhibition and alpha receptor blockade on the angiotensin pressor response in the American alligator. Gen Comp Endocrinol 1992;87:134–40.

137. Plumb DC. Pimobendan. In: Plumb's veterinary drug handbook. 6th edition. Ames (IA): Blackwell Publishing; 2008. p. 989–91.

138. Fuentes VL. Inotropes: inodilators. In: Ettinger SJ, Feldman EC, editors. Textbook of veterinary internal medicine. 7th edition. St Louis (MO): Elsevier Saunders; 2010. p. 1202–7.

139. Pedersoli WM, Ravis WR, Lee HS, et al. Pharmacokinetics of single doses of digoxin administered intravenously to ducks, roosters, and turkeys. Am J Vet Res 1990;51(11):1751–5.

140. Harrison LI, Gibaldi M. Pharmacokinetics of digoxin in the rat. Drug Metab Dispos 1976;4(1):88–93.

141. Ochs HR, Bodem G, Bales G, et al. Increased clearance of digoxin in rabbits during repeated administration. J Pharmacol Exp Ther 1978;205(2):516–24.

142. Plumb DC. Digoxin. In: Plumb's veterinary drug handbook. 6th edition. Ames (IA): Blackwell Publishing; 2008. p. 388–93.

143. de Wit M, Schoemaker NJ. Clinical approach to avian cardiac disease. Semin Avian Exot Pet Med 2005;14:6–13.

144. Miller MS. Electrocardiography. In: Harrison GJ, Harrison LR, editors. Clinical avian medicine and surgery. Philadelphia: Saunders; 1986. p. 286–92.

145. Summerfield NJ, Boswood A, O'Grady MR, et al. Efficacy of pimobendan in the prevention of congestive heart failure or sudden death in Doberman Pinschers with preclinical dilated cardiomyopathy. J Vet Intern Med 2012;26(6):1337–49.

146. Lewington J. Diseases of special concern. In: Lewington J, editor. Ferret husbandry, medicine and surgery. 2nd edition. Philadelphia: Elsevier Saunders; 2007. p. 258–88.

147. Plumb DC. Dobutamine. In: Plumb's veterinary drug handbook. 6th edition. Ames (IA): Blackwell Publishing; 2008. p. 422–4.

148. Ruffolo RR Jr, Messick K. Systemic hemodynamic effects of dopamine,($\pm$)-dobutamine and the (+)- and (−)-enantiomers of dobutamine in anesthetized normotensive rats. Eur J Pharmacol 1985;109(2):173–81.

149. Bradford KK, Deb B, Pearl RG. Combination therapy with inhaled nitric oxide and intravenous dobutamine during pulmonary hypertension in the rabbit. J Cardiovasc Pharmacol 2000;36(2):146–51.

150. Lichtenberger M. Shock and cardiopulmonary-cerebral resuscitation in small mammals and birds. Vet Clin North Am Exot Anim Pract 2007;10(2):275–91.

151. Plumb DC. Propranolol. In: Plumb's veterinary drug handbook. 6th edition. Ames (IA): Blackwell Publishing; 2008. p. 1048–51.

152. Plumb DC. Atenolol. In: Plumb's veterinary drug handbook. 6th edition. Ames (IA): Blackwell Publishing; 2008. p. 104–6.

153. Plumb DC. Carvedilol. In: Plumb's veterinary drug handbook. 8th edition. Ames (IA): Wiley-Blackwell; 2015. p. 163–5.

154. Plumb DC. Metoprolol. In: Plumb's veterinary drug handbook. 6th edition. Ames (IA): Blackwell Publishing; 2008. p. 817–9.

155. Gibbs CR, Davies MK, Lip GYH. ABC of heart failure. Management: digoxin and other inotropes, β blockers, and antiarrhythmic and antithrombotic treatment. BMJ 2000;320(7233):495–8.

156. Klapholz M. Beta-blocker use for the stages of heart failure. Mayo Clin Proc 2009;84(8):718–29.

157. Mann D, Bristow M. Mechanisms and models in heart failure: the biomechanical model and beyond. Circulation 2005;111:2837–49.

158. Williams JG, Graham JE, Laste NJ, et al. Tetralogy of Fallot in a young ferret (Mustela putorius furo). J Exot Pet Med 2011;20(3):232–6.

159. Cote E, Ettinger SJ. Electrocardiography and cardiac arrhythmias. In: Ettinger SJ, Feldman EC, editors. Textbook of veterinary internal medicine. 6th edition. St Louis (MO): Elsevier Saunders; 2005. p. 1040–76.

160. Plumb DC. Verapamil. In: Plumb's veterinary drug handbook. 6th edition. Ames (IA): Blackwell Publishing; 2008. p. 1236–9.

161. Plumb DC. Amlodipine besylate. In: Plumb's veterinary drug handbook. 6th edition. Ames (IA): Blackwell Publishing; 2008. p. 59–61.

162. Wagner RA. Ferret cardiology. Vet Clin North Am Exot Anim Pract 2009;12(1): 115–34.

163. Liao R, Carles M, Gwathmey JK. Animal models of cardiovascular disease for pharmacologic drug development and testing: appropriateness of comparison to the human disease state and pharmacotherapeutics. Am J Ther 1997;4: 149–58.

164. Fricke C, Schmidt V, Cramer K, et al. Characterization of atherosclerosis by histochemical and immunohistochemical methods in African grey parrots (Psittacus erithacus) and Amazon parrots (Amazona spp.). Avian Dis 2009;53:466–72.

165. Zandvliet MMJM, Dorrestein GM, van der Hage M. Chronic pulmonary interstitial fibrosis in Amazon parrots. Avian Pathol 2001;30:517–24.

166. Oyama MA, Sisson DD, Thomas WP, et al. Congenital heart disease. In: Ettinger SJ, Feldman EC, editors. Textbook of veterinary internal medicine. 7th edition. St Louis (MO): Elsevier Saunders; 2010. p. 1250–98.

167. MacDonald K. Myocardial disease, feline. In: Ettinger SJ, Feldman EC, editors. Textbook of veterinary internal medicine. 7th edition. St Louis (MO): Elsevier Saunders; 2010. p. 1328–41.

168. Künzel F, Mayer J. Endocrine tumours in the guinea pig. Vet J 2015;206(3): 268–74.

169. Crespo R, Shivaprasad H. Developmental, metabolic, and other noninfectious disorders. In: Saif Y, Fadly A, Glisson J, et al, editors. Diseases of poultry. 12th edition. Ames (IA): Blackwell Publishing; 2008. p. 1149–95.

170. Lichtenberger M. Determination of indirect blood pressure in the companion bird. Semin Avian Exot Pet Med 2005;14(2):149–52.

171. Beaufrere H. Avian atherosclerosis: parrots and beyond. J Exot Pet Med 2013; 22(4):336–47.

172. Snyder PS, Cooke KL. Management of hypertension. In: Ettinger SJ, Feldman EC, editors. Textbook of veterinary internal medicine. 6th edition. St Louis (MO): Elsevier Saunders; 2005. p. 477–9.

173. Zehnder AM, Hawkins MG, Pascoe PJ, et al. Evaluation of indirect blood pressure monitoring in awake and anesthetized red-tailed hawks (Buteo jamaicensis): effects of cuff size, cuff placement, and monitoring equipment. Vet Anaesth Analg 2009;36(5):464–79.

174. Johnston MS, Davidowski LA, Rao S, et al. Precision of repeated, Doppler-derived indirect blood pressure measurements in conscious psittacine birds. J Avian Med Surg 2011;25(2):83–90.

175. Julian RJ. Ascites in poultry. Avian Pathol 1993;22(3):419–54.

176. Kellihan HB. Pulmonary hypertension and pulmonary thromboembolism. In: Ettinger SJ, Feldman EC, editors. Textbook of veterinary internal medicine. 7th edition. St Louis (MO): Elsevier Saunders; 2010. p. 1138–41.

177. Powers LV. Pulmonary arterial hypertension in companion birds. In: Young K, editor. Proc Annu Assoc Avian Med. Teaneck (NJ): Association of Avian Veterinarians (AAV); 2014. p. 295–9.

178. Assi TB, Baz E. Current applications of therapeutic phlebotomy. Blood Transfus 2014;12:s75–83.
179. Fudge AM, Reavill DR. Pulmonary artery aneurysm and polycythaemia with respiratory hypersensitivity in a blue and gold macaw (Ara ararauna). In: Proc Europ Conf Avian Med Surg. 1993. p. 382–7.
180. Taylor M. Polycythemia in the blue and gold macaw: a report of three cases. In: Proc 1st Int Conf Zoo Avian Med. 1987. p. 95–104.
181. Plumb DC. Sildenafil. In: Plumb's veterinary drug handbook. 8th edition. Ames (IA): Wiley-Blackwell; 2015. p. 957–8.
182. Brown AJ, Davison E, Sleeper MM. Clinical efficacy of sildenafil in treatment of pulmonary arterial hypertension in dogs. J Vet Intern Med 2010;24:850–4.
183. Michelakis E, Tymchak W, Lien D, et al. Oral sildenafil is an effective and specific pulmonary vasodilator in patients with pulmonary arterial hypertension: comparison with inhaled nitric oxide. Circulation 2002;105:2398–403.
184. Fathi M, Haydari M, Tanha T. Effects of enalapril on growth performance, ascites mortality, antioxidant status and blood parameters in broiler chickens under cold-induced ascites. Poult Sci J 2015;3:121–7.
185. Hao XQ, Zhang SY, Cheng XC, et al. Imidapril inhibits right ventricular remodeling induced by low ambient temperature in broiler chickens. Poult Sci 2013;92:1492–7.
186. Hao XQ, Zhang SY, Li M, et al. Imidapril provides a protective effect on pulmonary hypertension induced by low ambient temperature in broiler chickens. J Renin Angiotensin Aldosterone Syst 2014;15:162–9.
187. Scagnelli A. Therapeutic review: pentoxifylline. J Exot Pet Med 2017;26:238–40.
188. Plumb DC. Pentoxifylline. In: Plumb's veterinary drug handbook. 8th edition. Ames (IA): Wiley-Blackwell; 2015. p. 836–8.
189. Sturkie PD. Heart: contraction, conduction, and electrocardiography. In: Sturkie PD, editor. Avian physiology. 4th edition. New York: Springer-Verlag; 1986. p. 130–66.
190. Schoemaker, NJ, van Zeeland YRA. Small mammal cardiology. In: Proc 2nd Int Conf Avian Herpetological Exotic Mammal Med. 2017. p. 192–8.
191. Powers LV. Evaluation and management of bradyarrhythmias in the domestic ferret. In: Bergman E, editor. Proc Annu Assoc Avian Med. Denver (CO): Association of Avian Veterinarians (AAV); 2011. p. 115–23.
192. Zandvliet MMJM. Electrocardiography in psittacine birds and ferrets. J Exot Pet Med 2005;14(1):34–51.
193. Rembert MS, Smith JA, Strickland KN, et al. Intermittent bradyarrhythmia in a Hispaniolan Amazon parrot (Amazona ventralis). J Avian Med Surg 2008;22(1):31–40.
194. Nap AM, Lumeij JT, Stokhof AA. Electrocardiogram of the African grey (Psittacus erithacus) and Amazon (Amazona spp.) parrot. Avian Pathol 1992;21(1):45–53.
195. Kushner LI. ECG of the month. Atrioventricular block in a Muscovy duck. J Am Vet Med Assoc 1999;214(1):33–6.
196. Mukai S, Noboru M, Nishimura M, et al. Electrocardiographic observation on spontaneously occurring arrhythmias in chickens. J Vet Med Sci 1996;58(10):953–61.
197. Plumb DC. Lidocaine (systemic). In: Plumb's veterinary drug handbook. 6th edition. Ames (IA): Blackwell Publishing; 2008. p. 721–4.
198. Guzman DSM, Mayer J, Melidone R, et al. Pacemaker implantation in a ferret (Mustela putorius furo) with third-degree atrioventricular block. Vet Clin North Am Exot Anim Pract 2006;9(3):677–87.

199. Kanfer S. Transvenous pacemaker implantation for complete heart block in a rabbit (Oryctolagus cuniculi). In: Proc Annu Conf Assoc Exotic Mammal Vet. 2013.

200. Plumb DC. Atropine sulfate. In: Plumb's veterinary drug handbook. 6th edition. Ames (IA): Blackwell Publishing; 2008. p. 112–6.

201. Martinez-Jimenez D, Hernandez-Divers SJ. Emergency care of reptiles. Vet Clin North Am Exot Anim Pract 2007;10:557–85.

202. Pace L. Atropine and glycopyrrolate, route of administration and response in the green iguana (Iguana iguana). In: Proc Annu Conf Assoc Rept Amph Vet. 2002. p. 79.

203. Jaensch SM, Cullen L, Raidal SR. The pathology of normobaric oxygen toxicity in budgerigars (Melopsittacus undulatus). Avian Pathol 2001;30:135–42.

204. Devi S, Jani RG. Review on nutritional management of cardiac disorders in canines. Vet World 2009;2(12):482–5.

205. Moneva-Jordan A. Dietary considerations for the cardiac patient. Practice 2012; 34(Suppl 1):28–9.

206. Elices M, Miguélez F, Morán C. Dietary management for dogs and cats with cardiac diseases. Argos-Informativo Veterinario 2011;128:44–8.

207. McCleery B, Jones MP, Manasse J, et al. Pericardial mesothelioma in a yellow-naped Amazon parrot (Amazona auropalliata). J Avian Med Surg 2015;29: 55–62.

208. Tobias AH. Pericardial disorders. In: Ettinger SJ, Feldman EC, editors. Textbook of veterinary internal medicine. 6th edition. St Louis (MO): Elsevier Saunders; 2005. p. 1104–18.

209. Straub J, Pees M, Krautwald-Junghanns ME. Diagnosis of pericardial effusion in birds by ultrasound. Vet Rec 2001;149:86–8.

210. Echols S. Collecting diagnostic samples in avian patients. Vet Clin North Am Exot Anim Pract 1999;2:621–49.

211. Hernandez-Divers SJ, McBride M, Hanley C. Minimally invasive endosurgery of the psittacine cranial coelom. Exotic DVM 2004;6:33–7.

212. Beaufrere H, Nevarez JG, Holder K, et al. Characterization and classification of psittacine atherosclerotic lesions by histopathology, digital image analysis, transmission and scanning electron microscopy. Avian Pathol 2011;40(5): 531–44.

213. Beaufrere H, Ammersbach M, Reavill DR, et al. Prevalence of and risk factors associated with atherosclerosis in psittacine birds. J Am Vet Med Assoc 2013; 242(12):1696–704.

214. Walsh AL, Shivaprasad HL. Unusual lesions of atherosclerosis in psittacines. J Exot Pet Med 2013;22(4):366–74.

215. Beaufrere H. Atherosclerosis: comparative pathogenesis, lipoprotein metabolism, and avian and exotic companion mammal models. J Exot Pet Med 2013;22(4):320–35.

216. Grosset C, Guzman DS, Keating MK, et al. Central vestibular disease in a blue and gold macaw (Ara ararauna) with cerebral infarction and hemorrhage. J Avian Med Surg 2014;28:132–42.

217. Jenkins JR. Use of computed tomography in pet bird practice. In: Proc Annu Conf Assoc Avian Vet. 1991. p. 276–9.

218. Elliott J, Soydan J. Characterisation of beta-adrenoceptors in equine digital veins: implications of the modes of vasodilatory action of isoxsuprine. Equine Vet J Suppl 1995;(19):101–7.

219. Belloli C, Carcano R, Arioli F, et al. Affinity of isoxsuprine for adrenoreceptors in equine digital artery and implications for vasodilatory action. Equine Vet J 2000; 32(2):119–24.

220. Plumb DC. Isoxsuprine. In: Plumb's veterinary drug handbook. 8th edition. Ames (IA): Wiley-Blackwell; 2015. p. 582–3.

221. Aarts PA, Banga JD, van Houwelingen HC, et al. Increased red blood cell deformability due to isoxsuprine administration decreases platelet adherence in a perfusion chamber: a double-blind cross-over study in patients with intermittent claudication. Blood 1986;67:1474–81.

222. Lewis JC, Storm J, Greenwood AG. Treatment of wing tip oedema in raptors. Vet Rec 1993;133(13):328.

223. Smith FM, West NH, Jones DR. The cardiovascular system. In: Whittow GC, editor. Sturkie's avian physiology. 5th edition. San Diego (CA): Academic Press; 2000. p. 141–231.

224. Wellehan JFX. Frostbite in birds: pathophysioloy and treatment. Compendium on Continuing Education for the Practicing Veterinarian 2003;25:776–81.

225. Martel-Arquette A, Mans C, Sladky K. Management of severe frostbite in a grey-headed parrot (Poicephalus fuscicollis suahelicus). J Avian Med Surg 2016;30: 39–45.

226. Wellehan JFX, Gunkel CI. Emergent diseases in reptiles. Semin Avian Exot Pet Med 2004;13:160–74.

227. Paoletti R, Bolego C, Cignerella A. Lipid and non-lipid effects of statins. In: von Eckarstein A, editor. Atherosclerosis: diet and drugs. Berlin: Springer Verlag; 2005. p. 365–88.

228. Elkin RG, Yan Z, Zhong Y, et al. Select 3-hydroxy-3-methylglutaryl-coenzyme A reductase inhibitors vary in their ability to reduce egg yolk cholesterol levels in laying hens through alteration of hepatic cholesterol biosynthesis and plasma VLDL composition. J Nutr 1999;129(5):1010–9.

229. Beaufrere H, Papich MG, Brandao J, et al. Plasma drug concentrations of orally administered rosuvastatin Hispaniolan Amazon parrots (Amazona ventralis). J Avian Med Surg 2015;29:18–24.

230. Bavelaar FJ, Beynen AC. Severity of atherosclerosis in parrots in relation to the intake of alpha-linolenic acid. Avian Dis 2003;47(3):566–77.

231. Petzinger C, Heatley JJ, Cornejo J, et al. Dietary modification of omega-3 fatty acids for birds with atherosclerosis. J Am Vet Med Assoc 2010;236(5):523–8.

232. Bavelaar FJ, Beynen AC. Atherosclerosis in parrots. A review. Vet Q 2004;26(2): 50–60.

Gonadotrophin-Releasing Hormone Agonists and Other Contraceptive Medications in Exotic Companion Animals

Nico J. Schoemaker, DVM, PhD, Dip ECZM (Small Mammal & Avian), Dipl ABVP-Avian

KEYWORDS

- Deslorelin • Neutering • HPG-axis • GnRH A-SRI • Small mammal • Avian • Reptile

KEY POINTS

- The gonadotrophin-releasing hormone agonist slow-release implant (GnRH A-SRI) containing deslorelin has a contraceptive action in ferrets, rats, parrots, chicken, quail, pigeons, and female iguanas.
- The use of the GnRH A-SRI containing deslorelin is associated with the development of histopathological changes to the uterus in rabbits and guinea pigs.
- The duration of action of the GnRH A-SRI containing deslorelin in birds is much shorter compared with those in ferrets, rats, and iguanas.
- The efficacy of the GnRH A-SRI containing deslorelin can best be established through hormone analysis and evaluation of the reproductive organs.

INTRODUCTION

Gonadotrophin-releasing hormone (GnRH) is a decapeptide that is produced in the hypothalamus. Through the hypothalamic–hypophysial portal system this hormone is transported to the anterior pituitary gland where it stimulates the release of the gonadotrophins, luteinizing hormone (LH) and follicle stimulating hormone (FSH). The gonadotrophins, in turn, stimulate the release of either testosterone or estradiol, depending on the gender of the animal. A negative feedback mechanism, whereby testosterone or estradiol suppress the release of both GnRH and the gonadotrophins, is in place to assure that only the required amount of hormones is released (**Fig. 1**).

More than 2000 different analogues of GnRH have been synthesised,[1] of which deslorelin ([d-Trp6, Pro9−des-Gly10–NH2]GnRH-ethylamide) is one of the more potent analogues.[2] This agonist is thought to have a potency 100 times greater than that of GnRH.[2] The other commonly used long-acting GnRH analogue in exotic

The author has nothing to disclose.
Division of Zoological Medicine, Utrecht University, Yalelaan 108, Utrecht 3584 CM, Netherlands
E-mail address: N.J.Schoemaker@uu.nl

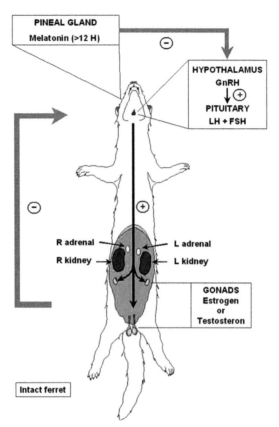

Fig. 1. Within the hypothalamus-pituitary-gonadal axis, GnRH is released in the hypothalamus and stimulates the secretion of the pituitary-derived gonadotrophins, LH and FSH. The gonadotrophins then stimulate the production of testosterone (male) or estradiol (female) in the gonads. The latter hormones insert a negative feedback action on the release of GnRH, LH, and FSH. L, left; R, right.

companion animals is leuprolide acetate. This analogue is registered for use in people with sex hormone–related disorders[3] and contains biodegradable microspheres, which continuously release leuprolide acetate over a certain amount of time.[4] In addition to stimulating the release of gonadotrophins, GnRH analogues may also suppress the release of gonadotrophins, which renders them potential agents to be used as contraceptive agents (see *Mode of Action of a Gonadotrophin-Releasing Hormone Agonist Slow Release Implant*).[2]

This review article mainly focuses on the use of the GnRH agonist slow-release-implant (GnRH A-SLI) containing deslorelin, describing its use in different animals. In case the GnRH A-SLI is not suitable for the species, and alternatives are available, these are briefly discussed. Surgical options for contraception are considered to be outside of the scope of this review and are, therefore, not reviewed.

GONADOTROPHIN-RELEASING HORMONE AGONIST SLOW RELEASE IMPLANT

Although the commercially available GnRH A-SLI containing deslorelin (Suprelorin) is the only one currently on the market, other pharmaceutical companies have developed similar implants. The former implant is widely accepted as an alternative to surgical neutering. In Europe, implants containing either 4.7 or 9.4 mg deslorelin are licensed as alternatives for surgical neutering in adult male dogs and ferrets (9.4 mg only) (European Medicines Agency 2012-06-05).[5] In the United States, only the implant containing 4.7 mg deslorelin is available. The latter implant is only registered for the treatment of hyperadrenocorticism in ferrets (Suprelorin F, United States). However, extralabel use is allowed, as no other animal drug registered for the intended use is available. Following an initial stimulation of gonadotrophin and testosterone, GnRH A-SRIs induce long-term suppression of fertility. However, a large individual variation in onset and duration of efficacy is seen.[5] In female animals, the initial increase in estradiol may result in a fertile estrus, thereby making it a less preferred option for contraception in dogs and cats.[5]

Aside from studies in dogs and cats, the GnRH A-SRIs have been used in a variety of species. Interestingly, the efficacy differs greatly between the different species. In boars, cheetahs, and flying foxes, for instance, spermatogenesis is suppressed after administration of a GnRH A-SRI.[6–9] In the bull, however, continuous administration of a GnRH analogue led to LH and testosterone concentrations that were higher than those in control animals.[10,11] In marmoset monkeys and wallabies, plasma testosterone concentrations remain within the normal range during the use of a GnRH A-SRI.[12,13] A GnRH A-SRI will, therefore, not be a suitable contraceptive drug in the last 3 species. In recent years, more and more information has become available on the potential use of GnRH A-SRIs in exotic animals kept as companion animals. The most recent information on the use of these implants is discussed here.

Mode of Action of a Gonadotrophin-Releasing Hormone Agonist Slow Release Implant

GnRH is physiologically secreted by the hypothalamus in a pulsatile pattern, similar to all hypothalamic and pituitary hormones. However, species-specific differences in amplitude and frequency of pulses may be seen. Application of a GnRH A-SRI initially induces a stimulatory effect on gonadotrophin and consequently gonadal hormone secretion, which is referred to as a flare-up.[5] This initial flare-up is followed by a significant decrease of plasma concentrations of gonadotrophins.[14,15] It has been hypothesized that the decrease in gonadotrophins and, consequently, gonadal hormone secretion may be due to downregulation of pituitary GnRH receptors via internalization and degradation.[16] Loss of the pulsatile release of GnRH, on the other hand, may have a similar effect on the release of gonadotrophins.[17]

SMALL MAMMALS

Neutering small mammals is most commonly performed to enable mixed-sex group housing. Surgical neutering is still considered the gold standard. However, the risk of anesthesia, especially in smaller exotic mammals, prevents some owners from choosing the surgical route. In these cases, the use of a GnRH A-SRI can be considered as an alternative method of contraception. Aside from the contraceptive use, GNRH A-SRIs are also used in the treatment of hyperadrenocorticism in ferrets[18] and adrenal tumors in male rabbits.[19] It has been hypothesized that the development of adrenal tumors in ferrets is stimulated by the elevation of gonadotrophins that occur after neutering.[20] The use of a GnRH A-SRI in ferrets as an alternative to surgical neutering may, therefore, also play a role in the prevention of the development of adrenal tumors in this species.[21] Similarly, these implants may also be helpful to prevent the development of mammary gland tumors in rats, uterine carcinoma in rabbits, and cystic ovaries in guinea pigs.

Ferret

Of all the small mammal species, ferrets are the species in which GnRH A-SRI use has been studied the best largely because the slow-release GnRH agonist, leuprolide acetate, was already used in the treatment of hyperadrenocorticism in ferrets[18] before GnRH A-SRI Suprelorin came onto the European market in 2007.

Location and technique of placement of the gonadotrophin-releasing hormone agonist slow-release implant in ferrets

According to the instructions of the manufacturer, the GnRH A-SRI Suprelorin should be placed subcutaneously (SC) between the shoulder blades while the ferret is under anesthesia. Personally, the author advises placing the implant somewhat further caudally, as the skin is extremely thick in the neck and gradually decreases in thickness in a cranial to caudal direction. The manufacturer also advises to place the implant under general anesthesia. Most ferrets, however, can easily be distracted by feeding them their favorite (liquid) food and allow placement without any struggle when they are preoccupied with eating (**Fig. 2**). Routine hygienic measures, similar to any SC injection, should be applied before placement of the implant. Some tissue glue may be applied on the injection site after placement of the implant to prevent (premature) loss of the implant.

Male

Just as in dogs, the first study on the use of GnRH A-SRIs as an alternative to surgical neutering was performed in male ferrets (hobs). In this study, hormonal effects, testis volume and histology, odor, as well as behavioral aspects were compared between ferrets receiving a placebo implant (control; n = 6), animals that were surgically neutered (n = 7), and those receiving an implant containing 9.4 mg deslorelin (n = 7).[15,22] After placement of the GnRH A-SRI, plasma concentrations of FSH and testosterone plasma were found to be significantly lower compared with the surgically neutered ferrets and those receiving a placebo implant after 2 and 4 weeks, respectively.[15]

Plasma FSH concentrations from this study clearly demonstrated that in surgically neutered ferrets, gonadotrophin concentrations are not only greater compared with

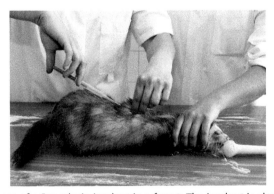

Fig. 2. SC placement of a Suprelorin implant in a ferret. The implant is placed over the back, instead of the neck, as the skin in the neck is much thicker, making placement a lot more difficult. Ferrets generally tolerate placement well without anesthesia when they are provided with their favorite food to distract them.

ferrets that had received the GnRH A-SRI but also compared with the control animals (**Fig. 3**). This finding serves as an extra indication that (surgical) neutering may indeed play a role in inducing the development of adrenal neoplasia. Because placement of a GnRH A-SRI results in significant suppression of the release of gonadotrophins, these implants may decrease the development of adrenal neoplasia in this species. Preliminary findings of a longitudinal study evaluating the adrenal volume of ferrets either surgically neutered or those receiving a GnRH A-SRI containing 4.7 mg deslorelin on a yearly basis are in support of this hypothesis (Schoemaker, unpublished data, 2018).

Similar to dogs and tomcats,[23,24] testes volume in ferrets decreases significantly after placement of a GnRH A-SRI.[15] The decrease in testicular size is particularly useful for owners to evaluate whether the implant is still functional. The decreased testicular volume can easily be explained when looking at histologic sections of these testes (**Fig. 4**). In addition to a severely decreased diameter of the seminiferous tubules, spermatogonia and spermatocytes were also absent, indicating cessation of fertility after placement of the GnRH A-SRI.[15]

An aspect that, to the author's knowledge, has not been studied in any other animal is the effect of a GnRH A-SRI on the odor produced by the sebaceous glands, typical for an intact male ferret. This typical musky odor is, for many owners, one of the major reasons to neuter a male ferret (in addition to inducing infertility). The GnRH A-SRI proved to be very effective in reducing the odor.[15] In addition, behavior changes were seen following placement of the GnRH A-SRI: intermale aggression was reduced, sexually motivated behavioral patterns decreased, and a higher incidence of play behavior was seen.[22] These findings led the researchers to conclude that the use of a GnRH A-SRI can be considered a suitable alternative for surgical neutering in male ferrets.[15,22]

Female

In female dogs and cats, the application of GnRH A-SRIs may result in a fertile estrus, irrespective of the stage in the reproductive cycle of the animal.[5] Especially in dogs, this is considered one of the main reasons why the GnRH A-SRI is not registered for use in female animals. Postimplant estrus is seen in ferrets as well.[25,26] In a study

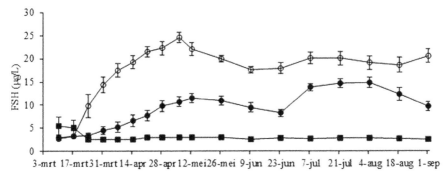

Fig. 3. Plasma FSH concentrations (± standard error of measurement; micrograms per liter) in male ferrets that were surgically castrated (*open circle*; n = 7), received a placebo implant (*closed circle*; n = 6), or received a depot-GnRH-agonist implant containing 9.4 mg deslorelin (*square*; n = 7) on March 17. (*From* Schoemaker NJ, van Deijk R, Muijlaert B, et al. Use of a gonadotropin releasing hormone agonist implant as an alternative for surgical castration in male ferrets [*Mustela putorius furo*]. Theriogenology 2008;70:164; with permission.)

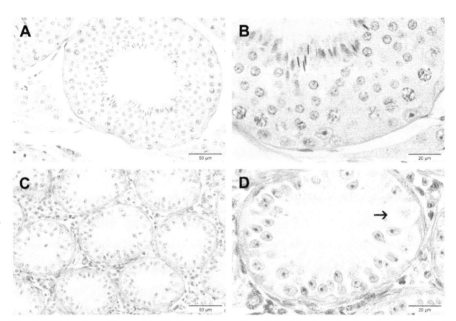

Fig. 4. Histologic sections of testis tissue from a ferret that had received a placebo implant (*A, B*) and a ferret that had received a depot GnRH-agonist implant containing 9.4 mg deslorelin (*C, D*). The seminiferous tubules in the testis of the latter ferret are much smaller and do not contain any functional germ cells. Only an occasional degenerated germ cell could be found (*arrow*). (*From* Schoemaker NJ, van Deijk R, Muijlaert B, et al. Use of a gonadotropin releasing hormone agonist implant as an alternative for surgical castration in male ferrets [*Mustela putorius furo*]. Theriogenology 2008;70:166; with permission.)

conducted in privately owned ferrets, almost 60% of nonestrus ferrets came into estrus within 3 days after placement of the GnRH A-SRI. This estrus, however, only lasted approximately 10 days, compared with an estrus that may last an entire season (up to 6 months). Pretreating the ferrets with medroxyprogesterone did not prevent this estrus from occurring.[26] Satisfaction among the owners of female ferrets was, nevertheless, greater than 93%.[26] The high percentage of satisfied owners is in large part because no serious side effects were seen, that is, generally these were limited to mild, local signs (eg, small scab or mild itch) and, in females, estrus induction, occasionally followed by pseudopregnancy (which responded well to treatment with cabergoline). Moreover, the duration of action of the GnRH A-SRI containing 4.7 mg deslorelin was at least 505 days but could last as long as 42 months.[26] This finding is comparable with the findings in 2 other (smaller) studies in which the duration of action of the same GnRH A-SRI varied between 17 and 35 months.[25,27]

As a result, the GnRH A-SRI containing either 4.7 or 9.4 mg deslorelin can also be considered a suitable contraceptive in female ferrets.

Other contraceptives used in ferrets
Historically, the most commonly used (nonsurgical) contraceptive in ferrets was the progestogen proligestone, which is given in a dose of 50 mg per ferret SC.[21] One injection was mentioned to be sufficient to prevent estrus for one season in 92% of the cases, whereas in the remainder of cases estrus would be successfully suppressed following a second injection.[28] However, when using proligestone in Dutch ferrets,

more than 2 injections were frequently needed and pseudopregnancy was often seen, leading to dissatisfied owners in more than 50% of cases (Schoemaker, unpublished, 2003). These findings are consistent with a study performed in Hungary where they administered 40 mg proligestone in mid-February to female ferrets (n = 5). The mean number of days (± standard deviation) between the treatment and first estrus was 99 ±40 days.[25] This number is, therefore, much less than what was previously reported[28] and explains the dissatisfaction of owners of ferrets that were given these injections.

GnRH vaccination has also been successfully used as contraceptive in ferrets.[29] Based on serum GnRH antibody titers, the researchers concluded that a single vaccination was sufficient to maintain adequate GnRH antibody titers for at least 3 years. Although the vaccine is not (yet) commercially available, more studies on the use of this vaccine are ongoing.[30] It should furthermore be noted that not all GnRH-vaccines may be safe to use in ferrets. In a vaccine study performed by the author approximately 20 years ago, more than 50% of the ferrets died with signs similar to myofasciitis in ferrets.[21,31] Caution is, therefore, advised before administering a new type of GnRH vaccine to ferrets to prevent the occurrence of the serious side effects previously seen with such vaccines.

Rabbit

Rabbits are the third most commonly kept companion animal, and housing them together with a mate is considered important for their welfare.[32] However, some rabbits can become extremely territorial either necessitating neutering or otherwise outplacement. Contraception would be another reason for neutering. Although anesthetic risks in rabbits are greater compared with those of the other companion animals,[33] studies on nonsurgical contraceptive methods are very limited, which may be, in part, because uterine adenocarcinomas are frequently diagnosed in intact rabbits and removal of the uterus will prevent carcinoma to develop in this organ.[34] However, because the development of these adenocarcinoma are under hormonal influence, the use of GnRH A-SRIs may be a suitable alternative.

Location and technique of placement of the gonadotrophin-releasing hormone agonist slow-release implant in rabbits

Two locations have been described for subcutaneous placement of the GnRH A-SRI containing 4.7 mg deslorelin. In one study the implants were placed lateral of the umbilicus to facilitate implant removal[35]; in the other study, the implants were placed in the neck region.[36]

Male

Indications for contraceptive use in male pet rabbits include reproduction control, reduction of intermale aggression and control of hypersexuality, territory marking, and aggression against humans.[36] The surgical approach is most commonly applied in practice, although a medical route may reduce the morbidity and mortality associated with any surgical procedure.

The use of a GnRH A-SRI containing 4.7 mg deslorelin as contraceptive in male rabbits was first described as a case report in 2001 and showed promising results. Testosterone concentrations were less than the detection limit of the assay (0.1 ng/mL) for 7 months, after seeing a flare-up for 14 days in which testosterone concentrations initially had increased.[37] Testes size had decreased to 50% of the original size during this period as well, and no sexual behavior toward the intact female rabbit companion was observed by the owner.[37]

In a research setting, however, these positive results could not be repeated. Of the 10 peri-pubertal (aged 4–5 months) rabbits that received a GnRH A-SRI containing 4.7 mg deslorelin, plasma testosterone concentrations remained identical to those of control rabbits over a period of 3 months. In addition, spermatogenesis, as evaluated on histologic evaluation of the testes 90 days after administration of the implant, remained present as well. The investigators of this study, therefore, concluded that application of this implant should not be considered as a reliable contraceptive method in male rabbits.[36]

Female

Just as in the male rabbits, the first report of the use of a GnRH A-SRI containing 4.7 mg deslorelin in 2.5- to 5.0-month-old female rabbits (n = 8) seemed promising. These rabbits were housed with an intact male rabbit. The rabbits from the control group, and those that had received a GnRH A-SRI containing 2.1 mg deslorelin (Ovuplant), became pregnant around the age of 3.5 months. In contrast, the rabbits with the GnRH A-SRI containing 4.7 mg deslorelin became pregnant at a later stage. Unfortunately, no information was provided by the researchers on the exact time frame with which pregnancy was delayed compared with the other groups.[38]

In recent studies, it was shown that with a GnRH A-SRI containing 4.7 mg deslorelin estrus could indeed be suppressed in 60-day-old female rabbits (n = 7).[35,39] Because rabbits ovulate after induction, efficacy of the implants was tested by administering buserelin (a short-acting GnRH agonist) after which progesterone was measured to confirm the presence of pseudopregnancy. A duration of estrus suppression was achieved for at least 9 months, after which the implants were removed and buserelin could induce estrus in all animals.[39] To investigate the total duration of estrus suppression in rabbits, further studies would be needed. However, the most important reason to use a GnRH A-SRI in female rabbits would be to prevent the development of uterine adenocarcinoma. Unfortunately, more than half of the rabbits that had received the GnRH A-SRI either developed endometritis or endometrial hyperplasia before 2 years of age.[39] These implants may, therefore, not be suitable to prevent the development of uterine pathology in rabbits.

Other contraceptives used in rabbits

A recent study describes the use of an anti-GnRH vaccine in 2-month-old intact male rabbits.[40] A booster vaccination was administered 15 days after vaccination. In all 20 rabbits, testes volume decreased as well as plasma testosterone concentrations. On histologic examination of the testes, sperm was absent in all seminiferous tubules of all rabbits.[40] This finding suggests that vaccination against GnRH might be a practical contraceptive for male rabbits. However, further studies are needed to evaluate how long animals remain infertile (ie, whether it is lifelong or not), and if and when a booster vaccination will be needed again to maintain continuous infertility.

Guinea Pig

Guinea pigs are highly social animals and are most frequently kept in (large) mixed-sex groups.[41] Contraception is, therefore, needed to manage population growth. In practice, this is most commonly achieved through surgical neutering of male guinea pigs. In addition, cystic ovaries are frequently seen and difficult to manage nonsurgically. Ovariectomy has, therefore, been suggested as a preventive measure.[42] The anesthetic risk of death while performing surgeries in guinea pigs (3.80 with a 95% confidence interval of 2.76–4.85), however, is even greater than those reported in rabbits (1.39 with a 95% confidence interval 1.14–1.64).[33] Nonsurgical neutering methods may, therefore, be warranted. However, to date, the number of studies on the use of a GnRH A-SRI as a contraceptive in guinea pigs has been extremely limited.

Location and technique of placement of the gonadotrophin-releasing hormone agonist slow-release implant in guinea pigs

In guinea pigs the GnRH A-SRIs have all been placed subcutaneously. In one study, the implants were placed near the umbilicus,[43] whereas in another study, the exact location was not described. Although the skin is thinner on the ventral surface of guinea pigs, the author prefers placement on the dorsal surface, as this is considered more practical as far less handling is needed.

Male

To the author's knowledge, the use of a GnRH A-SRI containing 4.7 mg deslorelin as a contraceptive in male guinea pigs has only been tested in 5 animals. In these animals, no effect of the GnRH A-SRI was seen on testicular volume, male behavior, or plasma testosterone concentrations. In addition, the males remained fertile and were all able to impregnate females they had mated with. Histologic evaluation of the testes further-more revealed normal spermatogenesis and spermatozoa in epididymal sections.[43] It may, therefore, be concluded that the GnRH A-SRI containing 4.7 mg deslorelin is not a suitable alternative for surgical neutering in male guinea pigs.

Female

Ovarian cysts are commonly diagnosed in guinea pigs.[44] The use of either human chorionic gonadotropin and/or GnRH has been described for the medical manage-ment of these cysts.[44] In a study performed in 11 nulliparous female guinea pigs (age range: 4–7 years) with confirmed cystic ovaries, 7 guinea pigs received a GnRH A-SRI containing 4.7 mg deslorelin (all guinea pigs had a cyst of at least 0.5 cm^2), whereas the other 4 guinea pigs served as controls (all had cysts with a maximum of 0.3 cm^2). In none of the guinea pigs did the size of the cyst change. It can, therefore, be concluded that the use of a GnRH A-SRI does not have any thera-peutic effect on ovarian cysts in this species.[44]

The contraceptive effects and/or preventive action on development of ovarian cysts have also been studied. An initial study in 15 female guinea pigs showed promising results with regard to the implant's contraceptive effects, as serum progesterone con-centrations dropped to less than the detection limit and cyclical variation of progester-one concentrations was lost within 15 days following placement of the implant. In addition, opening of the vaginal membrane was delayed.[45] These findings are sugges-tive that pregnancy may be prevented by using a GnRH A-SRI containing deslorelin. The contraceptive effect was later confirmed in 4 guinea pigs that had received a GnRH A-SRI containing 4.7 mg deslorelin while being group housed with intact males 161 days after placement of the implant. Whereas all control animals became preg-nant after mating, none of the guinea pigs that had received the implant did.[43] Despite the promising results on contraception, serious alterations to the ovaries and endome-trium have been described. In her PhD thesis, Kohutova[46] describes the ultrasono-graphic and histologic findings of the uterus and ovaries performed 10 months after placement of the GnRH A-SRI in the 15 guinea pigs described earlier. In these guinea pigs, ovarian cysts, cystic endometrial hyperplasia, adenomyosis, and uterine cervix hyperplasia and hypertrophy were found.[46] In contrast, in the 4 control animals used in that study, no abnormalities were found in the uterus and ovaries. Based on these findings, the use of the GnRH A-SRI containing 4.7 mg deslorelin may not be advisable in female guinea pigs.

Other contraceptives used in guinea pigs

In the same study that tested the effects of an anti-GnRH vaccine in rabbits (described in the rabbit section), the use of an anti-GnRH vaccine was tested in 1-month-old, intact male guinea pigs.[40] A booster was administered 15 days after the vaccination. Although testes volume decreased in all guinea pigs (n = 10), spermatogenesis remained present in 20% of the vaccinated animals. Plasma testosterone concentrations also did not decrease.[40] Vaccination against GnRH can, therefore, currently, not be considered a reliable form of contraception in male guinea pigs.

Rat

Just as many of the other rodents, rats are social animals that require group housing.[47] Ensuring some form of contraception (if males and females are housed together) is, therefore, recommended. Surgical neutering of the male rats is most commonly performed. Another important reason to neuter rats is to prevent the development of mammary gland tumors in female rats. Although a depot formulation of a GnRH agonist (goserelin) has already been used almost 30 years ago to determine to what extent the pituitary gonadal axis could be suppressed in male rats,[48] the use of these implants has, thus far, not become routine practice in rodent medicine.

Location and technique of placement of the gonadotrophin-releasing hormone gonadotrophin-releasing hormone agonist slow-release implant in rats

Similar to the other small mammals, GnRH A-SRIs containing deslorelin have been placed SC in rats, either near the umbilicus[49,50] or between the shoulder blades.[51,52] The author prefers the latter location, as the skin is looser in this area, making placement more easy.

Male

The use of the GnRH A-SRI containing deslorelin has been described in male rats.[51,53] In these studies, a specific formulation was used, whereby 1.1 mg deslorelin was used instead of the regular concentration of 4.7 mg. Within 6 weeks following placement of the implant, a suppression of testes volume and gonadotrophins, predominantly FSH, was found. The duration of action was at least 8 months.[51] Unfortunately, the studies were not continued after this period, thereby rendering it impossible to predict the total duration of action of these implants in male rats.

Female

Several studies describing the use of a GnRH A-SRI containing 4.7 mg deslorelin have been performed.[49,50,52] Based on vaginal smears, cyclic estrous periods disappeared following placement of the implant, which is consistent with the flare-up periods that have been described in other species.[52] Moreover, plasma concentrations of estradiol and progesterone were significantly lower in the deslorelin group compared with the control for up to 1 year after placement of the implant.[49] During this period, none of the rats that had received the GnRH A-SRI and were group housed with an intact male got pregnant either.[49,50]

Early studies have indicated that the long-acting GnRH agonist, leuprolide acetate, has a preventive effect on the development of mammary tumors in a 7,12-dimethyl-benz[a]anthracene–induced rat mammary carcinoma model.[54] Although the percentage of mammary tumors, 16 weeks after the start of the trial, decreased from 78% in the untreated rats to 30% in those receiving leuprolide acetate, this percentage did not decrease to 0% as was the case in those rats that had undergone oophorectomy.[54] To the author's knowledge, no preventive effect on the development of mammary gland tumors in rats after administration of a GnRH A-SRI containing 4.7 mg deslorelin has been scientifically reported.

Other contraceptives used in rats

In rats, GnRH vaccines have been used in experimental settings. In one study, a double-chain GnRH vaccine (GnRH3-hinge-MVP-Hsp65 protein) was used in both male and female rats.[55] This adjuvant-free vaccine induced degeneration of the reproductive organs in both male and female rats. In male rats, diminished spermatogenesis was seen, whereas in female rats, the uteri were reduced in size and the ovaries exhibited reduced follicular development.[55] Thus, based on the findings of this study, GnRH vaccines do possess a contraceptive capability in rats. Unfortunately, these vaccines are not commercially available (yet).

Mouse

Although mice are routinely kept in social groups, they are less frequently presented to veterinarians for neutering, most likely because of the cost involved. Castration of male mice, however, can be performed in a similar fashion as performed in other rodents.

To the author's knowledge, no studies have been published on the use of a GnRH A-SRI as a contraceptive in mice. The cost of the implant will most likely be a limiting factor for owners to be interested in this type of contraception. In a publication on the use of a GnRH A-SRI in rats, an unpublished finding in mice was reported, stating that gonadotrophins decreased after the application of a GnRH A-SRI containing 1.1 mg deslorelin in male mice. The suppression of testicular weight, however, was reported to be less in mice (75% of the testicular size of control animals) than those found in rats (33% of the testicular size of control animals).[51]

In a study in which the GnRH agonist buserelin was administered daily to mice, testicular weight and sperm numbers decreased with a maximum of 34%. These results indicate that, although fertility can be reduced after long-term treatment with a GnRH agonist, this does not result in full contraception.[56]

BIRDS

Neutering birds is not routinely recommended, as the gonads lie directly over the aorta thereby making ligation of their vessels extremely difficult.[57] In addition, incomplete removal of all testicular tissue may result in partial regrowth or hypertrophy of the remaining testicular tissues.[58] On the other hand, reproductive disorders (eg, excessive egg laying, egg binding, yolk coelomitis) and reproductive hormone-related undesired behavior are commonly seen by avian practitioners, rendering it necessary to consider medical management to limit these hormonally driven behaviors.[4,59,60] However, before considering medical and/or surgical intervention, evaluation and potential modification of environmental factors should be considered. If environmental modifications, such as decreasing caloric content of the diet, increasing foraging behavior, decreasing environmental humidity, decreasing the photoperiod, and removal of nesting material, are unsuccessful in decreasing reproductive behavior and egg laying, the use of the long-acting GnRH analogues leuprolide acetate and deslorelin may be considered.[57,61] Because of the considerable influence that environmental factors have on the hypothalamus-pituitary-gonadal (HPG)-axis in birds, these factors should always be addressed to optimize the effects of the slow-release GnRH agonists.[57] Leuprolide acetate needs to be administered in extremely high doses (approximately 1000 µg/kg) in birds.[62] In some cases, doses as high as 3500 µg/kg were used in the treatment of ovarian neoplasia in cockatiels.[63,64] The duration of action is usually no longer than 3 weeks.[62] Similarly, doses as high as 1000 μg/kg (intramuscularly [IM]) in racing pigeons (*Columbia livia domestica*) did not have any effect on plasma steroid hormone concentrations or on egg production.[65] As only a limited amount of studies have been published on the use of the GnRH-A-SRI containing deslorelin in species commonly kept as pets, no separate sections on specific avian species are described in this section.

Location and Technique of Placement of the Gonadotrophin-Releasing Hormone Agonist Slow-Release Implant in Birds

Although the GnRH A-SRI can be placed IM (eg, described in turkeys,[66] pigeons,[67] and Quaker parrots[68]), SC placement is considered the preferred technique in avian species. In budgerigars, the knee fold was used[69]; but the interscapular space is the most frequently used.[57] Because of the extremely limited amount of SC space in birds, placing the implant strictly SC can be challenging, especially in smaller birds. To facilitate placement of these implants, it is recommended to administer a small amount of fluid SC before placement of the implant (Y. van Zeeland, personal communication, 2017) (**Fig. 5**). Following placement, either tissue glue or placement of a suture can facilitate closure of the needle-made hole in the skin, thereby preventing accidental loss of the implant.

Male

The use of a GnRH A-SRI in male birds is not frequently reported. In one report, male turkeys (*Meleagris gallopavo*) received GnRH A-SRIs containing either 4.7 or 9.4 mg deslorelin IM.[66] The turkeys weighed approximately 18 kg and received 2 implants simultaneously at each occasion. The combined 4.7-mg deslorelin implants were effective in suppressing aggressive behavior and plasma testosterone concentrations for 3 to 5 months, whereas the combined 9.4-mg deslorelin implants had a similar effect for 7 months.[66] The author has used a single 4.7-mg deslorelin implant in a rooster but was unsuccessful in suppressing sexual behavior toward the hens. However, in other roosters, placement of similar implants has been successful to some extent to reduce crowing. Varying responses after the use of a deslorelin implant in aggressive male psittacines, pheasants, and a Harris hawk have also been described.[60,70] In a

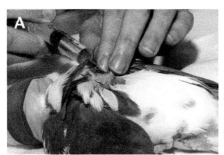
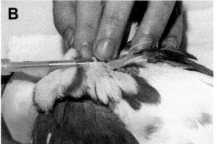

Fig. 5. As the SC space in birds is very limited and the implant is of reasonable size (especially in smaller birds), SC administration of a small amount of fluid is recommended before the placement of the implant (*A*). The injected fluid elevates the skin from the underlying tissues facilitating insertion of the implant (*B*). Preferably, insertion is performed in a craniocaudal direction to prevent the implant from exiting via the injection site. In addition, use of tissue glue or placement of a suture is recommended to close the needle-made hole in the skin.

sexually aggressive imprinted screech owl and an eclectus parrot with suspected hormonally driven feather-damaging behavior and hypersexual behavior (masturbation), a 4.7-mg deslorelin implant was successfully used, together with behavior modification. After the first implant had worn out in the eclectus parrot, a second implant did not result in the expected suppression of problem behavior. However, an additional implant given within a month after placement of the second did provide the desired response. Persistent exposure to environmental reproductive stimuli has been proposed as an explanation for lack of response to the exogenous pharmacologic action of the implant.[67]

In budgerigars diagnosed with Sertoli cell tumors, SC placement of a GnRH A-SRI containing 4.7 mg deslorelin resulted in clinical improvement, which lasted for approximately 20 weeks. After recurrence of the symptoms, placement of a new implant resulted in similar results also with a duration of approximately 20 weeks.[69] However, no blood was collected to confirm the actual effects on hormone concentrations. A similar effect to the placement of a GnRH A-SRI was seen in the author's clinic in a 12-year-old male budgerigar in which the ceres had turned brown; a slight lameness was seen in association with a decreased exercise tolerance. After placement of a 4.7-mg deslorelin containing implant the color of the ceres returned to light blue, the lameness resolved, and no respiratory distress was seen. Nine months after placement of the implant, the bird is still clinically fine.

In male pigeons, a GnRH A-SRI containing 4.7 mg deslorelin resulted in a significant suppression of plasma LH concentrations for a period of 2 months. Three months after placement of the implant, no significant difference was present in plasma LH concentrations.[67] No information on plasma testosterone or on fertility was reported. Therefore, the contraceptive effect in male pigeons has not been assessed and requires further studies in which at least intact, reproductive active female pigeons are used. Endoscopic evaluation of testicular size and measurement of plasma testosterone concentrations are also advised for future studies.[67]

Recently, a study has been published on the use of 1 and 5 mg/kg deslorelin, administered SC in the form of an implant in male Zebra finches. Although the deslorelin induced a reversible suppression of plasma concentrations of testosterone, little to no effect was seen on the song properties of the birds receiving deslorelin, which was found to be consistent with previous studies that demonstrated that testosterone had less influence on song in Zebra finches compared with other song birds.[71]

Female

In female birds, the GnRH A-SRIs have been used to suppress egg laying and managing ovarian tumors. In laying hens, a GnRH A-SRI containing 4.7 mg deslorelin was able to suppress egg laying for approximately half a year (range, 125–237 days), whereas a similar implant containing 9.4 mg deslorelin was able to suppress egg laying for a duration of a little more than 10 months (range, 229–357 days).[72]

In Japanese quail (*Coturnix coturnix japonica*) the duration of activity of the GnRH A-SRI containing 4.7 mg deslorelin was less consistent and only lasted for approximately 2 to 4 months, and egg laying was suppressed in only 60% to 90% of the animals.[73,74] Plasma estradiol concentrations were decreased for 1 month.[73] When two 4.7 mg deslorelin or one 9.4 mg deslorelin GnRH A-SRI was given to Japanese quails, these only worked in 7 out of 10 animals in suppressing egg laying for a period of 100 to 180 days.[75]

In pigeons, plasma LH concentrations were significantly suppressed after receiving a GnRH A-SRI containing 4.7 mg deslorelin for at least 7 weeks. During this period, also no eggs were produced. During the duration of the study (84 days), birds treated with deslorelin laid significantly fewer eggs (mean = 1.46, standard error of measurement [SEM] = 0.84) compared with females that had not received and implant (mean = 5.54, SEM = 0.88).[67]

A recent study described the use of a GnRH A-SRI containing 4.7 mg deslorelin in cockatiels (n = 13) that had proven to be egg laying animals in the period before placement of the implant. The birds were housed in the presence of a nest box and on a 16-hour light:8-hour dark light regime. The first egg was laid 192 days after placement of the implant, compared with day 12 in the control animals. Of the 13 birds that had received an implant, 8 did not lay an egg in the year following placement of the implant.[76] Similar results were found in Quaker parrots, in which administration of a GnRH A-SRI containing 4.7 mg deslorelin was found to suppress egg laying for at least 6 months.[68]

In love birds, the 4.7 mg deslorelin containing GnRH A-SRI was found to significantly suppress plasma progesterone concentrations. Whether these decreased concentrations would be enough to suppress ovarian activity was not published in this conference abstract.[77]

The first report on the use of a GnRH A-SRI-containing implant for the treatment of an ovarian carcinoma in an 18-year-old cockatiel was presented in 2012. It proved possible to maintain a clinically stable situation for 2 years by administering a new implant every 4 to 5 months. By taking radiographs at the time of placement of the implant and 1 month later, it could be demonstrated that on all occasions the ovary decreased in size compared with the size seen at time of placement of the implant.[64] A similar effect was later described in 2 cockatiels with ovarian neoplasia. In these cases, an implant containing 4.6 mg deslorelin was able to suppress reproductive activity for a duration of 4 months.[63] In the author's clinic, ascites associated with an ovarian neoplasia in a cockatiel could also be successfully managed for more than 2 years by administering deslorelin-containing implants every 3 to 5 months.

Other Contraceptives Used in Birds

Before the slow-release GnRH agonists were available for veterinary use, progesterone analogues were frequently used to suppress egg laying in birds. Of these analogues, medroxyprogesterone acetate was most commonly used.[59] Also the use of levonorgestrel has been described in Japanese quail.[78] However, serious side effects, such as excessive weight gain, hepatic lipidosis, and diabetes mellitus, were reported. Although these may potentially only be seen in the higher end of the wide dose range (5–50 mg/kg medroxyprogesterone acetate), this has not been accurately documented.[59] The general consensus, therefore, is not to use these drugs as contraceptives in birds, especially now that safer, more effective alternatives have become available.

REPTILES

In many reptile species, contraception is least on the priority list, as maintaining the captive population by reproduction in captivity is challenging. In some species, however, seasonal aggression and uncontrolled ovarian activity may lead to life-threatening disease.[79–81] In the latter cases, ovariectomy is the most common preventive and curative technique performed. Only a limited amount of studies has been performed on the use of nonsurgical contraceptives in reptiles. Some studies have been performed in lizards, and recently a study was published on the use of the GnRH A-SRI in terrapins. In a case report on the use of a GnRH A-SRI in a male bearded dragon, the investigator furthermore reported that he had been unsuccessful in controlling ovarian activity in female snakes using these implants.[79]

Location and Technique of Placement of the Gonadotrophin-Releasing Hormone Agonist Slow-Release Implant in Reptiles

In reptiles, the GnRH A-SRI can be placed SC, for example, on the flank, as described in bearded dragons[79]; in the neck area, as described in iguanas[82]; or in the right prefemoral fossa, as described in slider turtles.[81] Alternatively, the implant can be placed intracoelomically in the smaller animals that do not have enough SC space, as described in the leopard gecko.[83] As the skin in reptiles does not close easily, it is recommended to either place a suture over the insertion site or close it with tissue glue.

Lizards

Female lizards from the most commonly kept species (chameleons, bearded dragons, leopard geckos, and green iguanas) are commonly presented with either retained ovarian follicles or dystocia.[80] Limiting ovarian activity (in addition to optimization of the housing) may reduce the encountered reproductive morbidity and mortality. In studies performed in female iguanas, leopard geckos, and veiled chameleons, implants were only found to suppress ovarian activity in iguanas.[80,83] In the other species, no suppression of egg laying was observed. In most lizard species, preventive ovariectomy, therefore, currently remains the preferred method of preventing ovarian activity.

In a 6-month-old male bearded dragon that had displayed aggression toward the owner (ie, tendency to bite when being handled), reduction of this behavior was seen after administration of a GnRH A-SRI containing 4.7 mg deslorelin.[81] Plasma hormone concentrations, however, were not measured in this case. It is, therefore, difficult to interpret whether the change of behavior was due to placement of the implant or that the behavior had changed because of changes in husbandry that had also been applied.

Turtles

In turtles, to the author's knowledge, only 2 studies on the use of a GnRH A-SRI have been performed. One study was performed in 6 male yellow-bellied sliders (*Trachemys scripta* sp). In this study, testosterone was measured from April to September after placement of an implant containing 4.7 mg deslorelin.[81] Plasma testosterone concentrations were measured at the time of placement of the implant and at (or around) 2, 4, 8, 12, 17, and 22 weeks after placement of the implant. Significant differences in plasma testosterone concentrations were only seen 2 weeks following placement of the implant, at which time plasma testosterone concentrations in the animals receiving deslorelin exceeded those of the control. This finding corresponds with the flare-up effect that can be seen after placement of the GnRH A-SRI, thereby indicating that administration of a GnRH A-SRI containing 4.7 mg deslorelin is insufficient for contraception in slider turtles.

Similarly, in a second study, performed with 14 adult female red-eared sliders (*Trachemys scripta elegans*), the GnRH A-SRI containing 4.7 mg deslorelin failed to suppress progesterone and estrogens as well as cease ovarian activity.[84] Based on these findings, it may be concluded that a GnRH A-SRI containing deslorelin cannot be considered a good contraceptive agent to manage reproduction in this species of turtles. More studies will be needed in other turtle species to conclude that these results apply to all species of turtles or only a selection.

Table 1
Overview of the indication, its duration of action (if present), and potential side effects of the gonadotrophin-releasing hormone agonist slow-release implants containing deslorelin that have been reported in companion exotic animal species

Species	Indication	Duration of Action (4.7 mg)	Reported Side-Effects	Reference
Ferret	Contraception	Male: >300 d (mean: 2 y) Female: >500 d (mean: 2 y)	Mild, local reactions (eg, scab, pruritus); induction of (self-limiting) estrus, potentially followed by pseudopregancy in jills	15,22,26 25–27
	Hyperadrenocorticism	Mean: 16.5 mo	—	85
Rabbit	Contraception	Male: not reliable Female: >9 mo	— Development of endometritis and/or endometrial hyperplasia	36,37 35,38,39
Guinea pig	Contraception	Male: not effective Female: prevention of pregnancy for >160 d	— —	43 43,45,46
	Prevention ovarian cysts	No effect seen	Development of ovarian cysts and severe uterine pathology	44,46
Rat	Contraception	Male (1.1 mg): >8 mo Female: >1 y	— —	51,53 49,50,52
Budgerigar	Sertoli cell tumor	20 wk	—	69
Cockatiel	Suppress egg laying Ovarian neoplasm	At least 190 d 3–5 mo	— —	76 63,64
Quaker parrot	Suppress egg laying	At least 6 mo	—	68
Zebra finch	Song	No effect seen	—	71
Pigeon	Neutering Suppress egg laying	Male: 2 mo 8–10 wk	— —	67 67
Chicken	Suppress egg laying	4.7 mg deslorelin: 6 mo 9.4 mg deslorelin: 10 mo	— —	72 72
Japanese quail	Suppress egg laying	2–4 mo (60%–90% effective)	—	73–75
Turkey	Neutering (aggression)	Male (2.0 × 4.7 mg): 3–5 mo Male (2.0 × 9.4 mg): 7 mo	— —	66 66

(continued on next page)

Table 1
(continued)

Species	Indication	Duration of Action (4.7 mg)	Reported Side-Effects	Reference
Iguana	Ovarian activity	At least 1 y	—	80,82
Bearded dragon	Aggression	At least 2 mo	—	79
Veiled chameleon	Suppress egg laying	No effect seen	—	80
Leopard gecko	Suppress egg laying	No effect seen	—	83
Yellow-bellied slider	Contraception	No suppression of testosterone	—	81
Red-eared slider	Contraception	No effect seen	—	84

SUMMARY

Based on the HPG-axis, the role GnRH plays in hormonal regulation of reproduction, and the suppressive effect the deslorelin containing GnRH A-SRI has on the release of GnRH in many mammalian species, it seems logical that these implants can effectively be used as contraceptive agents in many species. Studies, however, have shown that these implants are ineffective in a variety of species from different orders and, in some cases, may even induce pathologic changes to the reproductive tract. An overview of companion exotic animal species in which the GnRH A-SRI has been used, the indication, its duration of action (if present), and potential side effects can be found in **Table 1**.

In many species, the effect of a GnRH A-SRI on the HPG-axis has not been evaluated. Based on the varying effect of these implants described in the various exotic companion species, it is important that further studies are performed to properly evaluate the effects of the implant in each species, so that more appropriate advice can be given to owners requesting contraception in their pets. Preferably, these studies include measurement of hormone concentrations, change of behavior, reproductive success (amount of eggs laid or amount of offspring produced), and duration of the effect. Although the reported side effects are only minimal (ie, local reaction at the site of placement), future studies preferably also contain information on side effects (if any) seen in the course of the study.

REFERENCES

1. Karten MJ, Rivier JE. Gonadotropin-releasing hormone analog design. Structure-function studies toward the development of agonists and antagonists: rationale and perspective. Endocr Rev 1986;7:44–66.
2. Padula AM. GnRH analogues—agonists and antagonists. Anim Reprod Sci 2005; 88:115–26.
3. Plosker GL, Brogden RN. Leuprorelin: a review of its pharmacology and therapeutic use in prostatic cancer, endometriosis and other sex hormone-related disorders. Drugs 1994;48:930–67.
4. Mans C, Pilny A. Use of GnRH-agonists for medical management of reproductive disorders in birds. Vet Clin North Am Exot Anim Pract 2014;17:23–33.
5. Goericke-Pesch S. Long-term effects of GnRH agonists on fertility and behaviour. Reprod Domest Anim 2017;52(Suppl 2):336–47.

6. Bertschinger HJ, Jago M, Nöthling JO, et al. Repeated use of the GnRH analogue deslorelin to down-regulate reproduction in male cheetahs (*Acinonyx jubatus*). Theriogenology 2006;66:1762–7.

7. Metrione LC, Verstegen JP, Heard DJ, et al. Preliminary evaluation of deslorelin, a GnRH agonist for contraception of the captive variable flying fox (*Pteropus hypomelanus*). Contraception 2008;78(4):336–45.

8. Kauffold J, Rohrmann H, Boehm J, et al. Effects of long-term treatment with the GnrH agonist deslorelin (Suprelorin®) on sexual function in boars. Theriogenology 2010;74(5):733–40.

9. Melville DF, O'Brien GMO, Crichton EG. Reproductive seasonality and the effect of the GnRH agonist deslorelin as a contraceptive in captive male Black Flying-foxes (*Pteropus alecto*). Theriogenology 2012;77(3):652–61.

10. D'Occhio MJ, Aspden WJ. Characteristics of luteinizing hormone and testosterone secretion, pituitary responses to LH releasing hormone (LHRH), and reproductive function in young bulls receiving the LHRH agonist deslorelin: effect of castration on LH responses to LHRH. Biol Reprod 1996;54:45–52.

11. D'Occhio MJ, Fordyce G, Whyte TR, et al. Reproductive responses of cattle to GnRH agonists. Anim Reprod Sci 2000;60–61:433–42.

12. Lunn SF, Cowen GM, Morris KD, et al. Influence of the gonad on the degree of suppression induced by an LHRH agonist implant in the marmoset monkey. J Endocrinol 1992;132:217–24.

13. Herbert CA, Trigg TE, Renfee MB, et al. Effects of a gonadotropin-releasing hormone agonist implant on reproduction in a male marsupial, *Macropus eugenii*. Biol Reprod 2004;70:1836–42.

14. Junaidi A, Williamson PE, Martin GB, et al. Pituitary and testicular endocrine responses to exogenous gonadotrophin-releasing hormone (GnRH) and luteinising hormone in male dogs treated with GnRH agonist implants. Reprod Fertil Dev 2007;19:891–8.

15. Schoemaker NJ, van Deijk R, Muijlaert B, et al. Use of a gonadotropin releasing hormone agonist implant as an alternative for surgical castration in male ferrets (*Mustela putorius furo*). Theriogenology 2008;70:161–7.

16. Rispoli LA, Nett TM. Pituitary gonadotropin-releasing hormone (GnRH) receptor: structure, distribution and regulation of expression. Anim Reprod Sci 2005;88: 57–74.

17. Schoemaker NJ, van Zeeland YRA. Disorders of the endocrine system. In: Johnson-Delaney CA, editor. Ferret medicine and surgery. Boca Raton (FL): CRC Press; 2016. p. 191–218.

18. Wagner RA, Bailey EM, Schneider JF, et al. Leuprolide acetate treatment of adrenocortical disease in ferrets. J Am Vet Med Assoc 2001;218:1272–4.

19. Lennox AM, Chitty J. Adrenal neoplasia and hyperplasia as a cause of hypertestosteronism in two rabbits. J Exot Pet Med 2006;15:56–8.

20. Schoemaker NJ, Teerds KJ, Mol JA, et al. The role of luteinizing hormone in the pathogenesis of hyperadrenocorticism in neutered ferrets. Mol Cell Endocrinol 2002;197:117–25.

21. Schoemaker NJ, Lumeij JT, Rijnberk A. Current and future alternatives to surgical neutering in ferrets to prevent hyperadrenocorticism. Vet Med 2005;100:484–96.

22. Vinke CM, van Deijk R, Houx BB, et al. The effects of surgical and chemical castration on intermale aggression, sexual behaviour and play behaviour in the male ferret (*Mustela putorius furo*). Appl Anim Behav Sci 2008;115:104–21.

23. Junaidi A, Williamson PE, Martin GB, et al. Dose–response studies for pituitary and testicular function in male dogs treated with the GnRH superagonist, deslorelin. Reprod Domest Anim 2009;44:725–34.

24. Goericke-Pesch S, Georgiev P, Antonov A, et al. Clinical efficacy of a GnRH-agonist implant containing 4.7 mg deslorelin, Suprelorin®, regarding suppression of reproductive function in tomcats. Theriogenology 2011;75(5):803–10.

25. Proháczik A, Kulcsár M, Trigg T, et al. Comparison of four treatments to suppress ovarian activity in ferrets (Mustela putorius furo). Vet Rec 2010;166:74–8.

26. van Zeeland YRA, Pabon M, Roest J, et al. Use of a GnRH agonist implant as alternative for surgical neutering in pet ferrets. Vet Rec 2014;175:66.

27. Goericke-Pesch S, Wehrend A. The use of a slow release GnRH-agonist implant in female ferrets in season for oestrus suppression. Schweiz Arch Tierheilkd 2012;154:487–91.

28. Oxenham M. Oestrus control in the ferret. Vet Rec 1990;126:148.

29. Miller LA, Fagerstone KA, Wagner RA, et al. Use of a GnRH vaccine, Gona-ConTM, for prevention and treatment of adrenocortical disease (ACD) in domestic ferrets. Vaccine 2013;31:4619–23.

30. Lennox A. Use of a GnRH Vaccine, Gonacon™, for prevention of adrenocortical disease (ACD) in domestic ferrets. Proc 2nd ICARE Conf. April 18-23, 2015, Paris. p. 365.

31. Garner MM, Ramsel K, Schoemaker NJ, et al. Myofasciitis in the domestic ferret. Vet Pathol 2007;44:25–38.

32. Schepers F, Koene P, Beerda B. Welfare assessment in pet rabbits. Anim Welf 2009;18:477–85.

33. Brodbelt DC, Blissitt KJ, Hammond RA, et al. The risk of death: the confidential enquiry into perioperative small animal fatalities. Vet Anaesth Analg 2008;35: 365–73.

34. Klaphake E, Paul-Murphy J. Disorders of the reproductive and urinary systems. In: Quesenberry K, Carpenter J, editors. Ferrets, rabbits, and rodents: clinical medicine and surgery. St Louis (MO): Elsevier; 2012. p. 217–31. https://doi.org/10.1016/B978-1-4160-6621-7.00017-8.

35. Geyer A, Daub L, Otzdorff C, et al. Reversible estrous cycle suppression in pre-pubertal female rabbits treated with slow-release deslorelin implants. Theriogenology 2016;85:282–7.

36. Goericke-Pesch S, Groegera G, Wehrend A. The effects of a slow release GnRH agonist implant on male rabbits. Anim Reprod Sci 2015;152:83–9.

37. Arlt S, Spankowski S, Kaufmann T, et al. Fertility control in a male rabbit using a deslorelin implant, a case report. World Rabbit Sci 2010;18:179–82.

38. Phungviwatnikul T, Tisyangkul V, Pagdepanichkit S, et al. Effect of GnRH-agonist deslorelin subcutaneously implantation on fertility in mixed breed female rabbits at the age of 2.5 months and 5 months. Thai J Vet Med Suppl 2011;41:179.

39. Geyer A, Poth T, Otzdorff C, et al. Histopathologic examination of the genital tract in rabbits treated once or twice with a slow-release deslorelin implant for reversible suppression of ovarian function. Theriogenology 2016;86:2281–9.

40. Aponte PM, Gutierrez-Reinoso MA, Sanchez-Cepeda EG, et al. Active immunization against GnRH in pre-pubertal domestic mammals: testicular morphometry, histopathology and endocrine responses in rabbits, guinea pigs and ram lambs. Animal 2017. https://doi.org/10.1017/S1751731117002129. First view.

41. Quesenberry K, Donnelly TM, Mans C. Biology, husbandry, and clinical techniques of guinea pigs and chinchillas. In: Quesenberry K, Carpenter J, editors.

Ferrets, rabbits, and rodents: clinical medicine and surgery. St Louis (MO): Elsevier; 2012. p. 279–94. https://doi.org/10.1016/B978-1-4160-6621-7.00017-8.

42. Pilny A. Ovarian cystic disease in guinea pigs. Vet Clin North Am Exot Anim Pract 2014;17(1):69–75.

43. Forman C, Wehrend A, Goericke-Pesch S. Deslorelin implants are suitable for contraception in female, but not male guinea pigs. Proc Int Symp Canine and Feline Reprod. Paris. June 22-24, 2016. p. 135.

44. Schuetzenhofer G, Goericke-Pesch S, Wehrend A. Effects of deslorelin implants on ovarian cysts in guinea pigs. Schweiz Arch Tierheilkd 2011;153:416–7.

45. Kohutova S, Jekl V, Knotek Z, et al. The effect of deslorelin acetate on the oestrous cycle of female guinea pigs. Vet Med (Praha) 2015;60(3):155–60.

46. Kohutova S. Diagnostika a terapia endokrinne aktívnych reprodukčných ochorení u morčaťa domáceho (*Cavia aperea f. porcellus*) [PhD thesis]. Czech Republic: Brno University; 2016.

47. Lennox A, Bauck L. Basic anatomy, physiology, husbandry, and clinical techniques. In: Quesenberry K, Carpenter J, editors. Ferrets, rabbits, and rodents: clinical medicine and surgery. St Louis (MO): Elsevier; 2012. p. 339–53. https://doi.org/10.1016/B978-1-4160-6621-7.00017-8.

48. Ward JA, Furr BJA, Valcaccia B, et al. Prolonged suppression of rat testis function by a depot formulation of Zoladex®, a GnRH agonist. J Androl 1989;10:478–86.

49. Alkis I, Cetin Y, Sendag S, et al. Long-term suppression of oestrus and prevention of pregnancy by deslorelin implant in rats. Bull Vet Inst Pulawy 2011;55:237–40.

50. Cetin Y, Alkis I, Sendag S, et al. Long-term effect of deslorelin implant on ovarian pre-antral follicles and uterine histology in female rats. Reprod Domest Anim 2013;48:195–9.

51. Edwards BS, Smith AW, Skinner DC. Dose and durational effects of the gonadotropin-releasing hormone agonist, deslorelin: the male rat (*Rattus norvegicus*) as a model. J Zoo Wildl Med 2013;44(4 Suppl):S97–101.

52. Grosset C, Peters S, Peron F, et al. 2012: Contraceptive effect and potential side-effects of deslorelin acetate implants in rats (*Rattus norvegicus*): preliminary observations. Can J Vet Res 2012;76:209–14.

53. Smith AW, Asa CS, Edwards BS, et al. Predominant suppression of follicle-stimulating hormone b-immunoreactivity after long-term treatment of intact and castrate adult male rats with the gonadotrophin-releasing hormone agonist deslorelin. J Neuroendocrinol 2012;24:737–47.

54. Hollingsworth AB, Lerner MR, Lightfoot SA, et al. Prevention of DMBA-induced rat mammary carcinomas comparing leuprolide, oophorectomy, and tamoxifen. Breast Cancer Res Treat 1998;47:63–70.

55. Jinshu X, Jingjing L, Duan P, et al. A synthetic gonadotropin-releasing hormone (GnRH) vaccine for control of fertility and hormone dependent diseases without any adjuvant. Vaccine 2005;23:4834–43.

56. Kehr R, Kalla NR. Antifertility effects of an LHRH agonist in male mice. Contraception 1996;53:299–306.

57. Lierz M, Petritz OA, Samour J. Reproduction. In: Speer BL, editor. Current therapy in avian medicine and surgery. St Louis (MO): Saunders-Elsevier; 2016. p. 531–49.

58. Mison M, Mehler S, Echols MS, et al. Selected coelomic surgical procedures. In: Speer BL, editor. Current therapy in avian medicine and surgery. St Louis (MO): Saunders-Elsevier; 2016. p. 645–57.

59. Mans C, Taylor WM. Update on neuroendocrine regulation and medical intervention of reproduction in birds. Vet Clin North Am Exot Anim Pract 2008;11:83–105.

60. Forbes NA. The use of GnRH implants in the treatment of sexual derived behavioural abnormalities in birds. Proc 10th EAAV Conf. Antwerp (Belgium). March 17-21, 2009. p. 119–22.
61. Klaphake E, Fecteau K, de Wit M, et al. Effects of leuprolide acetate on selected blood and fecal sex hormones in Hispaniolan Amazon parrots (Amazona ventralis). J Avian Med Surg 2009;23(4):253–62.
62. Hawkins MG, Barron HW, Speer BL, et al. Birds. In: Carpenter JW, editor. Exotic animal formulary. 4th edition. St Louis (MO): Saunders-Elsevier; 2012. p. 284.
63. Keller KA, Beaufrère H, Brandão J, et al. Long-term management of ovarian neoplasia in two cockatiels (Nymphicus hollandicus). J Avian Med Surg 2013; 27(1):44–52.
64. Nemetz L. Deslorelin acetate long-term suppression of ovarian carcinoma in a cockatiel (Nymphicus hollandicus). Proc 33rd AAV Conf. Louisville (KY). August 12-15, 2012. p. 37–42.
65. De Wit M, Westerhof I, Penfold L. Effect of leuprolide acetate on avian reproduction. Proc 25th AAV Conf. New Orleans (LA). August 17-19, 2004. p. 73–4.
66. Molter CM, Fontenot DK, Terrell SP. Use of deslorelin acetate implants to mitigate aggression in two adult male domestic turkeys (Meleagris gallopavo) and correlating plasma testosterone concentrations. J Avian Med Surg 2015;29:224–30.
67. Cowan ML, Martin GB, Monks DJ, et al. Inhibition of the reproductive system by deslorelin in male and female pigeons (Columba livia). J Avian Med Surg 2014; 28:102–8.
68. Winkel-Blair A, Berman J, Leal de Araujo J, et al. Deslorelin 4.7 mg implants reduce reproduction in quaker parrots (Myiopsitta monachus). Proc 3rd ICARE Conf. Venice (Italy). March 25-29, 2017. p. 507.
69. Straub J, Zenker I. First experience in hormonal treatment of sertoli cell tumors in budgerigars (Melopsittacus undulates) with absorbable extended release GnRH chips (Suprelorin®), Proc 1st ICARE Conf. Wiesbaden (Germany). April 20-26, 2013. p. 299–301.
70. Van Sant F, Sundaram A. Retrospective study of deslorelin acetate implants in clinical practice. Proc AAV Conf. Jacksonville (FL). August 4-7, 2013. p. 211–20.
71. Murphy K, Wilson DA, Burton M, et al. Effectiveness of the GnRH agonist deslorelin as a tool to decrease levels of circulating testosterone in zebra finches. Gen Comp Endocrinol 2015;22:150–7.
72. Noonan B, Johnson P, Matos D. Evaluation of egg-laying suppression effects of the GnRH agonist deslorelin in domestic chicken. Proc Annu Conf Ass Avian Vet. Louisville (KY). August 12-15, 2012. p. 321.
73. Petritz OA, Guzman DS, Paul-Murphy J, et al. Evaluation of the efficacy and safety of single administration of 4.7-mg deslorelin acetate implants on egg production and plasma sex hormones in Japanese quail (Coturnix coturnix japonica). Am J Vet Res 2013;74(2):316–23.
74. Schmidt F, Legler M, Einspanier A, et al. Influence of the GnRH slow-release agonist deslorelin on the gonadal activity of Japanese quail (Coturnix coturnix japonica). Proc 1st ICARE Conf. Wiesbaden (Germany). April 20-26, 2013. p. 501–2.
75. Petritz OA, Guzman D, Hawkins MG, et al. Comparison of two 4.7-milligam to one 9.4-milligram deslorelin acetate implants on egg production and plasma progesterone concentrations in Japanese quail (Coturnix coturnix japonica). J Zoo Wildl Med 2015;46(4):789–97.
76. Summa NM, Guzman D, Wils-Plotz EL, et al. Evaluation of the effects of a 4.7-mg deslorelin acetate implant on egg laying in cockatiels (Nymphicus hollandicus). Am J Vet Res 2017;78:745–51.

77. Montani A, Collarile T, Selleri P, et al. Evaluation of the efficacy and duration of single administration of 4.7-mg deslorelin acetate implant on follicular activity and plasma sex hormones in lovebird (*Agapornis* spp.) in a randomized controlled trial. Proc 3rd ICARE Conf. Venice (Italy). March 25-29, 2017. p. 508.
78. Tell L, Shukla A, Munson L, et al. A comparison of the effects of slow release, injectable levonorgestrel and depot medroxyprogesterone acetate on egg production in Japanese quail. J Avian Med Surg 1999;13(1):23–31.
79. Rowland MN. Use of a deslorelin implant to control aggression in a male bearded dragon (*Pogona vitticeps*). Vet Rec Case Rep 2013;1–2. https://doi.org/10.1136/vetreccr.d2007rep.
80. Knotek Z, Cermakova E, Oliveri M. Reproductive medicine in lizards. Vet Clin North Am Exot Anim Pract 2017;20:411–38.
81. Potier R, Monge E, Loucachevsky T, et al. Effects of deslorelin acetate on plasma testosterone concentrations in captive yellow-bellied sliders (*Trachemys scripta* sp.). Acta Vet Hung 2017;65:440–5.
82. Kneidinger N. GnRH implant in green iguana (*Iguana iguana*) [Diploma thesis]. University of Veterinary Medicine Vienna; 2010.
83. Cermakova E, Oliveri M, Knotek Z. Effect of GnRH agonist (deslorelin) on ovarian activity in leopard gecko (*Eublepharis macularius*). Proc 3rd ICARE Conf. Venice (Italy). March 25-29, 2017. p. 542.
84. Grundmann M, Möstl E, Knotkova Z, et al. The use of synthetical GnRH agonist implants (deslorelin) for the suppression of reptile endocrine reproductive activity. Proc 1st ICARE Conf. Wiesbaden (Germany). April 20-26, 2013. p. 248.
85. Lennox AM, Wagner RA. Comparison of 4.7-mg deslorelin implants and surgery for the treatment of adrenocortical disease in ferrets. J Exot Pet Med 2012;21:332–5.

Update on Cancer Treatment in Exotics

Ashley Zehnder, DVM, PhD, DABVP(avian)[a],*,
Jennifer Graham, DVM, DABVP(avian/exotic companion mammal), DACZM[b],
Gunther Antonissen, DVM, MSc, PhD[c,d]

KEYWORDS

- Exotics • Cancer • Therapeutics • Monitoring

KEY POINTS

- Cancer therapy in exotic species is heavily reliant on extrapolation from treatment recommendations for humans, dogs, and cats.
- The primary literature available for cancer in exotics is minimal and primarily comprises single case reports or small case series.
- The basic principles of cancer treatment do not vary across species and should be adhered to with modifications made for specific species requirements.
- Exotic clinicians should work closely with medical, surgical, and radiation oncologists to ensure the best care for their patients.
- There is an urgent need for exotic clinicians to be more collaborative and share their cancer cases to improve care for patients.

INTRODUCTION

Treatment options for animals with cancer are rapidly expanding, including in exotic animal medicine. Only limited information is available, however, about treatment effects in exotic pet species beyond individual case reports. Consequently, most cancer treatment protocols in exotic animals are extrapolated from those described in humans, dogs, and cats. Practical limitations, however, as well as anatomic or physiologic differences can complicate the application of certain cancer treatment modalities in exotic species. This review provides an overview and update on cancer treatment in exotic animal species, including the various considerations that are

The authors have nothing to disclose.
[a] Department of Biomedical Data Science, 1265 Welch Road, Stanford, CA 94305-5464, USA;
[b] Department of Clinical Sciences, Cummings School of Veterinary Medicine, Tufts University, 200 Westboro Road, North Grafton, MA 01536, USA; [c] Department of Pharmacology, Toxicology and Biochemistry, Faculty of Veterinary Medicine, Ghent University, Salisburylaan 133, Merelbeke 9820, Belgium; [d] Department of Pathology, Bacteriology and Avian Diseases, Faculty of Veterinary Medicine, Ghent University, Salisburylaan 133, Merelbeke 9820, Belgium
* Corresponding author.
E-mail address: azehnder.dvm@gmail.com

Vet Clin Exot Anim 21 (2018) 465–509
https://doi.org/10.1016/j.cvex.2018.01.012
1094-9194/18/© 2018 Elsevier Inc. All rights reserved.

important during the initial diagnosis, therapeutic planning, and monitoring of the exotic cancer patient.

TUMOR STAGING

Signalment, history, and thorough physical examination are important parts of the initial clinical evaluation of exotic patients with tumors. Because many tumors tend to affect animals of a particular age, gender, or species, collection of this information is vital. Diet history can help identify potential risk factors for neoplasia related to malnutrition; for example, in epidemiologic studies, the intake of carotenoid-rich fruits and vegetables has been correlated with protection from some forms of cancer[1] and it is suspected that chronic hypovitaminosis A may be a risk factor for development of squamous cell carcinoma (SCC) in pet birds.[2] Underlying viral disease is linked to cancers in a variety of species, for example, cholangiocarcinoma in Amazon parrot species with psittacid herpesvirus, lymphoproliferative disease in mice with murine leukemia virus, fibropapillomas in sea turtles with herpesvirus, and walleye dermal sarcoma retrovirus in fish, among others.[3–6] Ultraviolet light radiation has been linked to neoplastic disease in many species.[7–9] Reproductive history is important because chronic egg laying is a risk factor for development of ovarian/reproductive cancers.[10] Previous infection with *Macrorhabdus ornithogaster* may increase the risk of proventricular adenocarcinoma in budgerigars; therefore, a history of chronic macro rhabdiosis infection should not be overlooked.[11] Additionally, any chronic nonhealing wound or areas subject to repeated trauma or chronic inflammatory conditions may be at risk for development of neoplasia. In addition to revealing risk factors for neoplastic disease, patient evaluation is essential to determine the course of action. For example, it is important to rule out underlying (and potentially zoonotic) disease, such as chlamydiosis, salmonellosis, or mycobacteriosis, prior to the use of immunosuppressive agents. Similarly, underlying metabolic disease, including renal or hepatic disease; heart disease, including atherosclerosis; and other organ dysfunction may alter prognosis and a patient's ability to tolerate treatment.

For any exotic species with a suspected tumor, histologic or cytologic diagnosis of the tumor is recommended to determine (if possible) the tissue of origin and grade of tumor. Cytology can help differentiate neoplastic from non-neoplastic lesions and may broadly indicate tumor type, but accurate histogenesis and tumor grading require histology, with an exception of purely hematopoietic tumors, such as leukemias.[12] Special stains, including immunohistochemistry, may be needed to further determine various cellular antigens and cell of origin (discussed later). Mitotic index may can help determine tumor grade, but there is no clear evidence from the exotic species literature that mitotic index is prognostic.

The TNM approach, developed by the World Health Organization, is used in mammalian species to stage solid tumors and has been adapted for evaluation of disseminated tumors, such as lymphoma.[12] The TNM approach evaluates the primary tumor (T), presence or absence of metastatic disease in local and regional lymph nodes (N), and presence or absence of metastatic disease within the rest of the body (M). For exotic species that lack lymph nodes (birds, reptiles, and fish), this general concept can be adapted using a TM approach to evaluate tumors to best determine extent of disease and determine treatment options (**Fig. 1**). Because there is no clinical evidence to support the use of more precise tumor scales like those developed for specific tumors in human and companion animals, the authors recommend a more general staging technique that considers the overall health of the animal, in addition to details about the primary tumor and metastatic lesions. Once additional

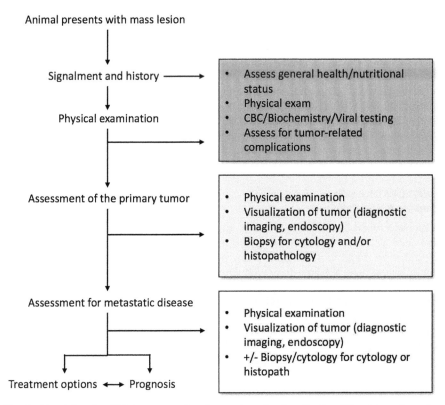

Fig. 1. Algorithm for TM tumor staging in exotic animal patients without lymph nodes. (*Adapted from* Zehnder A, Graham J, Reavill DR, et al. Neoplastic diseases in avian species. In: Speer B, editor. Current therapy in avian medicine and surgery. 1st edition. St Louis [MO]: Elsevier; 2016. p. 114; with permission.)

evidence on tumor types and outcome data are gathered, better predictions on prognosis based on tumors at their initial presentation can be made.

TM Approach

In evaluation of the primary tumor (T), the tumor is sampled by way of aspirates for cytologic diagnosis or biopsy for histologic diagnosis. In some situations, complete surgical excision of the mass may be the best option for diagnosis and treatment if disease is localized. The extent of the tumor can be evaluated by clinical examination of the patient but disease may extend beyond visible margins. Diagnostic imaging techniques, such as plain and contrast radiography, ultrasonography, CT, MRI, and endoscopy, can help assess extent of the tumor, depending on the tumor site. Objective tumor description, including specific location and measurement, in 3 planes whenever possible, should be recorded to monitor patient response. Two recent publications have provided avian body maps for use to describe more completely the location of tumors,[13,14] and maps for dogs and cats can often be adapted for many small mammal species.

In evaluation for metastatic disease (M), although the lung can be a common site for distant metastatic disease, other sites include the skin, liver, kidneys, bone, brain/nervous tissue, and spleen.[13] Physical examination may suggest metastases (for example, cutaneous masses), but diagnostic imaging techniques, as described previously, are generally required to evaluate for metastases. Multiple radiographic views can help evaluate for metastatic disease but CT scan is generally more sensitive for evaluation of metastatic disease compared with radiographs in many species. Radiographs may show changes in the size of shape of the liver, spleen, lymph nodes, and kidneys, but ultrasound-guided aspirates or endoscopic biopsies may be required to determine extent of disease into these organs. Bone marrow aspiration is recommended for staging and diagnosing disseminated diseases like lymphoma or leukemia. More advanced imaging modalities, including MRI, PET scan, and technetium (^{99m}Tc) bone scan, have been used to evaluate for metastatic disease in a variety of species.[13,15]

CLINICAL PATHOLOGY
Complete Blood Cell Count

A complete blood cell count (CBC) should be performed as part of a minimum database collection on any patient evaluated for cancer diagnosis or treatment. Anemia or leukopenia could indicate bone marrow or splenic disease. Leukocytosis with a neutrophilia or heterophilia with or without evidence of toxicity or a left shift may indicate a concurrent infection or infection related to the tumor itself, and appropriate antibiotic therapy should be instituted based on the site of the infection (if known) and, ideally, culture and sensitivity. Chemotherapy agents are generally most toxic to rapidly dividing cells so toxicity to the bone marrow and gastrointestinal (GI) tract is a concern. CBCs should be monitored and treatment should be delayed if the heterophil or neutrophil count is too low, that is, less than 2000 cells/μL, as recommended in dogs and cats.[15,16]

Biochemistry

Similar to CBC, biochemistry profile is recommended as part a minimum database collection. Renal or hepatic enzyme elevation may indicate organ involvement or dysfunction and may preclude use of certain chemotherapeutic drugs. Nevertheless, these tests rarely provide definitive information as to the type of cancer or whether metastasis is present.

IMAGING MODALITIES

Imaging often is essential in determining both the resectability of a primary tumor as well as identification of suspected metastatic lesions. This information is crucial for devising a rational treatment plan for a veterinary cancer patient. Radiographs of the thorax are valuable in determining the clinical stage of disease in mammals. To assess the lungs properly in mammals, 3 views should be obtained—both left and right lateral views as well as a ventrodorsal view, and these recommendations can be helpful for nonmammalian exotic patients as well. Conventional radiography, preferably with high-detail film, may provide adequate diagnostic imaging for nasal and oral tumors, although the extent of disease may not be fully elucidated. Ultrasonography allows evaluation of the architecture of abdominal viscera and has largely replaced radiographs in staging of mammalian cancer patients with abdominal neoplasia. CT has become more widely available for veterinary use, particularly at teaching institutions and large specialty practices. CT can be helpful to evaluate tumors within the nasal and oral cavities. CT is particularly useful when a veterinarian is trying to determine tumor margins prior to surgery or radiation therapy. CT imaging of the lungs, often accomplished with controlled ventilation, provides increased sensitivity in detecting small pulmonary nodules as well as enhanced discrimination of lesion location[17,18] compared with traditional radiography.

MRI is often the modality of choice for imaging tumors of the brain and spine. Lesions of the brainstem may require MRI for diagnostic quality. In addition to CT, MRI is useful when a veterinarian is trying to determine tumor margins prior to surgery or radiation therapy. MRI is often considered more sensitive in detecting tumor margins in soft tissues. Due to the slow speed of image acquisition, MRI has limited utility in imaging of the thorax in mammals and birds due to movement of the heart and lungs. PET is used to stage, plan surgery, evaluate response to therapy, and detect relapse of various neoplastic conditions. PET has been used to evaluate 2 cases of avian neoplasia, and normal PET image acquisition in Hispaniolan Amazon parrots has been described.[19]

TREATMENT MODALITIES

Although there are abundant articles on toxicity of chemotherapeutic agents in laboratory animals, these studies are generally performed in healthy animals at nontherapeutic doses in a laboratory setting and can be hard to extrapolate to pet species. Because information regarding the treatment effects in exotic pet species is scarce and generally limited to individual case reports, cancer treatment protocols in exotic animals are generally extrapolated from those described in humans, dogs, and cats.

There are some important differences, however, between exotic species versus dog and cat patients. Notably, many exotic patients presenting with tumors are small and vascular access is challenging for intravenous administration of chemotherapeutics. Nevertheless, the use of vascular access ports has been reported in exotic species, including ferrets, birds, rabbits, rodents, and reptiles, and can be considered in situations where repeated vascular access is necessary (eg, to administer medication or sample blood to monitor systemic response to therapy [**Fig. 2**]).[15,20] Due to their small size, vascular access ports in exotic patients are prone to clotting, and appropriate heparin locking is required to maintain function.

Depending on the type of neoplasia, a variety of treatment modalities can be considered for exotic species. Oral chemotherapeutics used in humans, dogs, and cats can be used in exotic animals, but compounding into appropriate doses may be necessary. If a medication needs to be swallowed whole versus crushed, use in exotic

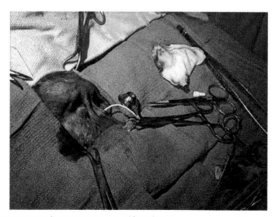

Fig. 2. Vascular access port placement in a wolf with a myxosarcoma. (Courtesy of Tara Harrison, DVM, MPVM, DACZM, DACVPM, North Carolina State University).

species may not be possible. Intratumoral chemotherapy consists of injecting antineo-plastic drugs into the tumor and nearby tissue and can be used in combination with surgery or radiation therapy. Slow-release formulations, such as sesame oil emulsions or collagen matrix, can optimize pharmacokinetics to allow for more prolonged exposure of the drug to tissue.

Radiation therapy is a common treatment modality in some exotic animal tumors, including thymoma in rabbits. Radiation therapies available for use in veterinary patients include teletherapy, plesiotherapy, brachytherapy, and systemic radiation therapy with radionucleotides.[21] In some situations, radiation therapy is combined with surgery or chemotherapy to maximize the chance for tumor response to therapy. Hormonal therapy, phototherapy, hyperthermia, immunotherapy, nonsteroidal therapy, antiangiogenic antibiotics, metronomic chemotherapy, and complementary and alternative therapy are other considerations for treatment of exotic neoplasia.

TRANSLATING CANCER THERAPIES TO EXOTICS
Metabolism

Birds have a high metabolic rate compared with most mammals but pharmacokinetic data has been obtained with some chemotherapeutics in a limited number of avian species. Results of these studies show that extrapolation of dosing regimens from mammals to avian species is at least a good starting point.[22] The opposite may be true for reptiles, and doses may need to be reduced or dosing intervals made less frequent as for other types of medications, such as antibiotics. Studies to determine appropriate metabolic scaling of chemotherapeutics for reptiles are, however, lacking. For poikilotherms, the ambient temperature and availability of appropriate temperature gradients within the enclosure are important for adequate drug metabolism. Better information is available in the laboratory animal literature for small mammals, but doses and dose intervals often still need to be adjusted from dog and cat doses.

Vascular Support, Renal/Hepatic Excretion

Birds and reptiles have a renal portal system and, in general, injection of chemotherapeutic drugs into leg vasculature should be avoided to prevent excretion of these agents before they enter the full circulatory system. Additionally, caution should be taken with the injection of any nephrotoxic agents into the leg vasculature for the same reason.

Risks of Corticosteroids and Immunosuppressive Agents

Any immunosuppressive therapy should be used with caution in most exotic species. Because of the high number of zoonotic diseases reported in exotic species, this issue must be taken into consideration when using immunosuppressive therapy in these patients or if owners are immunocompromised. Steroid therapy is not without risk of immunosuppression and secondary infection in exotic patients. Prophylactic antibiotic and antifungal therapy may be prudent whenever immunosuppressive drugs are used in these species. Certain species are known to harbor chronic infections that can exacerbate, flare up, or manifest clinically after use of steroids (eg, *Escherichia cuniculi* infections in rabbits). Thus, care should be taken before starting steroids in any exotic species. The exception to this is ferrets, which seem to tolerate steroid therapy well, and steroids can be used to help manage common diseases, like GI lymphoma.[23,24]

CHEMOTHERAPY

Although the use of chemotherapy in exotic animal oncology is increasing, the information in literature is limited and mainly based on case study findings and extrapolation from the human literature and the treatment of dogs and cats. Dosing of antineoplastic drugs should be done carefully because of their narrow therapeutic-toxic range. Therefore, it is of great importance to understand the basic mechanisms of action and potential toxicities before attempting to treat any animal species with chemotherapy (**Table 1**). Because recent reviews have discussed the basic pharmacology of common chemotherapeutics, this point is not be belabored in this article.[20] Currently, there is a growing interest in combining anticancer drugs aiming at maximizing efficacy while minimizing systemic toxicity through the delivery of lower drug doses. Combining 2 or more agents has a greater response than when used alone. The development of a multiagent chemotherapy protocol is based on selecting agents that act at different phases of the cell cycle (**Fig. 3**), have independent mode of actions, have synergistic effects to overcome drug resistance, and vary in their toxicities. Chemotherapy drugs can be administered by multiple routes, including orally, subcutaneously, intralesionally, intravenously, and intraosseously (**Fig. 4**). In particular, repeated intravenous administration might be difficult in many exotic animal species because of limited vascular access and because of the high vesicant and irritant properties of many chemotherapy drugs. In human medicine, there is a major trend in the development of oral chemotherapy, driven by pharmacoeconomic issues as well as patient convenience and quality of life. The availability of more oral chemotherapeutics will facilitate future usage of chemotherapy in exotic animals. Regardless of the route chosen, clinicians administering chemotherapy need to take appropriate precautions to protect themselves, patients, and owners from contact with potential toxic chemotherapeutics (**Fig. 5**).[20]

Chemotherapeutics are commonly dosed based on the body surface area (BSA) of a patient instead of the bodyweight (BW), because the BSA is considered a better indicator of the metabolic mass.[77] Because knowledge in exotic animal cancer treatment is limited, the use of BSA to derive interspecies equivalents for therapeutic dosages is opening treatment perspectives. Misunderstood and misinterpreted use of BSA conversions, however, may have unfavorable consequences, including underdosing, leading to treatment failure, and overdosing, inducing unexpected severe or even deadly adverse effects. Therefore, dose extrapolation between different animal species should be based on more advanced allometric and physiologically based pharmacokinetic modeling.[146] Recently, Antonissen and colleagues[22] demonstrated by allometric scaling a clear correlation ($R^2 > 0.97$) between BW and the elimination half-life ($T_{1/2el}$) of carboplatin in different avian species, expressed by the formula, $T_{1/2el\ carboplatin} = 0.1147$ (log value of BW)$^{0.3046}$. $T_{1/2el}$ could also be scaled with an acceptable correlation ($R^2 = 0.83$) in different mammalian species (rats, cats, dogs, and humans)[147–150] and different avian species (budgerigar, pigeons, ducks, cockatoos, and chickens).[22,137] Allometric scaling within 1 animal class is, however, preferred. Furthermore, carboplatin clearance is highly correlated with the animals' glomerular filtration rate. Taking into account the enormous differences in physiology between different exotic animal species, interanimal class dose extrapolation of chemotherapeutics is related to a major risk of therapy failure.

EMERGING MOLECULARLY TARGETED AGENTS

Most traditional chemotherapeutics have been drugs or other therapies that target cancer cells by killing rapidly dividing cells or killing all the cells in a particular area

Table 1
Chemotherapy agents that can be used in exotic animal medicine

Chemotherapy Agent	Mode of Action/Pharmacokinetics	Principal Indications	Toxicities/Side Effects	Administration Routes	Dosage	Case Reports
Nitrosoureas	Lomustine (CCNU) • Highly lipophilic, which enter cells through passive diffusion • Undergo bioactivation by cytochrome P450 enzymes in the liver • These metabolites cause alkylation and cross-linking of DNA (at the O_6-position of guanine-containing bases) and RNA, thus inducing cytotoxicity. • Also inhibit several key processes, such as carbamoylation and modification of cellular proteins • Urinary excretion, with minimal biliary excretion and GI reabsorption • Cell-cycle nonspecific	• Lymphoma • Mass cell tumor • Histiocytic sarcoma • Brain tumor	• Myelosuppression • GI toxicity • Sores in oral cavity • Pulmonary toxicity • Renal toxicity • Hepatotoxicity	PO	30–90 mg/m² Interval 3–8 wk[30-32]	[20,25-29]
	Carmustine (BCNU)	• Lymphoma • Neurologic tumor	• Myelosuppression • Pulmonary toxicity • GI toxicity	IV, local delivery	50 mg/m² Interval 6 wk[33,34]	N/A
Nitrogen mustard alkylating agents	Cyclophosphamide • Bifunctional alkylating agents • Mustards react with the N7 atom of purine bases, especially when they are flanked by adjacent guanines, inducing DNA strand breakage, cross-linking strands of DNA and ring cleavage. • Cell-cycle nonspecific • Well absorbed after PO administration • Excretion: small fraction a dose eliminated unchanged by urinary excretion, with minimal biliary excretion, majority eliminated by metabolic transformation[35-37] • Cyclophosphamide and ifosfamide: parent drug is relatively inactive, undergo bioactivation via hydroxylation by cytochrome P450 enzymes in the liver with formation of (iso)phosphoramide mustard • Chlorambucil and melphalan: direct alkylating ability • Sensitive to acquired tumor cell resistance by increased gluthatione conjugation[38]	• Lymphoma • Carcinoma • Sarcoma	• Myelosuppression[39] • GI toxicity • Renal toxicity • Urothelial toxicity (+ furosemide,[48] mesna[49]) • Feather abnormalities[51]	PO, IV, IO	10–80 mg/m² PO 3–4 consecutive d/wk[40,46,47] 100–200 mg/m² IV, IO Interval 1–3 wk 15 mg/m² PO daily (metronomic)[47,50]	[20,40-45]
	Ifosfamide	• Lymphoma • Sarcoma	• Myelosuppression • GI toxicity • Renal toxicity • Urothelial toxicity (+ furosemide,[54] mesna[55]) • Neurotoxicity	PO, IV	375–900 mg/m² IV Interval 3–4 wk[52,53]	N/A
	Chlorambucil	• Lymphocytic leukemia • Lymphoma • Mast cell tumor • Myeloma • Ovarian adenocarcinoma	• Myelosuppression • GI toxicity • Renal toxicity • Hepatotoxicity • Pulmonary toxicity • Alopecia	PO	10–20 mg/m² or 1–2 mg/kg Interval 0.5–2 wk[56,61] 4 mg/m² PO daily metronomic[62,63]	[26,40,42,56-60]
	Melphalan	• Myeloma • Lymphocytic leukemia • Lymphoma • Ovarian adenocarcinoma	• Myelosuppression[64] • GI toxicity • Pulmonary toxicity	PO	0.1 mg/kg daily for 10 d followed by 0.05 mg/kg per day or pulse dose administration of 3–7 mg/m² for 5 d in 3-wk cycle[65-67]	65

Antitumor antibiotics	Anthracyclines and anthracenediones: • Drugs first extracted from *Streptomyces* spp • Intercalation into DNA and disruption of topoisomerase-II–mediated DNA repair • Iron-mediated generation of free oxygen radicals that damage the DNA, proteins, and cell membranes • Cell-cycle nonspecific, although maximally cytotoxic during S phase • Low oral bioavailability • Doxorubicin is metabolized extensively to doxorubicinol by the ubiquitous aldo-keto reductase enzymes; by interfering with the iron and calcium regulation, this metabolite is important for doxorubicin cardiotoxicity,[68,69] • Biliary excretion, with minimal urinary excretion	Doxorubicin	• Cardiotoxicity[72] • Myelosuppression • GI toxicity • Renal toxicity • Hypersensitivity (mainly GI and skin related) • Alopecia • Perivascular damage with extravasation	IV, IO	20–60 mg/m² or 1–2 mg/kg Interval 2–3 wk[77–80]	20,40,41,43,68,73–76
		Epirubicin	• Less cardiotoxic than doxorubicin[81,82] • Similar to doxorubicin	IV	30 mg/m² Interval 3 wk[83]	N/A
		Mitoxantrone	• Less cardiotoxic than doxorubicin • More hepatotoxic than doxorubicin[87] • Myelosuppression • GI toxicity	IV, local delivery[84–86]	2.5–5 mg/m² IV Interval 3 wk[88,89]	N/A
	Chromomycins: • Drug first extracted from *Streptomyces* spp • Inhibit RNA synthesis by binding to guanine residues and inhibiting DNA-dependent RNA polymerase • Intercalation into DNA and disruption of topoisomerase-I and topoisomerase-II–mediated DNA repair[70] • Cell-cycle nonspecific • Biliary excretion, with minimal urinary excretion	Actinomycin D or dactinomycin	• Myelosuppression • GI toxicity • Perivascular damage with extravasation	IV	0.5–0.8 mg/m² Interval 3 wk[90,91]	N/A
	Miscellaneous: • Drug first extracted from *Streptomyces* spp • Forming an iron-oxygen-bleomycin complex that then forms free radicals, which cause single and double-stranded DNA breaks • Cell-cycle specific (G2 and M phase)	Bleomycin	• Pulmonary toxicity • Stomatitis • Hyperpigmentation of skin • Hypersensitivity	IV, IM, SC, local delivery	10–20 U/m² for 3–9 d, then weekly	20,92,93

(continued on next page)

Table 1 (continued)

Chemotherapy Agent	Mode of Action/Pharmacokinetics	Principal Indications	Toxicities/Side Effects	Administration Routes	Dosage	Case Reports
	• Metabolized by a cysteine protease hydrolase enzyme in normal tissues. The enzyme replaces a terminal amine with a hydroxyl, thereby inhibiting iron binding and cytotoxic activity. The low enzyme concentration in skin and lung may explain the unique sensitivity of these tissues to bleomycin toxicity.[71] • Mainly excreted with urine					
Antitubulin agents	**Vinca alkaloids** • Vincristine and vinblastine first extracted from periwinkle plant (*Catharanthus rosea*); vindesine and vinorelbine are semisynthetic derivatives of vinblastine. • Bind to the free tubulin-dimers, inhibiting the formation of microtubule—more specifically, the forming of the mitotic spindles—and thereby mitosis • Cell-cycle phase specific (M phase) • Metabolized in liver by cytochrome P450, and concomitantly administered drugs may either competitively inhibit or induce cytochrome P450 clearance of vinca alkaloids. • Largely excreted in the bile and feces, with little renal excretion[94,95]					
	Vincristine	• Lymphoma • Mast cell tumor	• GI toxicity • Myelosuppression • Neurotoxicity • Perivascular vesicant • Alopecia	IV, IO, local delivery	0.1–0.75 mg/m² Interval 1–2 wk	20,40,41,43,44,57,101,102
	Vinblastine	• Mast cell tumor[103] • TCC[104]	• GI toxicity • Myelosuppression • Perivascular vesicant	IV	2.0–3.5 mg/m² Interval 1–2 wk[103,147]	
	Vinorelbine	• Lymphoma • Mast cell tumor • TCC • Histiocytic sarcoma • Pulmonary carcinoma	• Myelosuppression • Perivascular vesicant[105] • Less neurotoxic than vincristine	IV	15 mg/m² Interval 1–2 wk[105,107,108]	105,106
	Taxanes • Complex diterpenes (hydrocarbons) originally identified from plants of the genus *Taxus* (yews) • As opposed to vinca alkaloids, taxanes increase microtubule stability and prevent dipolymerization, which causes tubulin bundling. • Cell-cycle phase specific, cells are arrested in G2/M phase, which is known to be the most radiosensitive phase of the cell cycle.					
	Paclitaxel	• Carcinoma • Sarcoma	• Myelosuppression • Hypersensitivity • Neurotoxicity • Alopecia • GI toxicity	IV, PO	130–150 mg/m² IV Interval 3 wk[96,109]	N/A
	Docetaxel	• Carcinoma • Sarcoma	• Myelosuppression • Hypersensitivity • GI toxicity	IV, PO	20–30 mg/m² or 1–2.5 mg/kg IV Interval 3 wk[111,112]	110

• Widely distribute into most tissues, except central nervous system • Substrates for the P-glycoprotein transporters, which interfere with their GI absorption—novel taxane analogs have been developed in human medicine that are poor substrates for P-glycoprotein and have higher oral bioavailability,[96] or taxane oral bioavailability increases by coadministration of competitive substrates for example, cyclosporine A.[97] • Largely excreted in the bile and feces, with little renal excretion					
Topoisomerase interactive agents • Semisynthetic derivatives of podophyllotoxin • Inhibit DNA synthesis by forming a complex with topoisomerase-II and DNA. This complex induces break in double-stranded DNA and prevents repair by topoisomerase-II binding. • Cell-cycle phase specific (late G2 and early S phases)	Etoposide	• Hemangiosarcoma[113] • Osteosarcoma[115] • Lymphoma[114] • Lung carcinoma	• Myelosuppression • Hypersensitivity • GI toxicity • Cardiotoxicity	IV, PO	50 mg/m² PO daily for 3 wk, 25 mg/m² for 4 consecutive days IV[113,114]	N/A
• Oral bioavailability is highly variable. Substrates for the P-glycoprotein transporters, which interfere with their GI absorption—oral bioavailability increases by coadministration of competitive substrates, for example, cyclosporine A.[98,99] • Converted to an O-demethylated metabolite by hepatic microsomal cytochrome P450, which has a similar potency at inhibiting topoisomerase-II and is more oxidatively reactive than the parent drug.[100] • Mainly excreted with urine	Teniposide	• Leukemia • Lymphoma • Lung carcinoma	• Myelosuppression • Hypersensitivity • GI toxicity • Cardiotoxicity	IV, PO	20 mg/kg IV or PO single administration 6.5 mg/kg IV Interval 3 d[116,117]	N/A

(continued on next page)

Table 1
(continued)

Chemotherapy Agent	Mode of Action/Pharmacokinetics	Principal Indications	Toxicities/Side Effects	Administration Routes	Dosage	Case Reports
Antimetabolites	General • Similar to endogenous metabolites, which are needed for normal biochemical activities involved in normal cell function and replication • Interfere directly with normal cell metabolism, interacting directly with specific enzymes by either inhibiting enzyme production or by producing a nonfunctional end product blocking cell processes dependent on that enzyme or end product, inhibiting protein, RNA or DNA synthesis • Cell-cycle phase specific (S phases)					
5-Flurouracil	Pyrimidine antagonists • Analogs of uracil or cytosine • 5-Fluoropyrimidines are structural pyrimidine base analog of uracil, inhibiting the enzymatic conversion of uracil to thymidine, inducing failure of normal DNA synthesis, faulty translation of RNA, and finally cytotoxicity of the rapidly dividing cancer cells. • Clearance of 5-fluoropyrimidines mediated by cytosolic enzyme dehydropyrimidine dehydrogenase–saturable enzyme process: impact on efficacy and safety bolus vs infusion administration • Gemcitabine is activated by being tri-phosphorylated on transport into the cell, which is catalyzed by the enzyme deoxycytidine kinase. Triphosporylated gemcitabine can masquerade as cytidine and is incorporated into new DNA strands. By masked chain termination	• Carcinoma	• Myelosuppression • GI toxicity • Cardiotoxicity[124,125] • Neurotoxicity	IV, local delivery	150–200 mg/m^2 IV Interval 1 wk[123] 1.47 mg/kg intralesionally Interval 3 wk[121,122]	121,122
Gemcitabine		• Lymphoma • Carincoma	• Myelosuppression • GI toxicity	IV	275–400 mg/m^2 Interval 2–3 wk Low dosage of 40 mg/m^2 as radiosensitizer[118,126]	20
Cytarabine		• Lymphoma • Leukemia	• Myelosuppression • GI toxicity	IV, SC	100–150 mg/m^2 IV or SQ for 4–5 consequent days repeat interval 3–4 wk[127,128]	44,127

by a normal nucleoside base aside gemcitabine, normal cell repair system not activated. Consequently, due to this irreparable DNA error, further DNA synthesis is inhibited and leads to cell death.[118]
- Cytosine arabinoside or cytarabine is a deoxycytidine base compound, which is phosphorylated in cells to the active metabolite arabinosylcytosine triphosphate, which is a competitive inhibitor of DNA polymerase α, and is incorporated into DNA and causes strand termination. Consequently, the cancer cell is unable to divide.[119]
- Low oral bioavailability
- Mainly excreted with urine[120]

Drug	Description	Indications	Side effects	Route	Dosage	Ref.
Methotrexate	Folate antagonist • Methotrexate is a competitive inhibitor of the enzyme folic acid reductase, preventing reduction of dihydrofolate to tetrahydrofolate, which is necessary for the synthesis of thymidylate, an essential component of DNA.[119] • High oral bioavailability • Largely excreted by urine but also substantial biliary excretion	• Lymphoma	• Myelosuppression • GI toxicity	PO, IV	2,5–5,0 mg/m² PO Interval 1–2 d[123] 0.3–0.8 mg/m² IV Interval 1–3 wk	40
Corticosteroids	Prednisolone/prednisone • Induce apoptosis of hematopoietic cancer cell by interaction with glucocorticoid receptor • Inhibit inflammatory and immune responses, most likely through alteration of cellular transcription and protein synthesis as well as through effects on lipocortins, which inhibit the release of arachidonic acid • Provide palliative appetite and anti-inflammatory support • Very high oral bioavailability	• Lymphoma • Mast cell tumor • Leukemia • Brain tumor • Insulinoma	• Polyuria/polydipsia • Polyphagia • GI toxicity • Hepatotoxicity • Hyperadrenocorticism • Dull hair coat • Pancreatitis	PO	0.5–2 mg/kg BW PO daily	20,26,41-44,58,76

(continued on next page)

Table 1
(continued)

Chemotherapy Agent	Mode of Action/Pharmacokinetics	Principal Indications	Toxicities/Side Effects	Administration Routes	Dosage	Case Reports
	• Avian patients: long-term usage predisposing for aspergillus infection or severe immune suppression • Do no use in combination with NSAIDs: increased toxicity • Cell-cycle nonspecific					
Platinum	Cisplatin					
	• Binding covalently to the N7 position of the imidazole ring of the purine bases of DNA, primarily guanine, and to a lesser extent adenine, forming monofunctional or bifunctional DNA intrastrand and interstrand adducts. This activates various signal-transduction pathways, such as those involved in DNA damage recognition and repair, cell-cycle arrest, and programmed cell death/apoptosis.[129]	• Carcinoma • Sarcoma	• Myelosuppression • GI toxicity • Nephrotoxicity • Ototoxicity • Pulmonary edema (species-specific, demonstrated in cats)[136]	IV, IO, local delivery	70 mg/m² IV Or 1 mg/kg BW IV Interval 3 wk[134] 1 mg/cm³ intratumoral[135]	20,132,133
	Carboplatin	• Carcinoma • Sarcoma	• Myelosuppression • GI toxicity • Less neurotoxic/ototoxic than cisplatin[142]	IV, IO, local delivery	125–300 mg/m² IV Or 5–10 mg/kg BW IV[22,137] Interval 3 wk 1.5 mg/cm³ intratumoral[143]	20,22,74,137–141
	• Platinum drugs (II), such as cisplatin, carboplatin, and oxaliplatin, are not orally bioavailable due to their chemical reactivity, poor absorption, and severe GI side effects. • Platinum (IV) compounds, such as satraplatin and tetraplatin, can be administered orally. These platinum compounds are prodrugs; once they enter cancer cells, they are reduced and activated by cellular reductants and form active complexes. These compounds are still under investigation.[130] • Mainly excreted with urine—platinum drug clearance is strongly associated with glomerular filtration rate. Carboplatin dosing using a pharmacologic formula is based on glomerular filtration rate and produces accurate targeting of the carboplatin AUC.[131] • Cell-cycle nonspecific					

Drug	Mechanism	Indications	Toxicity	Route	Dose	References
L-Asparaginase	• Enzyme purified from the bacterium *E coli* or *Erwinia carotovora* • Asparaginase hydrolyzes L-asparagine to L-aspartic acid and ammonia in leukemic cells, resulting in depletion of asparagine, inhibition of protein synthesis in leukemic cells, because these cells lack the enzyme asparagine synthase. • Pegaspargase: polyethylene glycol-conjugated asparaginase is slow-release form of *E coli* asparaginase • L-Asparaginase resistance in tumor cells, for example, by development of antiasparginase antibodies, or de novo biosynthesis of aspargine • No antigenic cross-reactivity between *E coli* and *E carotovora* asparaginase • No oral administration: denaturation and peptidase digestion within GI tract • Cell-cycle specific (G1 phase)[119]	• Lymphoma • Leukemia	• Hypersensitivity[144] • GI toxicity • Coagulopathies • Pancreatitis • Hepatotoxicity • Hyperglycemia	IM, SC	400 IU/kg BW IM/SQ Or 10,000–12,000 IU/m² Weekly interval	20,26,58
Hydroxyurea	• Inhibits DNA synthesis by inhibition of ribonucleotide diphosphate reductase. Hydroxyurea inhibits the conversion of DNA bases by blocking ribonucleotide reductase, thereby preventing conversion of ribonucleotides to deoxyribonucleotides. • Hydroxyurea also inhibits the incorporation of thymidine into DNA and may directly damage DNA. • Well absorbed after oral administration • Largely excreted by urine • Cell-cycle specific (S phase)	• Leukemia • Mast cell tumor • Meningioma	• Myelosuppression • GI toxicity	PO	30–60 mg/kg daily[145]	N/A

Abbreviations: IO, intraosseous; IV, intravenous; PO, oral; SC subcutaneous; N/A, Not Reported.

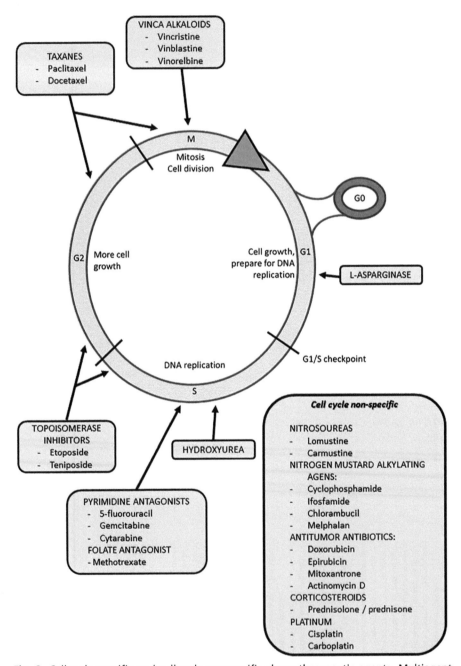

Fig. 3. Cell-cycle specific and cell-cycle nonspecific chemotherapeutic agents. Multiagent chemotherapy protocols should be based on selecting agents that act in at different phases of the cell cycle.

of the body affected by cancer. Although these treatments have certainly helped cure many patients, they also frequently have treatment-limiting side effects due to effects on normal cells. The holy grail of cancer therapy is to kill a cancerous cell while leaving

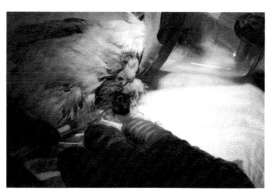

Fig. 4. Intralesional carboplatin administration to SCC in a cockatiel.

normal, healthy cells intact. New generations of targeted therapies attempt to achieve this goal through logically designed therapies targeting cancer specific mutations or cancer-specific pathways (**Fig. 6** and **Table 2**). Although many targeted agents actually affect many different receptors, with targeted therapies it becomes more important to know which particular mutations are present in a cancer cell or which cellular pathways it depends on for survival to rationally guide treatment. Although these therapies hold a great deal of promise for offering new, potentially less toxic treatments for exotic patients, it is unclear to what extent tumors in exotic species express the cellular receptors targeted by these agents. This may make it more difficult to translate new therapies emerging in human medicine (and for dogs and cats) without knowing how cancers in exotic species are alike and different. Some clinicians have begun to provide these therapies to patients when there are no other acceptable treatment options, but results from these cases are not yet available. These drugs also can have significant toxicities (see **Table 2**). Also, information on appropriate dosing for therapeutic efficacy is not at all known, and owners should always be made aware that use of these therapies in exotic species is experimental. Recording standardized

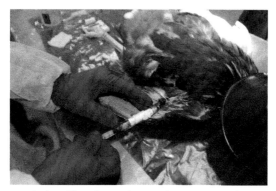

Fig. 5. Safety measures in handling chemotherapy: intravenous administration of carboplatin in a chicken. Veterinarians administering chemotherapy need to be familiar with the chemotherapeutic agents used and of safety issues for themselves, owners, and staff. Luer-Lok syringes should be used to avoid drug leakage, and all personnel handling drugs or patients receiving chemotherapeutic drugs should wear protective clothing, including gloves, eye protection, closed-toe shoes, and long sleeves.

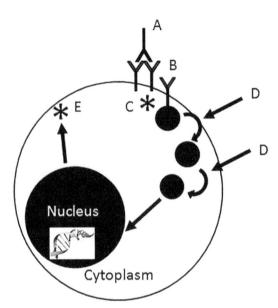

Fig. 6. Schematic of molecular targets for cancer therapy. A, antibody against cell surface receptor. B, cell surface receptor. C, small molecular inhibitor of cell surface receptor. D inhibitor of downstream pathway components. E, inhibitor of gene fusion product. (*Adapted from* Zehnder A, Graham J, Reavill DR, et al. Neoplastic diseases in avian species. In: Speer B, editor. Current therapy in avian medicine and surgery. 1st edition. St Louis [MO]: Elsevier; 2016. p. 132; with permission.)

case parameters (adverse effects and outcome information) for cases in which these agents are used is critical to evaluate their potential use in exotics species.

The types of therapies being developed for use in human and companion animals are summarized later and in **Table 2**, so that clinicians are aware of the types of therapies that may be available for treating exotic patients, with the caveat that little is known about the underlying cancer biology or the expression of certain cellular receptors in exotic species.

Tyrosine Kinase Inhibitors

There are 2 tyrosine kinase inhibitors that have been used in veterinary patients. Tyrosine kinases are cellular receptors that help normal cells and cancer cells interact with extracellular signals and are often mutated or overexpressed in multiple cancer types. The first is toceranib phosphate (Palladia), an inhibitor of the split-kinase family, which includes several growth factors implicated in cancer development: vascular endothelial growth factor receptor, platelet-derived growth factor receptor, c-kit, Flt-3, and others.[183] It was originally developed for use in mast cell tumors with an activating c-kit mutation but its role as an antiangiogenic therapy is also being studied, due to its inhibition of additional kinase family members. Toceranib has been used in a binturong (*Actictis binturong*) with renal carcinoma after nephrectomy with no discernible clinical effect but minimal adverse effects (mild inappetence).[184] In dogs, toceranib has been evaluated for safety in patients with a variety of solid tumor types[185] and found generally safe, with some mild GI effects requiring a treatment holiday. Reported side effects, however, can be as severe as GI perforation and can include other manifestations, such as lameness, hematochezia, pruritus, and localized edema (in a radiation patient).

Table 2
Summary of molecularly targeted agents

Toceranib

Combined with	Species	N	Tumor Type(s)	Clinical Effects	Adverse Events	Study Type	Citation
	Dogs	57	Various (MCT, lymphoma, STS, MMC, TCC, melanoma, OSCC, others)	ORR: 28% (highest in—55%)	Appetite loss, diarrhea, vomiting, neutropenia, grades 1 and 2, seen with daily dosing	Experimental, prospective, phase I	151
Single agent	Dogs	40	STS, TC, ASAGACA, NCA, SCC, OSA, carcinoma (various)	Clinical benefit: 90%	Majority grades 1 and 2, majority GI (52.5%), hematologic (42.5%), other effects: hypertension, PLN, lameness,	Experimental, prospective (phase I—evaluating effect of lower dose)	152
Prednisone/ hypofractionated radiation	Dogs	17	MCT	ORR: 86.7%, CR: 66.7%	GI and hepatic most common, mostly grades 1 and 2	Experimental, prospective clinical trial	153
Vinblastine	Dogs	14	MCT	ORR: 71%	Higher-grade neutropenia with combination than expected with single agent, improved with lower vinblastine doses	Experimental, prospective phase I clinical trial	154
Carboplatin/ cyclophosphamide	Dogs	126	OSA	No significant survival benefit	Grades 1 and 2 neutropenia and thrombocytopenia, trade 1 diarrhea, lethargy, vomiting most common	Experimental, prospective (randomized clinical trial)	155
Doxorubicin	Dogs	43	HSA	No significant survival benefit (compared with historical controls)	Grades 1 and 2 GI and grade 1 anemia most common	Experimental, prospective	156
Cyclophosphamide	Dogs	15	OSA, STS, HSA, LSA, MH, TCC, TC, ASAGACA, maxillary and perineum carcinoma	Decreased circulating Treg cells, increased serum concentration of IFN-γ	Grades 1 and 2, GI most common	Experimental, prospective	47

(continued on next page)

Table 2
(continued)

Toceranib

Combined with	Species	N	Tumor Type(s)	Clinical Effects	Adverse Events	Study Type	Citation
CCNU	Dogs	13	Multicentric LSA, OSA, PCA, STS, MLO, carcinoma/ adenocarcinoma (various)	Clinical benefit: 53.8%	Grades 3 or 4 effects: neutropenia, elevated ALT. AE more common in higher CCNU dose cohorts	Experimental, prospective (phase I—CCNU dose escalation)	[157]
Lomustine	Dogs	47	MCT	ORR: 46% (not increased over single agent studies)	Grades 1 and 2 GI, anemia, neutropenia most common, grade 4 neutropenia (n = 9)	Experimental, prospective (phase I—lomustine dose escalation)	[158]
Vinblastine	Dogs	10	TCC	No significant response (compared with historical single agent studies)		Experimental, prospective (pilot study, no internal control group)	[159]
Various	Dogs	85	ASAGACA, OSA, TC, HNCA, NCA	Clinical benefit: ASAGACA (87.5%), OSA (47.8%), TC (80%), HNCA (75%), NCA (71.4%)	AE in 77.6%, majority GI (AE not graded)	Observational, retrospective	[160]
Prednisone	Dogs	1	Chronic monocytic leukemia	Clinical remission	Not reported	Case report	[161]
Piroxicam or meloxicam	Cats	46	FOSCC	Significant increased survival rate compared with NSAID only controls	Grades 1 and 2 lethargy, anorexia, vomiting most common	Cohort, retrospective	[162]
Prednisolone or meloxicam	Cats	14	MCT, FOSCC, lymphoma, various carcinomas	Clinical benefit: 57.1%	Grade 1 neutropenia and GI AE most common, potential hepatotoxicity reported	Cohort, retrospective	[163]
Single agent	Cats	18	FISS	No measurable clinical response	Generally mild, grade 3 lymphopena and 4 ALT elevation managed with drug holidays	Experimental, prospective	[164]

	Species	N	Tumor Type(s)	Clinical Effects	Adverse Events	Study Type	Citation
Carboplatin, piroxicam	Cat	1	Tracheal adenocarcinoma	Survival: 755 d	None reported	Case report	165
Octreotide	Cat	1	Gastrinoma	Survival: 5 mo (euthanized)	Anorexia, treatment limiting	Case report	166
Single agent	Binturong	1	Renal carcinoma	Survival: 4 mo (euthanized)	Mild inappetence	Case report	184

Masatinib

Combination	Species	N	Tumor Type(s)	Clinical Effects	Adverse Events	Study Type	Citation
	Dogs	202	MCT	Increased time to progression 75–118 d, more significant in naive patients	Diarrhea, vomiting most common, generally grades 1 and 2	Experimental, Double-blind, randomized, placebo-controlled phase III clinical trial	167
	Dogs	132	MCT	Increased survival compared with placebo (617 vs 322d)	Not discussed	Experimental, placebo-controlled trial	168
	Dogs	26	MCT	ORR: 50%, response to treatment predictive of survival	Hepatic, proteinuria, hematologic and GI, majority mild and self-limiting	Experimental, placebo-controlled trial	169
	Dogs	10	CEL	Overall clinical response: 70%	myelosuppression (mild), vomiting/diarrhea (grade 4 in 1 dog), grade 3 anorexia, petechiae, elevated ALT	Experimental, prospective clinical trial	170
	Dogs	39	MCT	Overall clinical response: 82.1%	Elevated ALT (grade 3 or 4), anemia (grade 3 or 4) and vomiting (mild) most common	Observational, retrospective	171
	Cats	20	—	N/A	proteinuria and neutropenia noted, increased serum Cr, and GI effects (mild)	Experimental, prospective, randomized phase 1 clinical trial	172

Xenogeneic Melanoma Vaccines

Combination	Species	N	Tumor Type(s)	Clinical Effects	Adverse Events	Study Type	Citation
Surgery, radiation, ± chemotherapy	Dog	9	Oral, nail/footpad, intraocular	MST: 389 d	Mild injection site reactions	Experimental, prospective (phase I); antigen: huTyr	173

(continued on next page)

Table 2
(continued)

Xenogeneic Melanoma Vaccines

Combination	Species	N	Tumor Type(s)	Clinical Effects	Adverse Events	Study Type	Citation
Surgery, radiation, ± chemotherapy	Dog	170	Various	MST (stage II–IV): 389 d (huTyr), 153 (muGP75), 224 (muTyr)	Mild pain on injection	Experimental, prospective (phase I); antigens: huTry, muTyr, muGP75	174
Surgery alone ± steroids	Dog	111	Oral	Signficant improved survival over historical controls, MST could not be calculated	Mild injection site reactions, mild pain on injection	Experimental, prospective (phase II); antigen: huTyr	175
Amputation, radiation	Dog	58	Digit	MST: 476 d	Mild, local pain on injection, 9 dogs	Observational, retrospective; antigen: huTyr	176
Single agent or radiation	Dog	45	Oral	PFS (vaccinates): 199 d; (nonvaccinates): 247 d; no improvement in survival	Not discussed	Observational, retrospective; antigen: huTyr	177
Radiation, surgery	Dog	32	Oral	MST: 335 d	None observed	Observational, retrospective; antigen: huTyr	178
Surgical excision	Dog	38	Oral, digit, cutaneous	Oral: MST—26 mo; Digit: MST—36 mo; Other: 22 mo	None observed	Observational, retrospective; antigen: huTyr	179
Surgery, chemotherapy, radiation	Dog	11	Anal sac	MST: 107 d	None observed	Observational, retrospective; antigen: huTyr	180

Various chemotherapy, radiation	Dog	69	Oral	MST: 455 d	Not specified, stated as "minimal"	Observational, retrospective; antigen: huTyr	181
Various chemotherapy, radiation	Cat	24	Oral, ocular/periorbital, dermal, mucocutaneous, lip, subcutaneous	Not evaluated	Minimal, grades 1 and 2 anorexia, nausea, 2 cats grades 3 and 4 myelosuppression	Observational, retrospective; antigen: huTyr	182
Radiation, surgical excision	Lion	1	Oral	Complete response	None observed	Case report; antigen: huTyr	196
Radiation, strontium	African penguin	1	Nare	14-mo survival (previous reported mean of 7 mo)	None reported	Case report; antigen: huTyr	187

Clinical benefit: complete response, partial response, or stable disease.
Objective response rate (ORR): complete response, partial response.
Abbreviations: AE, adverse events; ALT, alanine transferase; ASAGACA, anal sac apocrine gland adenocarcinoma; CCNU, Lomustine; CEL, canine epitheliotropic lymphoma; Cr, creatinine; CR, complete response; FISS, feline injection-site sarcoma; FOSCC, feline oral SCC; HNCA, head and neck carcinoma; HSA, hemangiosarcoma; IFN, interferon; LSA, lymphosarcoma; MCT, mast cell tumor; MH, malignant histiocytosis; MLO, multilobulated osteochrondrosarcoma; MMC, mixed mammary carcinoma; MST, median survival time; N/A, not reported; NCA, nasal carcinoma; OR, objective response; OS, overall survival; OSA, osteosarcoma; OSCC, Oral Squamous Cell Carcinoma; PCA, prostatic carcinoma; PFS, progression-free survival; PLN, protein-losing nephropathy; STS, soft tissue sarcoma; TC, thyroid carcinoma; Treg, regulatory T Cells; TTP, time to progression.

The second is masitinib (Masivet), targeting primarily the mutated forms of the c-kit receptor, platelet-derived growth factor receptor, lymphocyte-specific kinase, Lck/Yes-related protein, fibroblast growth factor 3, and focal adhesion kinase.[183] It is being researched in human oncology for the treatment of multiple cancer types (including GI stromal tumors, pancreatic tumors, and melanoma). Masitinib was approved for use in veterinary medicine for the treatment of nonresectable canine mast cell tumors and represented one of the only drugs approved for veterinary cancer patients that is also used in clinical trials for human patients. There are no published reports of masitinib use in exotics species. Masitinib, however, lost conditional approval from the Food and Drug Administration on December 15, 2015, and it is no longer legal for this drug to be distributed in the United States. It is still available, however, in the United Kingdom and other European countries, according to the European Medicines Agency, as of October 2017.[186]

Tumor Vaccines

In addition to the tyrosine kinase inhibitors described previously, there is a vaccine (Oncept; Merial, Duluth, Georgia) developed to target canine melanoma that has been reported in sporadic proceedings case reports in exotic species.[187,188] This is a xenogeneic (cross-species) vaccine that targets an enzyme, tyrosinase, that is expressed in melanoma cells. It is xenogeneic because it uses human tyrosinase to trigger an immune response to canine tyrosinase in canine patients. It is the only US Department of Agriculture–approved cancer vaccine approved for dogs. The treatment protocol for canine melanoma involves a transdermal vaccine every 2 weeks for 4 treatments and then vaccine boosters every 6 months. The evidence for improved progression-free survival in dogs treated with vaccines compared with traditional radiation and chemotherapy protocols is inconclusive and it is unclear at this time that there is a significant survival benefit for animals treated with this vaccine. Also, the expression of tyrosinase in canine melanomas can be variable according to published reports.[189] The value of this therapy for exotic species remains to be seen, and more studies are needed to determine its potential efficacy.

RADIATION THERAPY IN EXOTIC SPECIES

For patients with confirmed local disease where complete surgical resection is not possible due to anatomic or other considerations, radiation therapy is a reasonable therapeutic modality. The 2 major types of radiation are external beam and strontium 90, both of which have been reported in exotic species. When clinicians are considering radiation therapy, the authors strongly recommend consultation with a radiation oncologist because there are frequent improvements in radiation oncology relating to the ability to accurately map tumor tissue and spare normal tissue.[190]

External Beam Radiation

Two different types of external beam radiation can be distinguished—orthovoltage and megavoltage radiation therapy. Each has its own characteristics, which render them useable for different tumor types. Orthovoltage (x-rays of 150–500 kilovolt [peak]) has lower energy and, therefore, lower penetration, making it more appropriate for tumors of the skin and subcutaneous tissues. This type of radiation has a preference for bone and the chances of late effects (necrosis) on bony tissues is high. Megavoltage (photons >1 million MeV) is higher energy and effects build up in tissue. The interaction of megavoltage rays with tissue is more predictable and this radiation type is used in computerized radiation planning schemes. Advances in radiation planning software and machine hardware allow for more contoured radiation plans, sparing more normal tissue (**Fig. 7**).

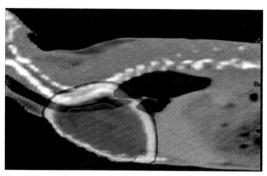

Fig. 7. Intensity-modulated radiation therapy planning in a rabbit for thymoma. (*Courtesy of* Tara Harrison, DVM, MPVM, Dipl. ACZM, Dipl. ACVPM, North Carolina State University.)

Tumors commonly treated with external beam radiation (in dogs and cats) include oral tumors, in particular melanoma and SCC, nasal tumors (sarcomas, carcinomas, and lymphomas), brain tumors, pituitary tumors, soft tissue sarcomas of the trunk and extremities, mast cell tumors, bone tumors (as part of multimodal therapy), and localized lymphomas. Recent reviews[14,21,191–193] have discussed the specific use of radiation in exotic species. Clinically, tumor types treated with radiation in exotics include a myxoma in a goldfish[191]; papilloma,[194] sarcoma,[195] and SCC[196] in reptiles; SCC,[197,198] melanoma,[199] hemangiosarcoma,[200] osteosarcoma,[201] lymphoma,[202] and fibrosarcoma in birds[203]; thymoma,[204] lymphoma, myeloma, seminoma, and nasal adenocarcinoma in rabbits[205–208]; preputial tumors[209]; chordoma[210]; SCC[211]; lymphoma[212]; and adenocarcinoma in ferrets.[213,214] In some cases, radiation can be used as a sole therapy, but it may also be combined with surgery or chemotherapy (in particular intralesional chemotherapy), depending on the tumor type/location and patient constraints (size and presence of comorbidities). Certain large tumors that cannot be resected may be treated with radiation to shrink them and make them more amenable to surgical resection. Also, radiation may be used after a surgical resection if the resection was determined to be incomplete on inspection of the margins.

Definitive versus palliative protocols
External beam radiation therapy can generally be broken into definitive and palliative protocols. The goal of definitive therapy is curative and involves an increased number of fractions and may provide higher gray/fraction. Definitive radiation is generally pursued if a patient is anticipated to live at least 1 year after therapy. These radiation protocols, however, may be associated with an increased risk of acute radiation side effects due to the increased number of fractions. Patients with an overall poor quality of life or a shorter life expectancy (generally <6 months) may be more appropriately treated with palliative protocols. These protocols have fewer fractions and have less frequent acute side effects.

Side effects and tolerance
The side effects of external beam radiation are divided into acute and chronic side effects. Acute side effects are related to the number of fractions provided as well as the area of the body being treated. Acute side effects may include mucositis, desquamation (dry or moist), and keratitis. Late radiation effects in mammals can include necrosis, fibrosis, nonhealing ulceration, central nervous system damage, and blindness, depending on the normal tissues being irradiated.[215] Although rare (1%–2% of cases) in humans and dogs, new tumors have been reported to develop at the site of radiation therapy. This has not yet been reported in avian oncology, but, given the long life span

of certain avian species, patients treated with radiation should be monitored for development of tumors at previous treatment sites.

The radiation tolerance of normal tissues in many species is not well defined and can be dramatically higher in some avian species. Quail and chickens are less radiosensitive compared with other animals, such as sheep, cattle, and swine, when whole-body irradiation effects on bone marrow are examined.[216–218] A study examined the tolerance dose of cutaneous and mucosal tissues in ring-necked parakeets (*Psittacula krameri*) for external beam megavoltage radiation and revealed minimal radiation-induced epidermal histologic changes in the high-dose group receiving 72 Gy in 4-Gy fractions.[219] A more recent study in macaws revealed that radiation delivered to the sinuses did not reach intended doses.[220] This implies that higher doses of radiation may be needed to produce equivalent response in avian patients compared with mammals, although the radiosensitivity of avian tumors has not yet been investigated. As in birds, studies examining the effects of radiation in other exotic species are mostly designed to effects of radiation contamination and not treatment efficacy.[14,21,191–193]

Strontium 90

Strontium 90 has specific indications for superficial tumors with less than 2 mm of depth. The level of radiation delivered decreases dramatically after 2 mm to 3 mm, so tumor staging is critical prior to choosing this modality. The circular area that can be treated with a strontium probe is approximately 8 mm and treated areas are arranged so they overlap to cover the entire tumor area. Common indications for strontium- 90 therapy include uropygial SCCs in birds, small tumors on the pinnal margin or nasal planum, and other superficial skin tumors as well as treating a tumor bed postexcision if there is concern regarding residual disease. Side effects of strontium 90 therapy are rare in the cases of it being been used and include local skin effects, such as alopecia, crusting, pruritus, leukotrichia, and thinning and depigmentation of the skin reported in cats.[221] Side effects in exotics have not been documented to the authors' knowledge.

OTHER/MISCELLANEOUS THERAPY TYPES
Hormonal/Steroidal Therapies

The most used hormones in veterinary medicine are corticosteroids, which are helpful in certain specific tumor types, including mast cell tumors, lymphomas, and lymphoid leukemias.[222] It is believed that steroids cause altered cellular transport of nutrients, apoptosis, and terminal differentiation in cancer cells. The effects are generally short lived, however, and there is concern of inducing multidrug resistance to chemotherapeutics in lymphoid cancers. Certain species are particularly susceptible to immunosuppression and secondary infection from the use of steroids, including birds and many small mammals, whereas others tolerate steroid therapy with few side effects (eg, ferrets). For steroid-sensitive species, prophylactic antibiotics and antifungals may be necessary when steroids are used as part of a cancer treatment protocol and patients should be closely monitored for signs of infection. Tamoxifen administration has not been evaluated for efficacy in cases of ovarian carcinoma, but antiestrogenic activity was suggested in 1 drug trial in budgerigars.[223] Gonadotropin-releasing hormone agonists (ie, leuprolide acetate) have been reportedly effective for ovarian carcinoma in birds in case reports in a small number of birds.[224,225]

Cryotherapy

Cryotherapy is reported infrequently in the exotic tumor literature.[132] It is a local therapy using extreme cold produced by liquid nitrogen or argon gas and is indicated in treating small, local lesions or residual disease postsurgical resection. Repeated treatments may be needed to achieve tumor control[226] and patients should be monitored closely for recurrence. Treatment areas should be monitored for any related skin effects, but such side effects are rarely reported. Care should be taken if used over areas of bone because it can cause necrosis.

Other Types of Therapy

Other therapy types that have been reported in exotic species include phototherapy, hyperthermia, immunotherapy, nonsteroidal therapy, antiangiogenic agents, metronomic chemotherapy, electrochemotherapy, and complementary and alternative therapies, and these have been discussed in recent reviews.[13,20,227,228] Because they have been recently reviewed and there are only sparse data on efficacy of these therapies, they are not discussed in depth in this review. A brief review of the use of nonsteroidal anti-inflammatory drugs (NSAIDs) in anticancer therapies is provided.

Epidemiologic studies in man have demonstrated a protective effect of chronic aspirin intake in the incidence of colorectal cancer.[229] Anti-inflammatory drugs to slow or stop tumor growth have shown promise in several animal model systems and clinical cancer cases. A majority of NSAIDs inhibit the isoforms of cyclooxygenase (COX-1 and COX-2) or are selective for 1 isoform. The NSAID piroxicam has activity against a variety of tumors in humans and dogs. Piroxicam is used in the treatment of transitional cell carcinomas (TCCs) of the urinary bladder and urethra in dogs and has also shown benefit in treatment of some SCCs and mammary adenocarcinomas. Canine patients receiving piroxicam or meloxicam seem to have an improved quality of life, with increased activity and alertness reported by owners.[229] Oral piroxicam has uncommonly been associated with GI ulceration and renal papillary necrosis in dogs. Meloxicam or other selective COX-2 inhibitors may be safer alternatives to piroxicam in the treatment of cancer, because they may reduce possible GI side effects due to increased COX-2 selectivity, but their effectiveness as an anticancer therapy is less well studied.

TREATMENT STRATEGIES FOR TUMORS

Often, deciding on the appropriate treatment regimen for a particular patient with cancer can be bewildering. Some general principles remain unchanged, regardless of species, and some are highly species specific. No 1 book chapter or journal article can address every clinical situation and the authors strongly recommend close consultation with a boarded veterinary oncologist to make individual-level treatment decisions.

General considerations that apply to every cancer patient are the resectability of the primary tumor, the presence of multiple or distant lesions, technical or logistical concerns, and patient comorbidities. Exotic practitioners are limited by some additional concerns, because basic issues like obtaining repeated, dedicated venous access may not be possible. Exotic patients can be very small, and they generally require repeated anesthetic episodes for treatments like chemotherapy, which poses more of a risk than for dogs and cats, which do not require multiple anesthetic episodes. Additionally, many exotic species may hide underlying illnesses and may be more susceptible to immunosuppressive effects of corticosteroids, a commonly component of treatment of dogs and cats with certain lymphoid tumors. Clinicians need to work closely with owners to make sure they understand that nearly all the treatment recommendations the authors make for exotic patients are extrapolated from treatments designed for human, dogs, or cats and there is only rare primary research examining the effectiveness of cancer therapy in exotic species. It is important to discuss with owners that necropsies at the time of death may provide additional information to expand the knowledge of behaviors of neoplasia in exotic species.

For every patient, the first question to ask of a diagnosed tumor is whether or not it is surgically resectable (**Fig. 8**). The first surgery represents the best chance of a cure and the surgeon needs to ask the following questions before planning a procedure: What is the histologic type and (to your best knowledge) the stage and grade of the cancer? What is the potential for local versus metastatic spread? Can a complete excision be performed and what are the cosmetic and functional trade-offs? and Are there any alternative options or plans for combined radiation or chemotherapy? This is the time when appropriate and interpretable diagnostics are key, to determine the true extent of the tumor and whether there is any evidence of distant disease because this would negate the reason for an extensive local surgical resection. Special considerations for exotic species include different healing capacities of skin types (mammal vs avian vs reptile) as well as elasticities for planning wound closures. Different species also tolerate different levels of surgical manipulations (eg, amputations) and knowledge of the normal anatomy and how well species can adapt to significant surgical alterations. Additionally, the planned "use" of the animal may guide therapy, in terms of whether this is a wild animal that needs to be released or a pet that can live with some level of disability.

For tumors where it is determined that surgical excision is feasible and indicated, basic oncological surgical principles apply. Appropriate surgical margins are not well defined for exotic species, and guidelines should be taken from histologically similar tumors in dogs, cats, or humans, where appropriate. The authors refer readers to recent excellent reviews on the topic and appropriate book chapters.[230,231] If surgical

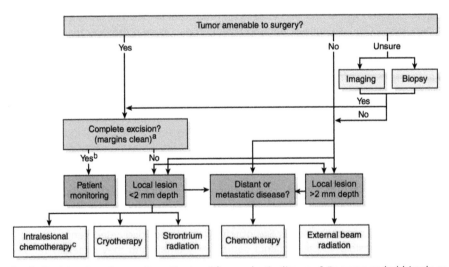

Fig. 8. Decision tree for exotic patients with neoplastic disease. [a] Recommended histology be performed on all excised tumors. [b] If tumor was high grade or there are metastases, adjunctive chemotherapy is indicated. [c] May be appropriate for lesions greater than 2 mm in depth depending on location and proximity to nearby vital structures. (*Adapted from* Zehnder A, Graham J, Reavill DR, et al. Neoplastic diseases in avian species. In: Speer B, editor. Current therapy in avian medicine and surgery. 1st edition. St Louis [MO]: Elsevier; 2016. p. 118; with permission.)

resection is not an option, if there is already distant disease detected, or if surgery is attempted but margins are not clean on histologic examination, additional therapies are determined by the lesion size, lesion depth, and presence of distant disease. For small local lesions or residual superficial tumor beds postsurgery, recommended treatments include intralesional chemotherapy, cryotherapy, or strontium 90 radiation. As discussed previously, strontium 90 is only important for lesions less than 2 mm in depth. For deeper but still local lesions, external beam radiation is considered more appropriate and the type and treatment protocol are guided by the histology. For distant lesions, chemotherapy or use of newer, molecularly targeted agents is appropriate. Again, the agent and protocol are guided by the type of disease as well as consultations with medical oncologists. The authors have attempted to discuss the indications for different chemotherapies as well as for newer molecular agents as a guide for clinicians. There is insufficient primary literature in exotic species, however, to be able to predict treatment efficacy or necessarily predict adverse events for specific patients, and owners need to be aware of these limitations.

NUTRITION/SUPPORTIVE CARE FOR EXOTIC CANCER PATIENTS

Appropriate nutritional support is vital for cancer patients. Cancer cachexia (CC) is a well-known phenomenon that has been described in both human and veterinary species.[232] CC causes significant changes in nutrient metabolism, leading to weight loss and muscle atrophy. CC is typically progressive and can have a significant impact on both length and quality of life if it is not appropriately managed.[233] Although no studies have been published on whether CC occurs in avian and reptile species, it is probable that they experience a similar syndrome, because progression of neoplasia in exotic species usually closely mirrors progression in other species.

Recommendations for management of CC include feeding a highly digestible diet that is limited in simple carbohydrates, contains moderate amounts of highly bioavailable amino acids, and contains increased amounts of fat. Supplementing the diet with omega-3 polyunsaturated fatty acids, eicosapentaenoic acid and docosahexaenoic acid, may be protective against some of the common metabolic abnormalities associated with CC and may improve response to treatment.[234] Omega-3 polyunsaturated fatty acids can be generally recommended as a healthy supplement for avian and other exotic patients, because they are also beneficial for cardiovascular, skeletal, and neurologic health.[235] Adequate insoluble fiber intake can improve GI health and promote normal GI flora, which may benefit patients undergoing cancer therapy.[236]

Unfortunately, there is no published information on the association of different dietary factors with cancer in exotic species. The impact of vitamins, minerals, and micronutrients on cancer risk and treatment has been extensively discussed in the human literature.[237] Carotenoids, selenium, folic acid, and vitamins A, C, E, and D have all been linked in certain studies to a reduction in cancer risk; however, many studies have produced conflicting information, and there is currently limited consensus on their correlation to cancer development.[238]

Regardless of which dietary supplements are elected for use in a cancer patient (if any), the patient must eat to benefit from nutritional support. The use of appetite stimulants, such as vitamin B complex or benzodiazepines, may be helpful.[239–241] Warming the food prior to offering it to a patient and decreasing stress in the surrounding environment may improve food acceptance. Appropriate medical management of pain and nausea is an extremely important factor. Metoclopramide may be used to help decrease nausea, improve appetite, and improve normal GI motility.[242] The efficacy and safety of other anti-nausea medications have not been critically evaluated in birds and other exotic species.

If necessary, supplemental gavage feeding or placement of an esophagostomy/ingluviotomy tube can be performed for long-term nutritional management. There are a variety of commercially available liquid critical care diets for exotic species that can be used for nutritional supplementation via these methods.

PATIENT MONITORING AND SIDE EFFECTS

In exotic animal practice, there is a lack of standardization for quantifying patient outcomes as well as adverse effects. This lack of consistency and quantitative patient information greatly hinders the ability to combine cases from different institutions as well as to assemble larger case series to analyze population-level data for different types of cancers. Within canine and feline oncology, as well as within human oncology, there are extensive tools for this type of patient monitoring and these should be adapted, as appropriate, for exotic patients. It is crucial for clinicians to convey to owners the importance of regular rechecks, even when patients are apparently doing well, and to inform veterinarians when patients die at home. Owners should be encouraged to allow necropsy whenever feasible, because it may be hard to know otherwise if therapies are truly effective or if there are subclinical side effects from therapy that may not otherwise be diagnosed.

Adverse Events

There is a range of adverse events that may occur secondary to chemotherapy administration, radiation treatment, or other cancer therapies. For patients undergoing chemotherapy, CBCs should be monitored weekly to biweekly, and treatment should be delayed if the heterophil/neutrophil count is too low. Based on information obtained in dogs and cats,[119,243] it is recommended that treatment should be delayed in patients with a heterophil (in birds and reptiles) or neutrophil (in mammals) counts less than 2000 cells/μL if a drug that is generally considered myelosuppressive is scheduled. If the drug is not considered myelosuppressive, it may be possible to administer therapy as long as the heterophil/neutrophil count is 1500 cells/μL. A conservative rule is to administer appropriate antimicrobial therapy to any avian or exotic patients with a heterophil count below 2000 cells/μL or less than 25% of the normal reference range for the species in question.

The Veterinary Cooperative Oncology Group (VCOG) has established common terminology criteria for adverse events after chemotherapy or biological antineoplastic therapy in dogs and cats.[184] These documents define an adverse event as "any unfavorable and unintended sign, clinical sign, or disease temporally associated with the use of a medical treatment that may or may not be considered related to the medical treatment." Adverse events are categorized by different body systems with a separate category for clinical pathology. There is a grading scale that quantifies the severity of the observed effects. Generally, grade 1 is mild and may be subclinical, grade 2 is moderate, grade 3 is severe, grade 4 is life-threatening, and grade 5 is death. Adverse events in exotic species being treated for cancer should be recorded and can be based on this information. A modified table for avian species is published in the recent review of avian oncology by 2 of the authors and the same authors are developing a more general version appropriate for additional exotic species.[13] It is important for clinicians to understand that they do not necessarily need to work out if the adverse event is a direct consequence of a treatment. For patients treated with combinations of therapies, it may not be clear which treatment is responsible for an observed event or an event may be due to an underlying disease process. It is important, however, to record any adverse events that are noted and make it clear in the medical record the doses, dosing intervals, and periods of time when treatments are administered so that cases can be accurately analyzed retrospectively for potential adverse events.

Assessing Response to Therapy

Human oncologists use Response Evaluation Criteria in Solid Tumors (RECIST) to objectively monitor primary tumors (target lesions) and lymph nodes and provide a standardized way to compare outcomes across multiple clinical trials and patient populations. These criteria received a major update in 2009 and are used in a majority of clinical trials.[244] The VCOG published an adapted version of these criteria for canine solid tumors in 2015.[245] Even in dog and cat oncology, these standards are not well established. There are a few basic guidelines, however, that clinicians can adopt into their practice to make their patient assessments more quantitative and allow accurate patient assessments over time.

Basic RECIST guidelines address the following points: baseline tumor measurements, methods of tumor assessments, evaluation of tumor response, and definitions of progression-free survival. Accurate, baseline tumor assessments (**Fig. 9**) are the key to objectively evaluating a patient's later response to therapy. It is recommended that measurements be taken as close as possible to the initiation of therapy. Lesions that are larger than 10 mm should be followed either with caliper measurements (for cutaneous lesions) or imaging modalities for internal lesions (where feasible). Ultrasonography is not recommended for repeated tumor assessments if other options are available. Due to the imprecise nature of radiographs and ultrasound, only lesions greater than 20 mm should be routinely monitored using these modalities. If patients have PET scans, they can be used to monitor response but not for accurate lesion measurements. Consistency is also important when tracking lesions. If caliper measurements are used, it is advisable for the same people to obtain those measurements at subsequent visits. CT scans are preferred over radiographs; however, these are not always feasible due to concerns over cost and longer anesthesia times. If ultrasound scans are used to follow lesions, it is important to use the same radiologist for the scans and use previous images to guide acquisition of new images so they are obtained in the same plane. In evaluation of patient response, clinicians should attempt to quantitate a patient's overall tumor burden in all measurable lesions. The longest diameters of target lesions (those that are measured repeatedly over time) are summed to obtain the "baseline sum diameters." This is the reference for assessing patient response.

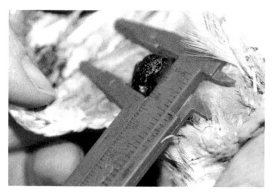

Fig. 9. Using calipers to measures a patagial SCC in a cockatiel prior to chemotherapy administration.

There are 4 different potential patient outcomes to any cancer treatment: complete response, partial response, progressive disease, and stable disease. Complete response describes the complete disappearance of all target (measured) lesions. Partial response describes at least a 30% reduction in the sum of diameters of target lesions (using the baseline sum as a reference). Progressive disease describes the appearance of new lesions or a 20% or greater increase in the sum of diameters of target lesions. Stable disease describes less than 30% decrease or less than 20% increase in tumor burden. There are additional details regarding nontarget or nonmeasurable lesions and the authors suggest reading the VCOG consensus document for more information.[245]

FUTURE DIRECTIONS

A recurring theme in every article and book chapter relating to cancer therapeutics in exotic and zoologic species is the extreme lack of remotely sufficient published knowledge regarding basic tenets of cancer biology and treatment of these species. Clinicians and researchers often are essentially guessing at the best therapies from 1, 2, or, in some cases, no published reports and every patient is an n of 1, particularly for more rare tumors in rarer species. The questions that remain to be asked are many. Do histologically similar tumors in these species behave like their counterparts in humans, dogs, or cats? Are the underlying genetic or molecular alterations similar and how do they affect patient prognosis? How long will a certain animal live with a particular tumor without treatments and which treatments actually prolong life? How do clinicians and researchers appropriately extrapolate therapies across species with widely different metabolisms, different dose tolerances, and potential species-specific toxicities? How can the level of case documentation, tumor quantification. and outcome and side effects reporting be improved to be able to better integrate clinical cases with those from other species?

How to do this is by better communicating cases to others and by accumulating cases in a central location with standardized clinical information, to start drawing statistically valid conclusions from clinical data. The Exotic Species Cancer Research Alliance is one such effort and has built a repository for clinical cases (Exotic Tumor Database) to try to answer some of these questions. Information regarding this effort is at www.escra.org, where there are resources to help clinicians find and enter their cases for the collective good of exotic clinicians and their patients.

REFERENCES

1. Bendich A, Olson JA. Biological actions of carotenoids. FASEB J 1989;3: 1927–32.
2. Schmidt RE, Reavill D. Respiratory system. In: Schmidt RE, Reavill D, editors. Pathology of pet and aviary birds. Ames (IA): John Wiley and Sons Inc; 2015. p. 21–54.
3. Hillyer EV, MS, Hoefer H, et al. Bile duct carcinoma in two out of ten parrots with with cloacal papillomas. J Assoc Avian Vet 1991;5:91–5.
4. Harkness JE, Turner PV, Wounde SC, et al. Specific diseases and conditions. In: Harkness JE, Turner PV, Wounde SV, et al, editors. Biology and medicine of rabbits and rodents. 5th edition. Ames (IA): Wiley-Blackwell; 2010. p. 249–394.
5. Jacobson ER, BC, Williams B, et al. Herpesvirus in cutaneous fibropapillomas of the green turtle Chelonia mydas. Dis Aquat Organ 1991;12:1–6.
6. Coffee LL, Casey JW, Bowser PR. Pathology of tumors in fish associated with retroviruses: a review. Vet Pathol 2013;50:390–403.

7. Watson M, Mitchell MA. Vitamin D and ultraviolet B radiation considerations for exotic pets. J Exot Pet Med 2014;24:369–79.

8. Ahmad M, Taqavi IH. Radiation induced leukemia and leukopenia in the lizard Uromastyx hardwickii. Radiobiol Radiother 1978;3:353.

9. Gallagher RP, Lee TK. Adverse effects of ultraviolet radiation: a brief review. Prog Biophys Mol Biol 2006;92:119–31.

10. Johnson PA, Giles JR. The hen as a model of ovarian cancer. Nat Rev Cancer 2013;13:432–6.

11. Garner MPL, Mitchell M. Does Macrorhabdus ornithogaster predispose budger-igars to proventricular adenocarcinoma? Proc Annu Conf Assoc Avian Vet. New Orleans, LA, 2014.

12. Blackwood L. Approach to the cancer case: staging–how and why. World Small Animal Veterinary Association World Congress Proceedings. Dublin, Ireland, 2008.

13. Zehnder A, Graham J, Reavill DR, et al. Neoplastic diseases in avian species. In: Speer B, editor. Current therapy in avian medicine and surgery. 1st edition. St Louis (MO): Elsevier; 2016. p. 107–41.

14. Robat C, Ammersbach M, Mans C. Avian oncology: diseases, diagnostics, and therapeutics. Vet Clin North Am Exot Anim Pract 2017;20:57–86.

15. Graham JE, Kent MS, Theon A. Current therapies in exotic animal oncology. Vet Clin North Am Exot Anim Pract 2004;7:757–81, vii.

16. Veterinary cooperative oncology group - common terminology criteria for adverse events (VCOG-CTCAE) following chemotherapy or biological antineo-plastic therapy in dogs and cats v1.1. Vet Comp Oncol 2016;14(4):417–46.

17. Krautwald-Junghanns ME, Schumacher F, Tellhelm B. Evaluation of the lower respiratory tract in psittacines using radiology and computed tomography. Vet Radiol Ultrasound 1993;34(6):382–90.

18. Tell L, Wisner E. Diagnostic techniques for evaluating the respiratory system of birds, reptiles, and small exotic mammals. Exotic DVM Vet Mag 2003;5:38–44.

19. Souza MJ, Wall JS, Stuckey A, et al. Static and dynamic (18) FDG-PET in normal hispaniolan Amazon parrots (Amazona ventralis). Vet Radiol Ultrasound 2011; 52:340–4.

20. Harrison TM, Kitchell BE. Principles and applications of medical oncology in exotic animals. Vet Clin North Am Exot Anim Pract 2017;20:209–34.

21. Kent MS. Principles and applications of radiation therapy in exotic animals. Vet Clin North Am Exot Anim Pract 2017;20:255–70.

22. Antonissen G, Devreese M, De Baere S, et al. Comparative pharmacokinetics and allometric scaling of carboplatin in different avian species. PLoS One 2015;10:e0134177.

23. Sinclair K, Eckstrand C, Moore PF, et al. Epitheliotropic gastrointestinal T-cell lymphoma with concurrent insulinoma and adrenocortical carcinoma in a do-mestic ferret (Mustela putorius furo). J Exot Pet Med 2016;25:34–43.

24. Hess L. Ferret lymphoma: the old and the new. Sem Av Exotic Med 2005;14: 199–204.

25. Goodnight AL, Couto G, Green E, et al. Chemotherapy and radiotherapy for treatment of cutaneous lymphoma in a ground cuscus (Phalanger gymnotis). J Zoo Wildl Med 2008;39:472–5.

26. Sinclair KM, Hawkins MG, Wright L, et al. Chronic T-cell lymphocytic leukemia in a black swan (Cygnus atratus): diagnosis, treatment, and pathology. J Avian Med Surg 2015;29:326–35.

27. Scheelings TF, Dobson EC, Hooper C. Cutaneous T-cell lymphoma in two captive tasmanian devils (Sarcophilus harrisii). J Zoo Wildl Med 2014;45: 367–71.

28. Onuma M, Kondo H, Ishikawa M, et al. Treatment with lomustine for mediastinal lymphoma in a rabbit. Journal of the Japan Veterinary Medical Association 2009; 62:69–71.

29. Onuma M, Kondo H, Ono S, et al. Lomustine for the treatment of alimentary lymphoma as a rescue protocol for ferrets. Journal of the Japan Veterinary Medical Association (Japan) 2008;717–9.

30. Rassnick KM, Williams LE, Kristal O, et al. Lomustine for treatment of mast cell tumors in cats: 38 cases (1999-2005). J Am Vet Med Assoc 2008;232:1200–5.

31. Musser ML, Quinn HT, Chretin JD. Low apparent risk of CCNU (lomustine)-associated clinical hepatotoxicity in cats. J Feline Med Surg 2012;14:871–5.

32. Risbon RE, de Lorimier LP, Skorupski K, et al. Response of canine cutaneous epitheliotropic lymphoma to lomustine (CCNU): a retrospective study of 46 cases (1999–2004). J Vet Intern Med 2006;20:1389–97.

33. Lucas SRR, Coelho BMP, Marquezi ML, et al. Carmustine, vincristine, and prednisone in the treatment of canine lymphosarcoma. J Am Anim Hosp Assoc 2004; 40:292–9.

34. Dimski DS, Cook JR. Carmustine-induced partial remission of an astrocytoma in a dog. J Am Anim Hosp Assoc 1990;26:179–82.

35. Boddy AV, Yule SM. Metabolism and pharmacokinetics of oxazaphosphorines. Clin Pharmacokinet 2000;38:291–304.

36. Holm KA, Kindberg CG, Stobaugh JF, et al. Stereoselective pharmacokinetics and metabolism of the enantiomers of cyclophosphamide. Preliminary results in humans and rabbits. Biochem Pharmacol 1990;39:1375–84.

37. Ma B, Zhang Y, Gu L, et al. Comparative pharmacokinetics of cyclophosphamide administration alone and combination with vitamin B6 in rats. Biomed Chromatogr 2015;29:62–7.

38. Black SM, Wolf CR. The role of glutathione-dependent enzymes in drug-resistance. Pharmacol Ther 1991;51:139–54.

39. Fulton RM, Reed WM, Thacker HL, et al. Cyclophosphamide (Cytoxan)-induced hematologic alterations in specific-pathogen-free chickens. Avian Dis 1996;40: 1–12.

40. Rassnick KM, Gould WJ, Flanders JA. Use of a vascular access system for administration of chemotherapeutic-agents to a ferret with lymphoma. J Am Vet Med Assoc 1995;206:500–4.

41. Folland DW, Johnston MS, Thamm DH, et al. Diagnosis and management of lymphoma in a green iguana (Iguana iguana). J Am Vet Med Assoc 2011;239: 985–91.

42. Hammond EE, Guzman DSM, Garner MM, et al. Long-term treatment of chronic lymphocytic leukemia in a green-winged macaw (Ara chloroptera). J Avian Med Surg 2010;24:330–8.

43. Ikpatt OF, Reavill D, Chatfield J, et al. Diagnosis and treatment of diffuse large B-cell lymphoma in an orangutan (Pongo pygmaeus). J Zoo Wildl Med 2014;45: 935–40.

44. Radcliffe RW, Paglia DE, Couto CG. Acute lymphoblastic leukemia in a juvenile southern black rhinoceros (Diceros bicornis minor). J Zoo Wildl Med 2000;31: 71–6.

45. Sacre BJ, Oppenheim YC, Steinberg H, et al. Presumptive histiocytic sarcoma in a great horned owl (Bubo-Virginianus). J Zoo Wildl Med 1992;23:113–21.

46. Burton JH, Mitchell L, Thamm DH, et al. Low-dose cyclophosphamide selectively decreases regulatory T cells and inhibits angiogenesis in dogs with soft tissue sarcoma. J Vet Intern Med 2011;25:920–6.

47. Mitchell L, Thamm DH, Biller BJ. Clinical and immunomodulatory effects of toceranib combined with low-dose cyclophosphamide in dogs with cancer. J Vet Intern Med 2012;26:355–62.

48. Rassnick KM, Rodriguez CO, Khanna C, et al. Results of a phase II clinical trial on the use of ifosfamide for treatment of cats with vaccine-associated sarcomas. Am J Vet Res 2006;67:517–23.

49. Ozcan A, Korkmaz A, Oter S, et al. Contribution of flavonoid antioxidants to the preventive effect of mesna in cyclophosphamide-induced cystitis in rats. Arch Toxicol 2005;79:461–5.

50. Elmslie RE, Glawe P, Dow SW. Metronomic therapy with cyclophosphamide and piroxicam effectively delays tumor recurrence in dogs with incompletely resected soft tissue sarcomas. J Vet Intern Med 2008;22:1373–9.

51. Ratnamohan N. Feather lesions in cyclophosphamide-treated chickens. Avian Dis 1981;25:534–7.

52. Payne SE, Rassnick KM, Northrup NC, et al. Treatment of vascular and soft-tissue sarcomas in dogs using an alternating protocol of ifosfamide and doxorubicin. Vet Comp Oncol 2003;1:171–9.

53. Rassnick KM, Frimberger AE, Wood CA, et al. Evaluation of ifosfamide for treatment of various canine neoplasms. J Vet Intern Med 2000;14:271–6.

54. Setyo L, Ma M, Bunn T, et al. Furosemide for prevention of cyclophosphamide-associated sterile haemorrhagic cystitis in dogs receiving metronomic low-dose oral cyclophosphamide. Vet Comp Oncol 2017;15(4):1468–78.

55. Vieira MM, Brito GAC, Belarmino JN, et al. Use of dexamethasone with mesna for the prevention of ifosfamide-induced hemorrhagic cystitis. Int J Urol 2003;10:595–602.

56. Newell SM, McMillan MC, Moore FM. Diagnosis and treatment of lymphocytic leukemia and malignant lymphoma in a Pekin duck (Anas platyrhynchos domesticus). Journal of the Association of Avian Veterinarians 1991;5(2):83–6.

57. Rivera S, McClearen JR, Reavill DR. Treatment of nonepitheliotropic cutaneous B-cell lymphoma in an umbrella cockatoo (Cacatua alba). J Avian Med Surg 2009;23:294–302.

58. Singleton CL, Wack RF, Zabka TS, et al. Diagnosis and treatment of chronic T-lymphocytic leukemia in a spotted hyena (Crocuta crocuta). J Zoo Wildl Med 2007;38:488–91.

59. Yu PH, Chi CH. Long-term management of thymic lymphoma in a java sparrow (Lonchura oryzivora). J Avian Med Surg 2015;29:51–4.

60. Malka S, Crabbs T, Mitchell EB, et al. Disseminated lymphoma of presumptive T-cell origin in a great horned owl (Bubo virginianus). J Avian Med Surg 2008;22:226–33.

61. Stein TJ, Pellin M, Steinberg H, et al. Treatment of feline gastrointestinal small-cell lymphoma with chlorambucil and glucocorticoids. J Am Anim Hosp Assoc 2010;46:413–7.

62. Leach TN, Childress MO, Greene SN, et al. Prospective trial of metronomic chlorambucil chemotherapy in dogs with naturally occurring cancer. Vet Comp Oncol 2012;10:102–12.

63. Schrempp DR, Childress MO, Stewart JC, et al. Metronomic administration of chlorambucil for treatment of dogs with urinary bladder transitional cell carcinoma. J Am Vet Med Assoc 2013;242:1534–8.

64. Page RL, Macy DW, Thrall DE, et al. Unexpected toxicity associated with use of body surface area for dosing melphalan in the dog. Cancer Res 1988;48: 288–90.

65. Scala C, Ortiz K, Nicolier A, et al. Lymphocytic leukemia in a captive dhole (Cuon alpinus). J Zoo Wildl Med 2013;44:204–7.

66. Fujino Y, Sawamura S, Kurakawa N, et al. Treatment of chronic lymphocytic leukaemia in three dogs with melphalan and prednisolone. J Small Anim Pract 2004;45:298–303.

67. Proulx DR, Ruslander DM, Dodge RK, et al. A retrospective analysis of 140 dogs with oral melanoma treated with external beam radiation. Vet Radiol Ultrasound 2003;44:352–9.

68. Gilbert CM, McGeary RP, Filippich LJ, et al. Simultaneous liquid chromatographic determination of doxorubicin and its major metabolite doxorubicinol in parrot plasma. J Chromatogr B Analyt Technol Biomed Life Sci 2005;826:273–6.

69. Cusack BJ, Young SP, Driskell J, et al. Doxorubicin and doxorubicinol pharmacokinetics and tissue concentrations following bolus injection and continuous infusion of doxorubicin in the rabbit. Cancer Chemother Pharmacol 1993;32: 53–8.

70. Wassermann K, Markovits J, Jaxel C, et al. Effects of morpholinyl doxorubicins, doxorubicin, and actinomycin D on mammalian DNA topoisomerases I and II. Mol Pharmacol 1990;38:38–45.

71. Dorr RT. Bleomycin pharmacology: mechanism of action and resistance, and clinical pharmacokinetics. Semin Oncol 1992;19:3–8.

72. Czarnecki CM. Doxorubicin (Adriamycin)-induced cardiotoxicity in Turkey poults - an animal-model. Comp Biochem Physiol C 1986;83:53–60.

73. McCain SL, Allender MC, Bohling M, et al. Thyroid neoplasia in captive raccoons (Procyon Lotor). J Zoo Wildl Med 2010;41:121–7.

74. Phalen DN, Frimberger AE, Peck S, et al. Doxorubicin and carboplatin trials in Tasmanian devils (Sarcophilus harrisii) with Tasmanian devil facial tumor disease. Vet J 2015;206:312–6.

75. Gilbert CM, Filippich LJ, Charles BG. Doxorubicin pharmacokinetics following a single-dose infusion to sulphur-crested cockatoos (Cacatua galerita). Aust Vet J 2004;82:769–72.

76. Harrison TM, Sikarskie J, Kitchell B, et al. Treatment of malignant lymphoma in an African lion (Panthera leo). J Zoo Wildl Med 2007;38:333–6.

77. Hahn KA. Chemotherapy dose calculation and administration in exotic animal species. Seminars in Avian and Exotic Pet Medicine 2005;14:193–8.

78. Kristal O, Lana SE, Ogilvie GK, et al. Single agent chemotherapy with doxorubicin for feline lymphoma: a retrospective study of 19 cases (1994-1997). J Vet Intern Med 2001;15:125–30.

79. Sorenmo KU, Baez JL, Clifford CA, et al. Efficacy and toxicity of a dose-intensified doxorubicin protocol in canine hemangiosarcoma. J Vet Intern Med 2004;18:209–13.

80. Lori JC, Stein TJ, Thamm DH. Doxorubicin and cyclophosphamide for the treatment of canine lymphoma: a randomized, placebo-controlled study. Vet Comp Oncol 2010;8:188–95.

81. Cave TA, Norman P, Mellor D. Cytotoxic drug use in treatment of dogs and cats with cancer by UK veterinary practices (2003 to 2004). J Small Anim Pract 2007; 48:371–7.

82. Yeung TK, Simmonds RH, Hopewell JW. A functional assessment of the relative cardiotoxicity of adriamycin and epirubicin in the rat. Radiother Oncol 1989;15: 275–84.

83. Kim SE, Liptak JM, Gall TT, et al. Epirubicin in the adjuvant treatment of splenic hemangiosarcoma in dogs: 59 cases (1997-2004). J Am Vet Med Assoc 2007; 231:1550–7.

84. DiMeco F, Li KW, Tyler BM, et al. Local delivery of mitoxantrone for the treatment of malignant brain tumors in rats. J Neurosurg 2002;97:1173–8.

85. Saini M, Roser F, Hussein S, et al. Intralesional mitoxantrone biopolymer-mediated chemotherapy prolongs survival in rats with experimental brain tumors. J Neurooncol 2004;68:225–32.

86. Ramirez LH, Zhao Z, Rougier P, et al. Pharmacokinetics and antitumor effects of mitoxantrone after intratumoral or intraarterial hepatic administration in rabbits. Cancer Chemother Pharmacol 1996;37:371–6.

87. Llesuy SF, Arnaiz SL. Hepatotoxicity of mitoxantrone and doxorubicin. Toxicology 1990;63:187–98.

88. Ogilvie GK, Moore AS, Obradovich JE, et al. Toxicoses and efficacy associated with administration of mitoxantrone to cats with malignant tumors. J Am Vet Med Assoc 1993;202:1839–44.

89. Ogilvie GK, Obradovich JE, Elmslie RE, et al. Efficacy of mitoxantrone against various neoplasms in dogs. J Am Vet Med Assoc 1991;198:1618–21.

90. Siedlecki CT, Kass PH, Jakubiak MJ, et al. Evaluation of an actinomycin-D-containing combination chemotherapy protocol with extended maintenance therapy for canine lymphoma. Can Vet J 2006;47:52–9.

91. Bannink EO, Sauerbrey ML, Mullins MN, et al. Actinomycin D as rescue therapy in dogs with relapsed or resistant lymphoma: 49 cases (1999–2006). J Am Vet Med Assoc 2008;233:446–51.

92. Lanza A, Baldi A, Spugnini EP. Surgery and electrochemotherapy for the treatment of cutaneous squamous cell carcinoma in a yellow-bellied slider (Trachemys scripta scripta). J Am Vet Med Assoc 2015;246:455–7.

93. Brunner CH, Dutra G, Silva CB, et al. Electrochemotherapy for the treatment of fibropapillomas in Chelonia mydas. J Zoo Wildl Med 2014;45:213–8.

94. Jordan MA, Thrower D, Wilson L. Mechanism of inhibition of cell proliferation by Vinca alkaloids. Cancer Res 1991;51:2212–22.

95. Leveque D, Jehl F. Molecular pharmacokinetics of catharanthus (vinca) alkaloids. J Clin Pharmacol 2007;47:579–88.

96. Khanna C, Rosenberg M, Vail DM. A review of paclitaxel and novel formulations including those suitable for use in dogs. J Vet Intern Med 2015;29:1006–12.

97. McEntee M, Silverman JA, Rassnick K, et al. Enhanced bioavailability of oral docetaxel by co-administration of cyclosporin A in dogs and rats. Vet Comp Oncol 2003;1:105–12.

98. Flory AB, Rassnick KM, Balkman CE, et al. Oral bioavailability of etoposide after administration of a single dose to tumor-bearing dogs. Am J Vet Res 2008;69: 1316–22.

99. Hande K, Anthony L, Hamilton R, et al. Identification of etoposide glucuronide as a major metabolite of etoposide in the rat and rabbit. Cancer Res 1988;48: 1829–34.

100. Yang J, Bogni A, Schuetz EG, et al. Etoposide pathway. Pharmacogenet Genomics 2009;19:552–3.

101. Phalen DN, Frimberger A, Pyecroft S, et al. Vincristine chemotherapy trials and pharmacokinetics in tasmanian devils with tasmanian devil facial tumor disease. PLoS One 2013;8(6):e65133.

102. Sandoval BJ, Amat AC, Sabri J, et al. Intralesional vincristine use for treatment of squamous cell carcinoma in a puma (Puma Concolor). J Zoo Wildl Med 2013;44: 1059–62.

103. Rassnick KM, Bailey DB, Flory AB, et al. Efficacy of vinblastine for treatment of canine mast cell tumors. J Vet Intern Med 2008;22:1390–6.

104. Arnold EJ, Childress MO, Fourez LM, et al. Clinical trial of vinblastine in dogs with transitional cell carcinoma of the urinary bladder. J Vet Intern Med 2011; 25:1385–90.

105. Kohno E, Murase S, Nishikata M, et al. Methods of preventing vinorelbine-induced phlebitis: an experimental study in rabbits. Int J Med Sci 2008;5: 218–23.

106. Cheng T, Si DY, Liu CX. Rapid and sensitive LC-MS method for pharmacokinetic study of vinorelbine in rats. Biomed Chromatogr 2009;23:909–11.

107. Wouda RM, Miller ME, Chon E, et al. Clinical effects of vinorelbine administration in the management of various malignant tumor types in dogs: 58 cases (1997-2012). J Am Vet Med Assoc 2015;246:1230–7.

108. Kaye ME, Thamm DH, Weishaar K, et al. Vinorelbine rescue therapy for dogs with primary urinary bladder carcinoma. Vet Comp Oncol 2015;13:443–51.

109. Poirier VJ, Hershey AE, Burgess KE, et al. Efficacy and toxicity of paclitaxel (Taxol) for the treatment of canine malignant tumors. J Vet Intern Med 2004; 18:219–22.

110. Wang J, Lan Z, Zhang L, et al. A rapid and sensitive UPLC-MS/MS method for determination of docetaxel in rabbit plasma: pharmacokinetic study of new lung-targeting docetaxel liposome at low dose. Cell Biochem Biophys 2015; 73:623–9.

111. Simon D, Schoenrock D, Baumgartner W, et al. Postoperative adjuvant treatment of invasive malignant mammary gland tumors in dogs with doxorubicin and docetaxel. J Vet Intern Med 2006;20:1184–90.

112. Shiu KB, McCartan L, Kubicek L, et al. Intravenous administration of docetaxel to cats with cancer. J Vet Intern Med 2011;25:916–9.

113. Lana S, U'Ren L, Plaza S, et al. Continuous low-dose oral chemotherapy for adjuvant therapy of splenic hemangiosarcoma in dogs. J Vet Intern Med 2007;21:764–9.

114. Hohenhaus AE, Matus RE. Etoposide (Vp-16) - retrospective analysis of treatment in 13 dogs with lymphoma. J Vet Intern Med 1990;4:239–41.

115. Ong SM, Saeki K, Kok MK, et al. Anti-tumour efficacy of etoposide alone and in combination with piroxicam against canine osteosarcoma in a xenograft model. Res Vet Sci 2017;113:130–5.

116. Zhang Z, Ma L, Jiang S, et al. A self-assembled nanocarrier loading teniposide improves the oral delivery and drug concentration in tumor. J Control Release 2013;166:30–7.

117. Broggini M, Colombo T, D'Incalci M. Activity and pharmacokinetics of teniposide in Lewis lung carcinoma-bearing mice. Cancer Treat Rep 1983;67:555–9.

118. Shipley LA, Brown TJ, Cornpropst JD, et al. Metabolism and disposition of gemcitabine, and oncolytic deoxycytidine analog, in mice, rats, and dogs. Drug Metab Dispos 1992;20:849–55.

119. Withrow SJ, Vail DM, Page R. General principles of cancer chemotherapy. In: Vail DM, editor. Small animal clinical oncology. St Louis (MO): Saunders; 2013. p. 157–79.

120. Heggie GD, Sommadossi JP, Cross DS, et al. Clinical pharmacokinetics of 5-fluorouracil and its metabolites in plasma, urine, and bile. Cancer Res 1987; 47:2203–6.

121. Karpinski LG, Miller CL. Fluorouracil as a treatment for corneal papilloma in a Malayan tapir. Vet Ophthalmol 2002;5:241–3.

122. Miller CL, Templeton RS, Karpinski L. Successful treatment of oral squamous cell carcinoma with intralesional fluorouracil in a Malayan tapir (Tapirus indicus). J Zoo Wildl Med 2000;31:262–4.

123. Chun R, Garret LD, Vail DM. Cancer chemotherapy. St Louis (MO): Saunders Elsevier; 2007.

124. Arellano M, Malet-Martino M, Martino R, et al. The anti-cancer drug 5-fluorouracil is metabolized by the isolated perfused rat liver and in rats into highly toxic fluoroacetate. Br J Cancer 1998;77:79–86.

125. Durak I, Karaayvaz M, Kavutcu M, et al. Reduced antioxidant defense capacity in myocardial tissue from guinea pigs treated with 5-fluorouracil. J Toxicol Environ Health A 2000;59:585–9.

126. Turner AI, Hahn KA, Rusk A, et al. Single agent gemcitabine chemotherapy in dogs with spontaneously occurring lymphoma. J Vet Intern Med 2006;20:1384–8.

127. Jankowski G, Sirninger J, Borne J, et al. Chemotherapeutic treatment for leukemia in a bearded dragon (Pogona vitticeps). J Zoo Wildl Med 2011;42:322–5.

128. Marconato L, Bonfanti U, Stefanello D, et al. Cytosine arabinoside in addition to VCAA-based protocols for the treatment of canine lymphoma with bone marrow involvement: does it make the difference? Vet Comp Oncol 2008;6:80–9.

129. Kelland L. The resurgence of platinum-based cancer chemotherapy. Nat Rev Cancer 2007;7:573–84.

130. Cheng Q, Shi H, Huang H, et al. Oral delivery of a platinum anticancer drug using lipid assisted polymeric nanoparticles. Chem Commun (Camb) 2015;51: 17536–9.

131. Millward MJ, Webster LK, Toner GC, et al. Carboplatin dosing based on measurement of renal function - experience at the Peter MacCallum Cancer Institute. Aust N Z J Med 1996;26:372–9.

132. Ferrell ST, Marlar AB, Garner M, et al. Intralesional cisplatin chemotherapy and topical cryotherapy for the control of choanal squamous cell carcinoma in an African penguin (Spheniscus demersus). J Zoo Wildl Med 2006;37:539–41.

133. Jaensch SM, Butler R, O'Hara A, et al. Atypical multiple, papilliform, xanthomatous, cutaneous neoplasia in a goose (Anser anser). Aust Vet J 2002;80:277–80.

134. Filippich LJ, Bucher AM, Charles BG. Platinum pharmacokinetics in sulphur-crested cockatoos (Cacatua galerita) following single-dose cisplatin infusion. Aust Vet J 2000;78:406–11.

135. Theon AP, Wilson WD, Magdesian KG, et al. Long-term outcome associated with intratumoral chemotherapy with cisplatin for cutaneous tumors in equidae: 573 cases (1995-2004). J Am Vet Med Assoc 2007;230:1506–13.

136. Barabas K, Milner R, Lurie D, et al. Cisplatin: a review of toxicities and therapeutic applications. Vet Comp Oncol 2008;6:1–18.

137. Filippich LJ, Charles BG, Sutton RH, et al. Carboplatin pharmacokinetics following a single-dose infusion in sulphur-crested cockatoos (Cacatua galerita). Aust Vet J 2004;82:366–9.

138. Sander SJ, Hope KL, McNeill CJ, et al. Metronomic chemotherapy for myxosarcoma treatment in a kori bustard (Ardeotis kori). J Avian Med Surg 2015;29: 210–5.

139. Childs-Sanford SE, Rassnick KM, Alcaraz A. Carboplatin for treatment of a Sertoli cell tumor in a mallard (Anas platyrhynchos). Vet Comp Oncol 2006;4:51–6.

140. Macwhirter PPD, Wayne J. Use of carboplatin in the treatment of renal adenocarcinoma in a budgerigar. Exotic DVM 2002;4:11–2.

141. Sutherland-Smith M, Harvey C, Campbell M, et al. Transitional cell carcinomas in four fishing cats (Prionailurus viverrinus). J Zoo Wildl Med 2004;35:370–80.

142. Taudy M, Syka J, Popelar J, et al. Carboplatin and cisplatin ototoxicity in guinea-pigs. Audiology 1992;31:293–9.

143. Theon AP, VanVechten MK, Madewell BR. Intratumoral administration of carboplatin for treatment of squamous cell carcinomas of the nasal plane in cats. Am J Vet Res 1996;57:205–10.

144. Blake MK, Carr BJ, Mauldin GE. Hypersensitivity reactions associated with L-asparaginase administration in 142 dogs and 68 cats with lymphoid malignancies: 2007-2012. Can Vet J 2016;57:176–82.

145. Rassnick KM, Al-Sarraf R, Bailey DB, et al. Phase II open-label study of single-agent hydroxyurea for treatment of mast cell tumours in dogs. Vet Comp Oncol 2010;8:103–11.

146. Blanchard OL, Smoliga JM. Translating dosages from animal models to human clinical trials–revisiting body surface area scaling. FASEB J 2015;29:1629–34.

147. Bailey DB, Rassnick KM, Kristal O, et al. Phase I dose escalation of single-agent vinblastine in dogs. J Vet Intern Med 2008;22:1397–402.

148. Gaver RC, George AM, Duncan GF, et al. The disposition of carboplatin in the beagle dog. Cancer Chemother Pharmacol 1988;21:197–202.

149. van der Vijgh WJ. Clinical pharmacokinetics of carboplatin. Clin Pharmacokinet 1991;21:242–61.

150. Siddik ZH, Jones M, Boxall FE, et al. Comparative distribution and excretion of carboplatin and cisplatin in mice. Cancer Chemother Pharmacol 1988;21:19–24.

151. London CA, Hannah AL, Zadovoskaya R, et al. Phase I dose-escalating study of SU11654, a small molecule receptor tyrosine kinase inhibitor, in dogs with spontaneous malignancies. Clin Cancer Res 2003;9:2755–68.

152. Bernabe LF, Portela R, Nguyen S, et al. Evaluation of the adverse event profile and pharmacodynamics of toceranib phosphate administered to dogs with solid tumors at doses below the maximum tolerated dose. BMC Vet Res 2013;9:190.

153. Carlsten KS, London CA, Haney S, et al. Multicenter prospective trial of hypofractionated radiation treatment, toceranib, and prednisone for measurable canine mast cell tumors. J Vet Intern Med 2012;26:135–41.

154. Robat C, London C, Bunting L, et al. Safety evaluation of combination vinblastine and toceranib phosphate (Palladia(R)) in dogs: a phase I dose-finding study. Vet Comp Oncol 2012;10:174–83.

155. London CA, Gardner HL, Mathie T, et al. Impact of toceranib/piroxicam/cyclophosphamide maintenance therapy on outcome of dogs with appendicular osteosarcoma following amputation and carboplatin chemotherapy: a multi-institutional study. PLoS One 2015;10:e0124889.

156. Gardner HL, London CA, Portela RA, et al. Maintenance therapy with toceranib following doxorubicin-based chemotherapy for canine splenic hemangiosarcoma. BMC Vet Res 2015;11:131.

157. Pan X, Tsimbas K, Kurzman ID, et al. Safety evaluation of combination CCNU and continuous toceranib phosphate (Palladia((R))) in tumour-bearing dogs: a phase I dose-finding study. Vet Comp Oncol 2016;14:202–9.

158. Burton JH, Venable RO, Vail DM, et al. Pulse-administered toceranib phosphate plus lomustine for treatment of unresectable mast cell tumors in dogs. J Vet Intern Med 2015;29:1098–104.

159. Rippy SB, Gardner HL, Nguyen SM, et al. A pilot study of toceranib/vinblastine therapy for canine transitional cell carcinoma. BMC Vet Res 2016;12:257.

160. London C, Mathie T, Stingle N, et al. Preliminary evidence for biologic activity of toceranib phosphate (Palladia((R))) in solid tumours. Vet Comp Oncol 2012;10: 194–205.

161. Perez ML, Culver S, Owen JL, et al. Partial cytogenetic response with toceranib and prednisone treatment in a young dog with chronic monocytic leukemia. Anticancer Drugs 2013;24:1098–103.

162. Wiles V, Hohenhaus A, Lamb K, et al. Retrospective evaluation of toceranib phosphate (Palladia) in cats with oral squamous cell carcinoma. J Feline Med Surg 2017;19:185–93.

163. Harper A, Blackwood L. Toxicity and response in cats with neoplasia treated with toceranib phosphate. J Feline Med Surg 2017;19:619–23.

164. Holtermann N, Kiupel M, Hirschberger J. The tyrosine kinase inhibitor toceranib in feline injection site sarcoma: efficacy and side effects. Vet Comp Oncol 2017; 15:632–40.

165. Azevedo C, Brawner W, Schleis Lindley S, et al. Multimodal non-surgical treatment of a feline tracheal adenocarcinoma. JFMS Open Rep 2017;3. 2055116916689630.

166. Lane M, Larson J, Hecht S, et al. Medical management of gastrinoma in a cat. JFMS Open Rep 2016;2. 2055116916646389.

167. Hahn K, Ogilvie G, Rusk T, et al. Masitinib is safe and effective for the treatment of canine mast cell tumors. J Vet Intern Med 2008;22(6):1301–9.

168. Hahn KA, Legendre AM, Shaw NG, et al. Evaluation of 12- and 24-month survival rates after treatment with masitinib in dogs with nonresectable mast cell tumors. Am J Vet Res 2010;71:1354–61.

169. Smrkovski OA, Essick L, Rohrbach BW, et al. Masitinib mesylate for metastatic and non-resectable canine cutaneous mast cell tumours. Vet Comp Oncol 2015; 13:314–21.

170. Holtermann N, Kiupel M, Kessler M, et al. Masitinib monotherapy in canine epitheliotropic lymphoma. Vet Comp Oncol 2016;14(Suppl 1):127–35.

171. Grant J, North S, Lanore D. Clinical response of masitinib mesylate in the treatment of canine macroscopic mast cell tumours. J Small Anim Pract 2016;57:283–90.

172. Daly M, Sheppard S, Cohen N, et al. Safety of masitinib mesylate in healthy cats. J Vet Intern Med 2011;25:297–302.

173. Bergman PJ, McKnight J, Novosad A, et al. Long-term survival of dogs with advanced malignant melanoma after DNA vaccination with xenogeneic human tyrosinase: a phase I trial. Clin Cancer Res 2003;9:1284–90.

174. Bergman PJ, Camps-Palau MA, McKnight JA, et al. Development of a xenogeneic DNA vaccine program for canine malignant melanoma at the Animal Medical Center. Vaccine 2006;24:4582–5.

175. Grosenbaugh DA, Leard AT, Bergman PJ, et al. Safety and efficacy of a xenogeneic DNA vaccine encoding for human tyrosinase as adjunctive treatment for oral malignant melanoma in dogs following surgical excision of the primary tumor. Am J Vet Res 2011;72:1631–8.

176. Manley CA, Leibman NF, Wolchok JD, et al. Xenogeneic murine tyrosinase DNA vaccine for malignant melanoma of the digit of dogs. J Vet Intern Med 2011;25: 94–9.

177. Ottnod JM, Smedley RC, Walshaw R, et al. A retrospective analysis of the efficacy of Oncept vaccine for the adjunct treatment of canine oral malignant melanoma. Vet Comp Oncol 2013;11:219–29.

178. Treggiari E, Grant JP, North SM. A retrospective review of outcome and survival following surgery and adjuvant xenogeneic DNA vaccination in 32 dogs with oral malignant melanoma. J Vet Med Sci 2016;78:845–50.

179. McLean JL, Lobetti RG. Use of the melanoma vaccine in 38 dogs: the South African experience. J S Afr Vet Assoc 2015;86:1246.

180. Vinayak A, Frank CB, Gardiner DW, et al. Malignant anal sac melanoma in dogs: eleven cases (2000 to 2015). J Small Anim Pract 2017;58:231–7.

181. Verganti S, Berlato D, Blackwood L, et al. Use of Oncept melanoma vaccine in 69 canine oral malignant melanomas in the UK. J Small Anim Pract 2017;58:10–6.

182. Sarbu L, Kitchell BE, Bergman PJ. Safety of administering the canine melanoma DNA vaccine (Oncept) to cats with malignant melanoma - a retrospective study. J Feline Med Surg 2017;19:224–30.

183. London CA. Tyrosine kinase inhibitors in veterinary medicine. Top Companion Anim Med 2009;24:106–12.

184. Thompson KA, Patterson J, Fitzgerald SD, et al. Treatment of renal carcinoma in a binturong (Arctictis binturong) with nephrectomy and a tyrosine kinase inhibitor. J Zoo Wildl Med 2016;47:1109–13.

185. Chon E, McCartan L, Kubicek LN, et al. Safety evaluation of combination toceranib phosphate (Palladia(R)) and piroxicam in tumour-bearing dogs (excluding mast cell tumours): a phase I dose-finding study. Vet Comp Oncol 2012;10:184–93.

186. European Medicines Agency. Available at: http://www.ema.europa.eu. Accessed October 15, 2017.

187. Mangold BJ, Flower JE, Burgess K, et al. A novel therapeutic approach to management of malignant melanoma in an African penguin. IAAAM. Cancun, Mexico, 2017.

188. Krause K. Malignant melanomas in domestic rabbits (Oryctolagus cuniculus): 27 cases. AEMV. Orlando, FL, 2014.

189. Smedley RC, Lamoureux J, Sledge DG, et al. Immunohistochemical diagnosis of canine oral amelanotic melanocytic neoplasms. Vet Pathol 2011;48:32–40.

190. LaRue S, Gordon IK. Radiation therapy. In: Withrow S, Vail DM, Page RL, editors. Withrow and MacEwen's small animal clinical oncology. St Louis (MO): Elsevier; 2013. p. 180–97.

191. Stevens B, Vergneau-Grosset C, Rodriguez CO Jr, et al. Treatment of a facial myxoma in a goldfish (Carassius auratus) with intralesional bleomycin chemotherapy and radiation therapy. J Exot Pet Med 2017;26:283–9.

192. Christman F, Devau M, Wilson-Robles H, et al. Oncology of reptiles: diseases, diagnosis, and treatment. Vet Clin North Am Exot Anim Pract 2017;20:87–110.

193. van Zeeland Y. Rabbit oncology: diseases, diagnostics, and therapeutics. Vet Clin North Am Exot Anim Pract 2017;20:135–82.

194. Gull J, Lange CE, Favrot C, et al. Multiple papillomas in a diamond python, Morelia spilota. J Zoo Wildl Med 2012;43:946–9.

195. Sharpe S, Lamm CG, Killick R. Intracoelomic anaplastic sarcoma in a Maragascar tree boa (Sanzinia madagascariensis). J Vet Diagn Invest 2013;25:153–7.

196. Steeil JC, Schumacher J, Hecht S, et al. Diagnosis and treatment of a pharyngeal squamous cell carcinoma in a Madagascar ground boa (Boa madagascariensis). J Zoo Wildl Med 2013;44:144–51.

197. Manucy T, Bennett RA, Greenacre CB, et al. Squamous cell carcinoma of the mandibular beak in a Buffon's Macaw (Ara ambigua). J Avian Med Surg 1998; 12:158–66.

198. Swisher SD, Phillips KL, Tobias JR, et al. External beam radiation therapy of squamous cell carcinoma in the beak of an African Grey Parrot (Psittacus timneh). J Avian Med Surg 2016;30:250–6.

199. Guthrie AL, Gonzalez-Angulo C, Wigle WL, et al. Radiation therapy of a malignant melanoma in a thick-billed parrot (Rhynchopsitta pachyrhyncha). J Avian Med Surg 2010;24:299–307.

200. Kimberly P, Freeman KAH, Adams WH, et al. Radiation therapy for an hemangiosarcoma in a budgerigar. J Avian Med Surg 1993;13:40–4.

201. Fordham M, Rosenthal K, Durham A, et al. Case Report: intraocular osteosarcoma in an umbrella cockatoo (Cacatua alba). J Avian Med Surg 2010;15:23–30.

202. Paul-Murphy J, Lowenstine L, Turrel JM, et al. Malignant lymphoreticular neoplasm in an African gray parrot. J Am Vet Med Assoc 1985;187:1216–7.

203. Lamberski N, Theon AP. Concurrent irradiation and intratumoral chemotherapy with cisplatin for treatment of a fibrosarcoma in a blue and gold macaw (Ara ararauna). J Avian Med Surg 2002;16:234–8.

204. Sanchez-Migallon D, Mayer J, Gould J, et al. Radiation therapy for the treatment of thymoma in rabbits (Oryctolagus cuniculus). J Exot Pet Med 2006;15:138–44.

205. Nakata M, Miwa Y, Tsuboi M, et al. Surgical and localized radiation therapy for an intranasal adenocarcinoma in a rabbit. J Vet Med Sci 2014;76:1659–62.

206. Varga M. Neoplasia. In: Meredith A, Lord B, editors. BSAVA manual of rabbit medicine. Quedgeley (United Kingdom): BSAVA; 2014. p. 264–73.

207. Mauldin G, Shiomitsu K. Principles and practice of radiation therapy in exotic and avian species. Semin Av Exotic Med 2005;14:168–74.

208. Antinoff N. Mediastinal masses in rabbit: another therapeutic option. Proc of the Ann Assoc of Exotic Mammal Veterinarians. Milwaukee, WI, 2009. p. 65.

209. van Zeeland Y, Lennox A, Quinton JF. Prepuce and partial penile amputation for treatment of preputial gland neoplasia in two ferrets. J Small Anim Pract 2014;55:593–6.

210. Graham J, DeCubellis J, Keyerleber MA, et al. Radiation therapy to manage cervical chordoma in two ferrets (Mustela putorius furo). Proc Ann Assoc Exotic Mammal Veterinarians. Indianapolis, IN, 2013.

211. Graham J, Fidel J, Mison M. Rostral maxillectomy and radiation therapy to manage squamous cell carcinoma in a ferret. Vet Clin North Am Exot Anim Pract 2006;9:701–6.

212. Hudson C, Kopit MJ, Walder EJ. Combination doxorubicin and orthovoltage radiation therapy, single-agent doxorubicin, and high-dose vincristine for salvage therapy of ferret lymphosarcoma. J Am Anim Hosp Assoc 1992;28:365–8.

213. Nakata M, Miwa Y, Nakayama H, et al. Localised radiotherapy for a ferret with possible anal sac apocrine adenocarcinoma. J Small Anim Pract 2008;49:476–8.

214. Miller T, Denman DL, Lewis DC. Recurrent adenocarcinoma in a ferret. J Am Vet Med Assoc 1985;187:839–41.

215. Moore AS. Radiation therapy for the treatment of tumours in small companion animals. Vet J 2002;164:176–87.

216. von Zallinger C, Tempel K. The physiologic response of domestic animals to ionizing radiation: a review. Vet Radiol Ultrasound 1998;39:495–503.

217. Eisele GR. Bacterial and biochemical studies on gamma-irradiated swine. Am J Vet Res 1974;35:1305–8.

218. Broerse J, Macvittie TJ. Response of different species to total-body irradiation. Boston: Nijhoff; 1984.

219. Barron HW, Roberts RE, Latimer KS, et al. Tolerance doses of cutaneous and mucosal tissues in ring-necked parakeets (Psittacula krameri) for external beam megavoltage radiation. J Avian Med Surg 2009;23:6–9.

220. Cutler DNJ, Shiomitsu K. Measurement of therapeutic radiation delivery in military macaws. Association of Avian Veterinarians Conference. Jacksonville, FL, 2013.

221. Turrel JM, Farrelly J, Page RL, et al. Evaluation of strontium 90 irradiation in treatment of cutaneous mast cell tumors in cats: 35 cases (1992-2002). J Am Vet Med Assoc 2006;228:898–901.

222. Kitchell B. Practical chemotherapy–an overview. Proceeding World Small Animal Veterinary Association World Congress. Mexico City, Mexico, 2005.

223. Lupu C. Evaluation of Side Effects of Tamoxifen in Budgerigars (Melopsittacus undulatus). J Avian Med Surg 2000;14:237–42.

224. Keller KA, Beaufrere H, Brandao J, et al. Long-term management of ovarian neoplasia in two cockatiels (Nymphicus hollandicus). J Avian Med Surg 2013; 27:44–52.

225. Nemetz L. Deslorelin acetate long-term suppression of ovarian carcinoma in a cockatiel (Nymphicus hollandicus). Louisville, KY: Association of Avian Vets; 2012.

226. McLaughlin A, RD, Maas AK. Management of recurrent cutaneous squamous cell carcinoma in a cockatiel (Nymphicus hollandicus). Proc Assoc Avian Vet. New Orleans, LA, 2014.

227. Suedmeyer W, McCaw D, Turnquist S. Attempted photodynamic therapy of squamous cell carcinoma in the casque of a great hornbill. J Avian Med Surg 2001;15:44–9.

228. Suedmeyer WK, Henry C, McCaw D, et al. Attempted photodynamic therapy against patagial squamous cell carcinoma in an African rose-ringed parakeet (Psittacula krameri). J Zoo Wildl Med 2007;38:597–600.

229. Argyle D, Brearley M, Turek M, et al. Cancer treatment modalities. In: Decision making in small animal oncology. Ames (IA): Wiley-Blackwell; 2008. p. 69–128.

230. Steffey M. Principles and applications of surgical oncology in exotic animals. Vet Clin North Am Exot Anim Pract 2017;20:235–54.

231. Farese JP, Withrow SJ. Surgical oncology. In: Withrow S, VD, Page R, editors. Withrow and MacEwen's small animal clinical oncology. St Louis (MO): Elsevier; 2013. p. 149–56.

232. Nitenberg G, Raynard B. Nutritional support of the cancer patient: issues and dilemmas. Crit Rev Oncol Hematol 2000;34:137–68.

233. Ogilvie GK, Fettman MJ, Mallinckrodt CH, et al. Effect of fish oil, arginine, and doxorubicin chemotherapy on remission and survival time for dogs with lymphoma: a double-blind, randomized placebo-controlled study. Cancer 2000; 88:1916–28.

234. Barber MD, Ross JA, Voss AC, et al. The effect of an oral nutritional supplement enriched with fish oil on weight-loss in patients with pancreatic cancer. Br J Cancer 1999;81:80–6.

235. Petzinger C, Heatley JJ, Cornejo J, et al. Dietary modification of omega-3 fatty acids for birds with atherosclerosis. J Am Vet Med Assoc 2010;236:523–8.

236. Ogilvie GK. Interventional nutrition for the cancer patient. Clin Tech Small Anim Pract 1998;13:224–31.

237. Gonzalez CA, Riboli E. Diet and cancer prevention: contributions from the European Prospective Investigation into Cancer and Nutrition (EPIC) study. Eur J Cancer 2010;46:2555–62.

238. Greenwald P, Anderson D, Nelson SA, et al. Clinical trials of vitamin and mineral supplements for cancer prevention. Am J Clin Nutr 2007;85:314S–7S.

239. Hawkins M, Ljung BH, Speer BL, et al. Nutritional/mineral support used in birds. In: JW C, editor. Exotic animal formulary. 4th edition. St Louis (MO): Elsevier; 2013. p. 306.

240. Gaskins L, Massey JG, Ziccardi MH. Effect of oral diazepam on feeding behavior and activity of Hawaii amakihi (Hemignathus virens). Appl Anim Behav Sci 2008;112:384–94.

241. Suarez D. Appetite stimulation in raptors. In: Redig P, Hunter B, editors. Raptor biomedicine. Minneapolis (MN): University of Minnesota Press; 1993. p. 225–8.

242. Carpenter J, Marion CJ. Exotic animal formulary. 4th edition. St Louis (MO): Elsevier; 2013.

243. Kent M. The use of chemotherapy in exotic animals. Vet Clin North Am Exot Anim Pract 2004;7:807–20.

244. Eisenhauer EA, Therasse P, Bogaerts J, et al. New response evaluation criteria in solid tumours: revised RECIST guideline (version 1.1). Eur J Cancer 2009;45: 228–47.

245. Nguyen SM, Thamm DH, Vail DM, et al. Response evaluation criteria for solid tumours in dogs (v1.0): a Veterinary Cooperative Oncology Group (VCOG) consensus document. Vet Comp Oncol 2015;13(3):176–83.

Nontraditional Therapies (Traditional Chinese Veterinary Medicine and Chiropractic) in Exotic Animals

Jessica A. Marziani, DVM, CVA, CVC, CCRT

KEYWORDS

- Nontraditional therapies • Traditional Chinese Veterinary Medicine • Acupuncture
- Chiropractic • Complementary therapies • Alternative therapies
- Integrative therapies

KEY POINTS

- Nontraditional therapies can be used in conjunction with conventional Western therapies to enhance patient outcome.
- Nontraditional therapies are often sought out by exotic pet owners; therefore, overall understanding is important for general practitioners.
- Exotic animal species can benefit from the application of nontraditional therapies.
- Traditional Chinese Veterinary Medicine is tailored to the individual patient to optimize health.
- Chiropractic care can be used as preventative form of treatment and for chronic conditions.

INTRODUCTION

In the broadest definition, nontraditional therapies are therapies that currently are not conventionally used in Western practice. Other terms, such as alternative, integrative, and complementary, are commonly used to categorize nontraditional therapies. However, no matter what nomenclature is used, all are considered the practice of veterinary medicine.[1]

According to the National Center for Complementary and Integrative Health, a division of the National Institute of Health (NIH), approximately 38% of adults in 2007 were using some sort of complementary therapy.[2] Those same adults may seek similar complementary therapies for their pets. Therefore, even if complementary therapies are not a core part of a veterinarian's skill set, it is still prudent to be grounded in

CARE Veterinary Services PLLC, PO Box 132082, Houston, TX 77219, USA
E-mail address: marzianidvm@gmail.com

Vet Clin Exot Anim 21 (2018) 511–528
https://doi.org/10.1016/j.cvex.2018.01.013
1094-9194/18/© 2018 Elsevier Inc. All rights reserved.
vetexotic.theclinics.com

general knowledge, treatment options, and how and when nontraditional therapies can be used effectively.

This general working knowledge of the subject will help veterinarians better educate clients in nontraditional therapies. Without a referral from their veterinarian, clients may research nontraditional therapies on their own if they believe that the treatments will be beneficial. A recent survey of competitive horse riders and trainers showed that of the 37% of the respondents that were seeking nontraditional therapies for their horses, only 7% were doing so in collaboration with their veterinarian.[3]

Practitioners who integrate nontraditional therapies and Western medicine can take advantage of the strengths of each. This integration of methodologies can deliver overall better results than Western medicine or nontraditional therapies alone. A working knowledge of nontraditional therapies and open dialogue can also enhance the veterinarian-owner relationship.

This article is intended to expose the general practitioner to the 2 most common and sought out nontraditional therapies: Traditional Chinese Veterinary Medicine (TCVM) and chiropractic treatments. The descriptions of each are intended to provide a basic understanding of what additional therapies are available and how they can be effectively utilized. The article is not intended to train the general practitioner on how to perform these therapies. Attending a specialized training course is highly recommended. These are listed in **Table 1**. Alternatively, practitioners who are trained in nontraditional therapies but have not practiced on exotic animals will also find this article useful as a reference for species comparisons and differences.

INTRODUCTION TO TRADITIONAL CHINESE VETERINARY MEDICINE

Traditional Chinese Medicine (TCM) used in Western culture is relatively new. TCM was first introduced to the United States when an aide to President Nixon became ill while Nixon was visiting China in the 1970s. This aide was treated successfully with TCM and thus TCM was prominently introduced to Western culture. Because it

Table 1 Certification training opportunities	
TCVM	**Chiropractic**
Chi Institute www.tcvm.com (800) 860–1543	Healing Oasis Wellness Center www.healingoasis.edu (262) 898–1680
International Veterinary Acupuncture Society www.ivas.org (970) 266–0666	Options for Animals www.optionsforanimals.com (309) 658–2920
	Parker University https://ce.parker.edu/courses/doctor-of-chiropractic/animal-chiropractic-program/ (800) 266–4723
	Veterinary Chiropractic Learning Center (Canada) www.veterinarychiropractic.ca (519) 756–1597
	Backbone Academy for Veterinary Chiropractic and Healing Arts (Germany) www.backbone-academy.com +49–4282–590688

Disclaimer: This is not an endorsement; these are the training programs the author is aware of.

has been practiced in the United States only in the last 40 years, TCM is considered a nontraditional or complementary therapy. However, it is among the oldest recorded forms of medical practice.

Thousands of years ago, ancient farmers began identifying methods to treat their sick livestock and horses. Without horses, they would lose battles, be limited in travel, and unable to plow their fields. Without livestock, they would go hungry. Effective methods of treatment were passed down from generation to generation and, in this way, TCVM was born.

As TCVM was introduced to the Western world, modern advances were also added to the implementation of TCVM. Western practitioners changed from multiple-use needles to reusable sterile needles, and added electrical current and laser light stimulation to acupoints.[4] Western society also expanded TCVM to fit other species beyond livestock and horses.

TCM and TCVM are often difficult for the Western practitioner to understand because both take an entirely different approach to health and treatment of disease. The general overriding principle in Western medicine is control. If the spread of the bacteria can be controlled, the infection can be treated. In TCVM, the prevailing principle is balance. If the body is in balance, it is in good health. The diagnostics in Western medicine range from an examination to advanced imaging. Diagnostics in TCVM are limited to observation and examination of the tongue, pulse, and palpation of points throughout the body. Western medicine treats a disease, whereas TCVM treats an individual's imbalance pattern. TCVM is so individualized that it is not effective in herd-health medicine. For example, 2 Netherland dwarf rabbits with radiologically similar spinal arthritis are treated with the same approach in Western medicine, probably with nonsteroidal antiinflammatories and/or a centrally acting opiate agonist.[5] In TCVM, those same 2 Netherland dwarf rabbits will be treated differently based on their individual disease pattern, not solely based on the diagnosis of the spinal arthritis.

Explanation of Traditional Chinese Veterinary Medicine Pattern Diagnosis

An overarching tenant of TCVM is that the absence of disease means that the body is in harmony and balanced. Illness occurs when the body is out of harmony and out of balance. To establish balance, the practitioner must first ascertain what is out of balance. Is the patient too hot or too cold? Is there too much (an excess) of something or too little (a deficiency) of something? Are there multiple deficiencies and excesses? TCVM treatments revolve around what is referred to as a pattern diagnosis. For a patient with a complicated chronic disease condition, that pattern diagnosis may change numerous times throughout treatment while working through each layer of the imbalance. A TCVM practitioner must constantly be reassessing the patient's pattern as the treatment continues to achieve better results.

The essentials of balance start with Yin and Yang. The Yin and Yang are 2 supporting opposites. Without the other to balance the scale, either can get out of control. Yin characteristics are cold, rest, slowness, weakness, and night. Yang characteristics are the opposite of Yin: warmth, activity, speed, strength, and day. If there is not enough warmth to balance the cold, then cold wins out and the leading characteristic exhibited is cold. In TCVM, this is considered Yang deficient because the body is deficient of warmth. The opposite of Yang deficient is Yin deficient, which is described as being too hot because there is not enough Yin, or cold, to counteract the warmth from the Yang. There is species variability in how much Yin or Yang is possessed, especially when it comes to exotics. For example, reptiles and amphibians are naturally more Yin than most animals, whereas avians are more Yang than most animals.[6]

After identifying the Yin-Yang pattern, the practitioner must also identify the Zang-Fu pattern to know which organ system is deficient or in excess. The Zang organ systems are heart, kidney, liver, lung, pericardium, and spleen. The Fu organ systems are bladder, gall bladder, large and small intestines, stomach, and triple heater (similar to the Western circulatory system). The zang-fu organ systems are similar to the Western organs they are named after; however, in TCVM principles, each has additional or slightly different jobs than considered in a Western sense.

For instance, in TCVM principles, the kidney system not only functions as the kidney organ but also regulates bone, controls energy, and stores the essence of the body.[7] If a patient is diagnosed by an acupuncturist as kidney deficient, that does not necessarily mean that they have abnormal renal values. The kidney deficiency may be diagnosed based on the presence of arthritis, which suggests that the kidney system is not controlling the growth of bone. It is a good idea to support the kidneys in these patients with normal renal values but they are diagnosed as kidney deficient because they may have renal insufficiency later in life. The zang-fu organ system is very detailed and complicated beyond the scope of this introduction.

The basis of a TCVM examination is the evaluation of the tongue and pulse. A TCVM practitioner uses the quality and symmetry of pulses, and the color, shape, and texture of the tongue, to identify the disease pattern or come to a TCVM diagnosis. In most species, the tongue has round edges and is relatively flat, pink, moist, and smooth. For example, tongues that are coated in yellow and are dark red and swollen indicate too much heat in the body, or a Yin deficiency. When tongues vary in shape, color, and texture, using the tongue color for pattern diagnosis becomes more of a challenge. Reptiles, amphibians, and avians, for example, are not suitable species for tongue diagnosis. For birds, an alternative to tongue evaluation is to assess the color and characteristics of the vent and cloaca.[8]

In most species the pulse is taken bilaterally, comparing the contralateral pulse. The artery used depends on which is most assessable, usually the carotid or femoral artery. For most avian species, the brachial artery on ventral surface of the wing as it crosses the ventral surface of the humerus provides the most assessable palpable pulse.[8]

Pattern diagnosis in certain exotic species poses unique problems. Reptiles are particularly challenging because, typically, there is not a palpable pulse and their tongues do not follow the general TCVM characteristics. Therefore, pattern diagnosis is based more for general observations about their behavior; changes in quality, quantity, or color of feces; discharges; skin lesions; body odor; and so forth.[9] The same observations are used for pattern diagnosis in amphibians.

After the pattern is identified, treatment is focused on correction of the excess or deficiency. The course of treatment is modified because the excess or deficiency changes.

Explanation of Acupuncture

While TCVM encompasses many different types of treatments, the most common type of treatment is acupuncture. Acupuncture works through acupoints, which are stimulated to have an effect on the nervous and circulatory system. The acupoints are located on meridians or channels that run throughout the body. Point selection is based on the pattern diagnosis and correcting the identified imbalance. The location of acupoints in exotic animals is not as well studied as it is in domestic animals. An experienced acupuncturist uses anatomic correlation between species to identify the possible locations of the acupoints. Careful palpation around those areas may reveal active acupoints, which are perceived as vague depressed areas. When those areas feel cool, it signifies a deficiency. When there is warmth, or areas that are raised and swollen, it signifies excess.[9]

After the point is selected and located, it can be stimulated in a variety of ways. The classic method is using an acupuncture needle. This type of stimulation is termed dry needle acupuncture (**Fig. 1**). These needles are malleable and range in thickness from 0.12 mm to 0.25 mm. Each needle requires a guide tube for placement because they will bend during insertion. This flexibility is important because muscle contraction in response to stimulation of the acupoint can bend and twist the needles. The needles can be used alone or can be stimulated with electrical current at frequencies based on the pattern being treated. This method is called electroacupuncture (**Fig. 2**). Needles can also be stimulated with heated herbs, a process called moxibustion, which is useful in cases in which heat is needed in the body. In addition to dry needle acupuncture, hypodermic needles can be used to inject a substance, usually vitamin B12, into an acupoint. This method is termed aquapuncture. Injecting the patient's own blood into an acupoint is termed hemopuncture.

Acupoints do not need to be stimulated by needles, they can also be stimulated with pressure, or acupressure. Laser can also be used to stimulate the acupoint[10,11] (**Fig. 3**). Acupressure and laser acupuncture have advantages in exotic animal patients that would not tolerate needle placement, cannot be touched, need to be handled in protected contact, or are at risk of needle placement depth, such as over the air sacs in birds. Laser acupuncture has an advantage over dry needle acupuncture because there is no perception of the needle entering the skin, it can be used without contact

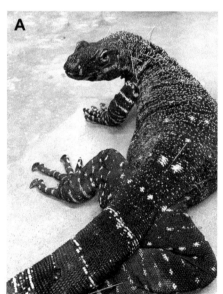
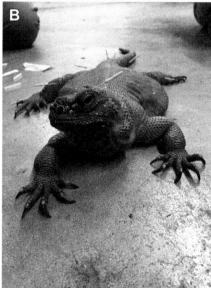

Fig. 1. Acupuncture needles are made out of stainless steel. The handles of the needles can be coated in copper, plastic, or rubber. Dry needle acupuncture in reptiles is practiced with needles placed along edges of scales. (*A*) Lace monitor (*Varanus varius*) with diagnosis of gout and arthritis was treated with dry needle acupuncture for kidney Yin deficiency and kidney and spleen Qi deficiency. (*B*) Chuckwalla (*Sauromalus*) presenting with inactivity and weight gain was treated with dry needle acupuncture for Qi deficiency and phlegm. (© Stephanie Adams, Houston Zoo, Houston, Texas; with permission.)

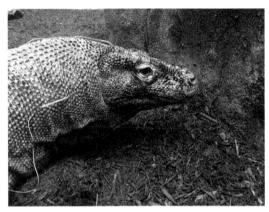

Fig. 2. Electroacupuncture requires stainless steel acupuncture needles without plastic or rubber coating. Komodo dragon (*Varanus komodensis*) with forelimb lameness, decreased cervical range of motion, and cervical torticollis on radiographs was treated with dry needle and electroacupuncture for kidney Yin deficiency and blood stagnation and Bi syndrome in the cervical spine. (© Stephanie Adams, Houston Zoo, Houston, Texas; with permission.)

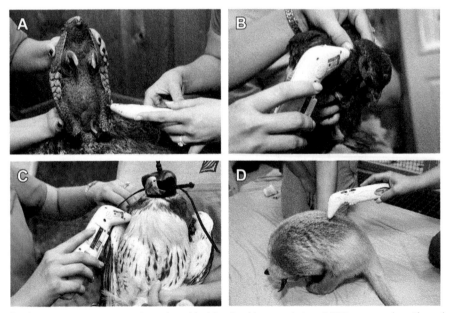

Fig. 3. Laser acupuncture using a hand-held pulsed laser pointer at 650 nw wavelength and 5 mW power. (*A*) Three-banded armadillo (*Tolypeutes tricinctus*) with hind limb ataxia treated with laser acupuncture for kidney Qi deficiency. (*B*) Congo peafowl (Afropavo congensis) with wryneck or torticollis was treated with laser acupuncture for blood stagnation in the cervical spine. (*C*) Red tailed hawk (*Buteo jamaicensis*) with inability to use wing due to chronic muscle wasting from traumatic fracture was treated with laser acupuncture for kidney Jing and spleen Qi deficiency. (*D*) Tamandua (*Tamandua*) with severe spondylosis and decreased activity and tail motion was treated with laser acupuncture for kidney Yin and Qi deficiency and Bi syndrome. (© Stephanie Adams, Houston Zoo, Houston, Texas; with permission.)

and even at a distance and also decreases acupoint stimulation time.[10,12] Functional MRI studies in humans are being completed with laser acupuncture verses dry needles to eliminate any placebo effect from sensing needle placement.[11] **Table 2** contains some examples of acupoints that are easily stimulated at a distance with laser acupuncture.

Explanation of Traditional Chinese Veterinary Medicine Food Therapy

Another approach TCVM practitioners use to restore their patients to a balanced state is food therapy. Sun Si Miao, a famous TCM practitioner from the Tang Dynasty (AD 618–907), said "dietary therapy should be the first step when one treats a disease. Only when this is unsuccessful should one try medicines. Without the knowledge of proper diet, it is hardly possible to enjoy good health."[13]

Western nutritional principles rely on categorization into carbohydrates, fat, protein, vitamins, minerals, and trace elements. For TCVM, food therapy considers the energy, or thermal nature of the food, and uses the food as a form of treatment.[14] The most practical principle of TCVM food therapy to apply to exotic practice is using the thermal nature of the food to balance the Yin-Yang pattern. Feed cooling foods to patients who are overheated (Yin deficient) and warming foods to patients that are too cold (Yang deficient). Diet change in exotic medicine can be limited, but subtle application of TCVM food therapy can be straightforward and just as effective as herbal medicine. **Tables 3–5** serve as general references for introducing TCVM food therapy into an exotic animal practice.

Explanation of Traditional Chinese Veterinary Medicine Herbal Therapy

Herbs should be treated like medications and only be used when assured of the patient's pattern diagnosis. Herbs are not necessarily safe because they are natural. When the correct herb is chosen, it can be of great benefit to the patient. Because

Table 2
Basic acupuncture points for the general practitioner

Acupoint	Anatomic Location	Uses
Governing vessel (GV)-1	On midline under tail and above anus	Diarrhea and/or constipation
GV-20	On dorsal midline on a line drawn from the level of the ear canals	Calming point
GV-27	On midline at junction of nose and upper lip in the philtrum	Shock
Bladder-60	On the lateral side of the hock in the thin skin between the calcaneus and the lateral malleolus	General pain point
Er-jian	At tip on ear on the convex side	Fever
Shan-gen	On midline on top of nose in depression at junction of hairline	Anorexia
Da-feng-men	On dorsal midline on a line drawn from the cranial rim of the ears	Epilepsy
Er-jian	On the convex surface of the ear tip	Fever
Wei-jian	Tip of tail	Heatstroke

Data from Xie H. Canine transpositional acupoints and canine classical acupoints. In: Xie H, Preast V, editors. Xie's veterinary acupuncture. Ames (IA): Blackwell Publishing; 2007. p. 129–234.

Table 3
Basic Traditional Chinese Veterinary Medicine food therapy for the general practitioner (fruits and vegetables)

Warming	Neutral	Cooling
Papaya	Apple	Mango
Tangerine	Pineapple	Orange
Coconut	Lemon	Strawberry
Peach	Carrots	Watermelon rind
Cherry	Cauliflower	Banana
Sweet potato	Potato	Broccoli
Pumpkin	Yam	Eggplant
Squash	Asparagus	Cucumber
Mustard	Cabbage	Lettuce

Data from Xie H. Food and herbology. In: Xie H, editor. TCVM atlas Dr. Xie's masterpieces. Reddick (FL): Chi Institute; 2015. p. s. 5-1.

TCVM treats the individual patient and not a disease, it is not advisable to always use herb A to treat arthritis in a bird. In TCVM, arthritis in that bird may be due to several different TCVM pattern diagnoses. The bird could be Yin or Yang deficient. It could also have a Qi deficiency, kidney deficiency, and so forth. Each of these circumstances would call for a different herbal formula. Therefore, consultation with a Chinese herbalist is highly encouraged. In exotic medicine, it is even more difficult to give guidelines on herbs due to patient size, limited information on dosages, and differences in absorption. This is an area in which more studies are needed in exotic animals and domestic species. Herbal therapies also pose additional complications because the product consistency varies with growth cycles, harvest, storage, and processing practices, making them not as reliable as pharmaceuticals. It is also important to be sure that products are coming from a reputable company with ethically sourced herbs.

Cases That Could Benefit from Traditional Chinese Veterinary Medicine

TCVM has a wide scope of potential uses. Because TCVM is a complementary therapy, any TCVM treatment modalities can be used alongside Western treatments to enhance the Western therapy; decrease side effects; or, in some cases, prolong the need for Western therapy intervention.

TCVM can be used as preventative care in healthy patients. Patients that, based on species or breed, may be predisposed to conditions later in life can benefit from

Table 4
Basic Traditional Chinese Veterinary Medicine food therapy for the general practitioner (meats)

Warming	Neutral	Cooling
Venison	Pork	Rabbit
Chicken	Goose	Turkey
Lamb	Beef	Duck

Data from Xie H. Food and herbology. In: Xie H, editor. TCVM atlas Dr. Xie's masterpieces. Reddick (IA): Chi Institute; 2015. p. s. 5-1.

Table 5
Basic Traditional Chinese Veterinary Medicine food therapy for the general practitioner (grains)

Warming	Neutral	Cooling
Oats	Corn	Barley
White rice	Sweet rice	Brown rice
Maltose	Rice bran	Wheat bran, buckwheat
Sweet feed	Beet pulp	Grass, grass hay, alfalfa

Data from Xie H. Food and herbology. In: Xie H, editor. TCVM atlas Dr. Xie's masterpieces. Reddick (IA): Chi Institute; 2015. p. s. 5-2.

preventative TCVM therapies. Examples include supporting heart function in parrots and hedgehogs that are predisposed to cardiovascular disease, boosting the endocrine function of ferrets, and supporting renal and liver function across all species.

TCVM can also be used for acute and chronic diseases that are being treated with or without Western medical therapies. In cases of acute emergencies, Western medicine provides a faster response. When stable, TCVM can be added to help complement the Western therapies. Additionally, there is an acupoint that can be stimulated to help with resuscitation. However, the author recommends that cardiopulmonary resuscitation be initiated first and the acupoint only be stimulated if there is an extra person who can do so without interfering with the resuscitation efforts (see **Table 2**). TCVM is also beneficial when there is no definitive diagnosis, cause, or course of treatment. A study performed by Brady and colleagues[15] found a positive response to treatment of owl monkey wasting disease (OMWD) using acupuncture with vitamin B12. Before this study, there was no known treatment of OMWD.

Examples of cases involving exotic animals treated with acupuncture are in **Box 1**.

Treatment Protocols

TCVM works to restore balance, which is a gradual process in the face of a chronic condition. The author recommends that owners commit to at least 5 treatments before making a decision on treatment effectiveness or assessing patient response. Treatments are typically spaced 1 to 2 weeks apart for most cases. For severe cases, there may be a need for 2 treatments a week. After the initial 3 to 5 treatments at 2 weeks apart, if the patient is responding, then the treatment intervals are gradually spread out to get to a maintenance treatment schedule of 3 to 4 times a year. If using TCVM to treat an acute illness, then only a few treatments may be necessary.

Side Effects, Precautions, and Contraindications

TCVM generally is considered safe with relatively few side effects. Acupuncture side effects include the release of endogenous endorphins that can cause patients to be sleepy or tired. In some cases, acupuncture temporarily worsens symptoms before gradual improvement. For exotic patients, there could be bruising around needle placement in thinner-skinned species and possibly soreness in the muscle from needle insertion. Side effects of using TCVM food therapy are gastrointestinal related. Herbal therapy can have varying side effects, depending on the potency of the herb.

Precautions should be taken when using acupuncture, especially on a new species in which the practitioner has no prior experience. A veterinarian experienced with the species should work closely with the acupuncturist to ensure that species variables

---

Box 1
Examples of some exotic animal cases treated by the author with acupuncture

- Ferret (*Mustela putorius furo*) with an insulinoma
- Flamingo (*Phoenicopterus chilensis*) recovering from ulnar fracture repair
- Lace monitor (*Varanus varius*) with gout
- Mandrill (*Mandrillus sphinx*) with neurologic deficits
- Spectacled bear (*Tremarctos ornatus*) with mammary carcinoma
- Red tailed hawk (*Buteo jamaicensis*) with inability to use wing due to chronic muscle wasting from traumatic fracture
- Holland Lop (*Oryctolagus cuniculus*) with decreased activity and constipation
- Green sea turtle (*Chelonia mydas*) with dislocated shoulder
- Babirusa (*Babyrousa*) with immune-mediated polyarthritis
- Komodo dragon (*Varanus komodensis*) with forelimb lameness, decreased cervical range of motion, and cervical torticollis on radiographs
- Aracari (*Pteroglossus viridis*) with decreased use of pelvic limbs and pelvic limb ataxia
- Chuckwalla (*Sauromalus*) with inactivity and weight gain
- Tamandua (*Tamandua*) with severe spondylosis, decreased activity and tail motion
- Congo peafowl (*Afropavo congensis*) with wryneck or torticollis
- Three-banded armadillo (*Tolypeutes tricinctus*), Damaraland mole-rat (*Fukomys damarensis*), Guinea hog (*Sus scrofa domesticus*), and opossum (*Didelphimorphia*) with hind limb ataxia
- White-tailed deer (*Odocoileus virginianus*), various breeds of goats (*Capra aegagrus hircus*) with osteoarthritis
- Black-and-white ruffed lemur (*Varecia variegate*), grizzly bear (*Ursus arctos*), ocelot (*Leopardus pardalis*), coati (*Nasua nasua*), leopards (*Panthera pardus*), chimpanzees (*Pan troglodytes*), jaguars (*Panthera onca*), gorillas (*Gorilla gorilla gorilla*), Malayan tiger (*Panthera tigris jacksoni*) with osteoarthritis (all with laser acupuncture and protected contact)

---

are known, for the safety of both the patient and the acupuncturist. An acupuncturist also needs to understand the diet of the species before suggesting any changes for using TCVM food therapy.

Contraindications for TCVM food and herbal therapy include unknown source of herb or food, unknown pattern diagnosis, and unfamiliarity with species digestion and absorption. Considerations for acupuncture include avoiding certain points during pregnancy, avoiding points around a tumor, and not using acupuncture needles in open wounds. Electroacupuncture should be used with caution in the weak or debilitated patient or patients with history of seizures. Additionally, electrical leads should not cross the heart in a patient in poor cardiovascular health.[16]

INTRODUCTION TO CHIROPRACTIC

Chiropractic-type therapies can be traced back to multiple ancient civilizations, including Chinese, Roman, Greek, and Egyptian. Modern day chiropractic attributes its founding to D.D. Palmer, with Palmer School of Chiropractic being the first official training institution in the 1800s. Unlike TCVM, which seems to be more easily accepted by Western practitioners, chiropractic typically has more difficulty gaining broader acceptance. There is also frequently limited knowledge regarding the safety and education level of a trained chiropractor. Only 15% of people can correctly answer how much education is required to be a chiropractor.[17]

Chiropractic care in humans is widely requested. A Gallop poll from 2015 showed that over 50% of adults had sought chiropractic care at some point in their life.[17] Chiropractic care in animals may be sought out by those who have experienced chiropractic for themselves. Although well-intentioned, a problem can arise when these owners cannot find appropriate chiropractic care for their animals and seek treatment by laypersons or other underqualified practitioners.

Dr Sharon Willoughby was a veterinarian who also became a doctor of chiropractic in order to apply it to companion animals. Her endeavors lead to the formation of the first animal chiropractic training courses in the late 1980s. Since that time, several schools have been established that train both human chiropractors and veterinarians in chiropractic care for animals. In most states, animal chiropractic must be performed by a licensed veterinarian or a licensed chiropractor. A licensed chiropractor needs written consent from the patient's attending veterinarian before performing any animal chiropractic. Despite this legal requirement, there are still many lay people who inaccurately refer to themselves as animal chiropractors and who have caused injury to the animals and problems for the image of the profession. Clients seeking chiropractic for their animals, if not educated by their veterinarian about how to find a certified animal chiropractor or, for that matter, why they should, will often find a lay or untrained person to provide the treatment. **Table 6** can be used to help seek certified animal chiropractors.

Table 6
Where to find a certified veterinary acupuncturist and chiropractor

Certified Veterinary Acupuncturist (CVA)	Certified Veterinary Chiropractor (CVC)
American Holistic Veterinary Medical Association https://www.ahvma.org/find-a-holistic-veterinarian/	American Veterinary Chiropractic Association http://animalchiropractic.org/avca-doctor-search.htm
Chi Institute http://www.tcvm.com/Resources/FindaTCVMPractitioner.aspx	International Veterinary Chiropractic Association https://ivca.de/veterinary-chiropractor-search/
American Academy of Veterinary Acupuncture http://www.aava.org/search/custom.asp?id=1530	Options for Animals https://optionsforanimals.com/find-a-doctor/#student-businesses-map/
College of Integrative Veterinary Therapies http://www.civtedu.org/directory/	Parker University https://ce.parker.edu/courses/doctor-of-chiropractic/animal-chiropractic-program/
Association of British Veterinary Acupuncturist http://www.abva.co.uk/find-a-vet/	College of Animal Chiropractors http://www.collegeofanimalchiropractors.org/en/members/find-members/
Association of Veterinary Acupuncturist of Canada https://www.avacanada.org/vetfinder.htm	Veterinary Chiropractic Learning Center https://veterinarychiropractic.ca/our-grads

Disclaimer: This is not an endorsement; these are the find a vet sites the author is aware of.

As with any new skill, a veterinarian should be properly trained in chiropractic techniques before providing these services to patients. The purpose of this article is to broadly educate the general practitioner regarding chiropractic, not necessarily to teach specific chiropractic techniques.

Explanation of Chiropractic

Dating back to ancient civilizations, with energy and balance as principles of health, chiropractic, like acupuncture, directly affects the circulatory and nervous systems. Most Western thinkers consider chiropractic relevant for only musculoskeletal type issues because that is the focus of most research and studies. This is a common misconception. The musculoskeletal component and influence of chiropractic on the body is profound. The impact on the nervous system is an overlooked benefit of chiropractic care and modern research has shown the imprint chiropractic can have on the body as a whole.

When describing chiropractic care, some of the confusion is due to terminology. The term chiropractic subluxation typically raises the most uncertainty. In Western training, a subluxation is a partial dislocation of a joint. A chiropractic subluxation refers to 2 adjacent joints that are lacking normal motion and/or alignment but are within the normal joint space. It is this lack of normal motion or alignment that causes interference with the nervous and circulatory system and, therefore, generates decreased function and pain. This is referred to as the vertebral subluxation complex (VSC). Modern advances in imaging have supported the VSC, which is now widely accepted and taught in chiropractic university training programs. VSC encompasses a variety of issues that can arise from a subluxation.

A trained chiropractic practitioner assesses a patient with the understanding of normal joint motion. A normal or healthy joint has a springy end feel and subluxated joints have a hard or restricted end feel when put through normal range of motion. Within the normal joint space, there are varying degrees of motion. Joints move through passive range of motion to active range of motion. At the end of the active range of motion of a joint there is an elastic barrier that stops the joint from going all the way to the end of its anatomic barrier. The chiropractic adjustment occurs in the space between the elastic barrier and the physical barrier to restore both passive and active range of motion.

To carry out the adjustment, the practitioner must know the directional plane in which the joint normally moves. This correct directional plane is determined by knowing the facet angle of the joint, which provides the practitioner the line of correction (LOC). The LOC is the guideline for the correction of the subluxation or the adjustment. Within a normal spine, the LOC changes with each segment and, in the case of the thoracic spine, it changes with each vertebra. A chiropractic practitioner can make adjustments in their LOC for each individual patient due to unique anatomic differences.

Recognizing differences in LOC within the same species will allow a practitioner to be more comfortable adapting to new species in which the practitioner has no prior experience. Training courses for animal chiropractic focus on the dog and horse. Extrapolating from those species, a skilled practitioner can move on to different species but only after becoming well-practiced and proficient (**Fig. 4**). The size of smaller exotic species puts a premium on chiropractic finesse because the correction of the VSC does not stop at finding the LOC. After the LOC of the joint that is lacking normal motion is found, the adjustment is made by thrusting into the LOC. This thrust is a low-amplitude, high-velocity motion that, if not well practiced, could be particularly dangerous on a species in which the practitioner has no prior experience or training.

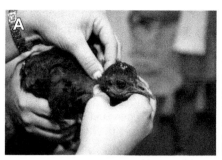
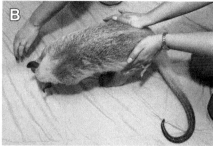
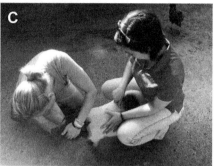

Fig. 4. (*A*) Chiropractic adjustment of the cervical spine of a Congo peafowl (*Afropavo congensis*) with wryneck or torticollis. (*B*) Chiropractic adjustment of the pelvis of a Tamandua (*Tamandua*). (*C*) Chiropractic adjustment of the lumbar spine of a Juliana pig (*Sus scrofa*). (© Stephanie Adams, Houston Zoo, Houston, Texas; with permission.)

The thrust that makes the adjustment is usually performed manually; however, new adjustment devices in the human field are slowly being introduced to animal chiropractic techniques.[18]

Cases That Could Benefit from Chiropractic

The *Journal of the American Medical Association* published a study in 2017 that supports the use of spinal manipulative therapy as a first-line treatment of acute low back pain.[19] The American College of Physicians released new guidelines in 2017 that recommended spinal manipulation among the first-line of treatments for acute and chronic low back pain.[20] Acute and chronic low back pain cases have a high rate of positive response to chiropractic care in humans and in animals. However, for animals, chiropractic is not yet the first-line of treatment of back pain. Ettinger's *Textbook of Veterinary Internal Medicine* lists exercise restriction and pain medication as treatments for back pain in animals.[21] More veterinary studies are needed to know if chronic back pain, spinal osteoarthritis, intervertebral disc degeneration, and advanced spondylosis could be prevented if chiropractic was introduced as an initial defense. Many clients are not waiting for these studies and are pursuing veterinary chiropractic on their own to potentially prevent these types of long-term issues.

Thirty-one percent of pet rabbits have vertebral column deformities and degenerative back lesions.[22] Chiropractic care can be initiated early in life to help prevent these issues by maintaining normal joint range of motion throughout the spine. Later in life, chiropractic can still be used to restore motion, even with an arthritic spine. Any motion that can be returned will help improve function. A series of animal experiments on nerve root compression found that only 10 mm Hg (which is about the weight of a dime) of compression on a nerve decreased the conduction of that nerve by 40% in the first 15 minutes and by 50% at 30 minutes.[23] Other studies have suggested this decrease in function to be 60% to 75%. After the compression is removed, recovery to near normal function occurred in 15 to 30 minutes.

Torticollis or wryneck has been documented in several species. In the human literature, there are many case reports of chiropractic improving or resolving torticollis.[24–29] In the veterinary literature, there is a case of successful management of acute-onset torticollis acquired during shipping in a 2-year-old giraffe (*Giraffa camelopardalis reticulate*).[30] The author has also successfully treated wryneck in a Congo peafowl (*Afropavo congensis*) and numerous canines (**Fig. 4**A). After fractures are ruled out, any species with an abnormal neck position should be considered for chiropractic care.

Nutritional deficiencies are common in exotic practice and several nutritional deficiencies can lead to joint inflammation. Examples include iguanas with metabolic bone disease and Guinea pigs with scurvy.[31] An inflamed joint can easily become fixated and lack normal motion. Once nutritional deficiencies have been treated, patients should be evaluated by a professional chiropractor.

Chiropractic can also be used as part of a preventative health care plan because it maintains a healthy nervous system and encourages normal gate patterns and weight-bearing to decrease the likelihood of extremity injury and maximize overall performance.[32] Many human athletes attest long careers in part to chiropractic care as a key component of overall physical conditioning. National Football League players often receive chiropractic adjustments before, during, and after a game.[33]

Examples of cases involving exotic animals treated with chiropractic are given in **Box 2**.

Treatment Protocols

The recommended frequency of chiropractic adjustments depends on the condition, if it is acute or chronic, and if the goals are preventative or maintenance of a chronic condition. The recommended treatment frequency also varies between practitioners. For most cases, the author sees patients every 1 to 2 weeks for 2 to 3 treatments, in total. If the patient is responding well, then the time between treatments can gradually disperse to assess efficacy. Each situation is unique. One patient with spinal arthritis may walk better if adjusted every 4 weeks, whereas another may benefit with treatments every 12 weeks. Because the spine is constantly in motion and subject to strain, the author does not recommend longer than 4 to 6 months between adjustments. In acute cases, several adjustments may completely resolve the issue and ongoing chiropractic for that particular issue may no longer be needed. However, one must keep in mind that spinal nerve root compression can be present without causing the sensation of pain and, therefore, the absence of clinical signs.[34]

Side Effects, Precautions, and Contraindications

When used skillfully and appropriately, chiropractic therapy is safe and effective.[35] The most common side effect to chiropractic is muscular soreness. Changing the way that the joint moves also changes the muscles engagement. This muscle soreness is similar to a new workout routine when muscles are stressed beyond typical restful conditions. Some patients are noticeably sore 24 to 48 hours after their first adjustment, whereas other patients do not show any signs of soreness. In the author's experience, patients that do exhibit soreness do so for only 24 to 48 hours and generally do not require any medical intervention. Using damp or moist heat therapy over

---

Box 2
Examples of some exotic animal cases treated by the author with chiropractic

- Rabbit (*Oryctolagus cuniculus*) with decreased activity and constipation
- Ferret (*Mustela putorius furo*) dragging 1 hind limb
- Alpaca (*Vicugna pacos*) with forelimb lameness
- Pot-bellied pig (*Sus scrofa domesticus*) with back pain
- Green sea turtle (*Chelonia mydas*) with dislocated shoulder
- Cheetahs (*Acinonyx jubatus*) with impacted anal glands (under general anesthesia)
- Llama (*Lama glama*) with pelvic limb lameness
- Babirusa (*Babyrousa*) with immune-mediated polyarthritis
- Juliana pig (*Sus scrofa*) with behavioral change and aggression
- Aardvark (*Orycteropus afer*), Capybara (*Hydrochoerus hydrochaeris*), Damaraland mole-rat (*Fukomys damarensis*), Guinea hog (*Sus scrofa domesticus*), and opossum (*Didelphimorphia*) with hind limb ataxia
- Komodo dragon (*Varanus komodensis*) with forelimb lameness, decreased cervical range of motion, and cervical torticollis on radiographs
- Andalusian rooster (*Gallus gallus domesticus*) with decreased activity
- St. Vincent Amazon parrot (*Amazona guildingii*) with inability to use right pelvic limb
- Aracari (*Pteroglossus viridis*) with decreased use of pelvic limbs and pelvic limb ataxia
- Chuckwalla (*Sauromalus*) with inactivity and weight gain
- Great horned owl (*Bubo virginianus*) with inability to close digits on 1 pelvic limb
- Tamandua (*Tamandua*) with severe spondylosis and decreased activity and tail motion
- Leopard (*Panthera pardus*) with self-mutilation of distal end of tail
- Congo peafowl (*Afropavo congensis*) with wryneck
- White-tailed deer (*Odocoileus virginianus*), various breeds of goats (*Capra aegagrus hircus*) with osteoarthritis
- Leopards (*Panthera pardus*), chimpanzees (*Pan troglodytes*), jaguar (*Panthera onca*), gorillas (*Gorilla gorilla gorilla*), Malayan tiger (*Panthera tigris jacksoni*) with osteoarthritis (adjustment performed while under general anesthesia for other procedures)

---

sore, tight muscles will help a patient improve faster and provide relief (**Fig. 5**). Damp heat also prevents the drying effect on skin and muscles that can come from dry heat therapy. To apply damp heat, a moist warm towel is used. To increase duration of treatment a heating pad or hot rice bag maybe added.

Precautions should be made whenever undertaking treatment on a new species. Having an understanding of species anatomy and normal motion is important. It is difficult to assess abnormal motion without a baseline definition of normal motion. Chiropractors (DC or DVMs) who are not familiar with particular exotic species should be assisted by an experienced exotic veterinarian. This helps to ensure the safety of the patient as well as the practitioner, who may not be aware of the dangers of working with certain exotic species.

Chiropractic is contraindicated if there is a history of trauma or disease in which bone integrity could be compromised. This case history could include fractures, congenital anomalies, acute infections (eg, osteomyelitis and septic discs), spinal

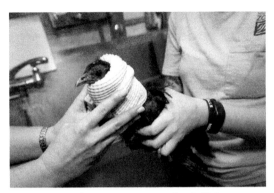

Fig. 5. Damp heat therapy used on a Congo peafowl (*Afropavo congensis*) following chiropractic adjustment of the cervical spine. (© Stephanie Adams, Houston Zoo, Houston, Texas; with permission.)

tumors or malignancies, dislocation of vertebra, internal fixation or stabilization devices, and other diseases causing instability of the spine.[35] In cases of focal spine lesions, a chiropractic adjustment may still be performed on other areas of the spine.

SUMMARY

Studies on applying nontraditional therapies in exotic animal practice are very limited. However, the research being done in the human and companion animal fields support the safe application of nontraditional therapies into exotic animal practice.

Integrating nontraditional therapies into general practice requires advanced training and skills. Attending an advanced training course or coordinating with a practitioner who is already trained in nontraditional therapies will provide a practitioner additional tools to complement Western therapies and work together toward the goal of prevention and relief of animal suffering.

REFERENCES

1. Model Veterinary Practice Act July 2017. Available at: https://www.avma.org/KB/Policies/Pages/Model-Veterinary-Practice-Act.aspx. Accessed November 28, 2017.

2. Barnes PM, Bloom B, Nahin R. CDC National Health Statistics Report #12. Complementary and Alternative Medicine Use Among Adults and Children: United States, 2007. 2008. Available at: https://nccih.nih.gov/research/statistics/2007/camsurvey_fs1.htm. Accessed November 16, 2017.

3. Meredith K, Bolwell CF, Rogers CW, et al. The use of allied health therapies on competition horses in the North Island of New Zealand. N Z Vet J 2011;59(3): 123–7.

4. Xie H. Preface. In: Xie H, Preast V, editors. Xie's veterinary acupuncture. Ames (IA): Blackwell Publishing; 2007. p. xi–xiii.

5. Conference Proceedings: Pacific Veterinary Conference: PacVet 2015. Peter G. Fisher "Exotic Mammal Geriatrics". Available at: http://www.vin.com/members/cms/project/defaultadv1.aspx?id=6789820&pid=11768 11/26. Accessed November 16, 2017.

6. Xie H. How to start traditional Chinese veterinary medicine in exotic animal practice. In: Xie H, Trevisanello L, editors. Application of traditional Chinese veterinary medicine in exotic animals. Reddick(FL): Jing Tang Publishing; 2011. p. 3–28.

7. Xie H. Zang-Fu physiology. Traditional Chinese veterinary medicine fundamental principles, vol. 1. Reddick(FL): Chi Institute; 2007. p. 105–48.

8. West C. TCVM for avian species: introduction, general overview, acupuncture point locations, indications and techniques. In: Xie H, Trevisanello L, editors. Application of traditional Chinese veterinary medicine in exotic animals. Reddick(FL): Jing Tang Publishing; 2011. p. 53–72.

9. Eckermann-Ross C. Traditional Chinese veterinary medicine in reptiles. In: Xie H, Trevisanello L, editors. Application of traditional Chinese veterinary medicine in exotic animals. Reddick(FL): Jing Tang Publishing; 2011. p. 159–92.

10. Law D, McDonough S, Bleakley C, et al. Laser acupuncture for treating musculoskeletal pain: a systemic review with meta-analysis. J Acupunct Meridian Stud 2015;8(1):2–16.

11. Quah-Smith I, Sachdev PS, Wen W, et al. The brain effects of laser acupuncture in healthy individuals: an fMRI investigation. PLoS One 2010;5(9):e12619.

12. Petermann U. The components of the pulse controlled laser acupuncture. American Journal of TCVM 2012;7(1):57–67.

13. Kastner J. Theory. Chinese Nutritional Therapy Dietetics in Traditional Chinese Medicine (TCM). 2nd edition. New York: Thieme; 2009. Kindle edition Chapter 1, section 5, paragraph 10–11.

14. Kastner J. Theory. Chinese Nutritional Therapy Dietetics in Traditional Chinese Medicine (TCM). 2nd edition. New York: Thieme; 2009. Kindle edition Chapter 1, section 7, paragraph 1–2.

15. Brady A, Wilkerson G, Williams L, et al. Characterization and treatment of a new wasting disease of owl monkeys (Aotus sp.). In: Joint AAZV/EAZWV/IZW Conference Proceedings, Atlanta (GA), July 16–22, 2016.

16. Xie H. General rules of acupuncture therapy. In: Xie H, Preast V, editors. Xie's veterinary acupuncture. Ames(IA): Blackwell Publishing; 2007. p. P245–6.

17. Daly J. Gallup-Palmer College of Chiropractic Inaugural Report: American's Perception of Chiropractic. 2015. http://www.palmer.edu/uploadedFiles/Pages/Alumni/gallup-report-palmer-college.pdf. Accessed November 29, 2017.

18. Duarte FC, Kolberg C, Barros RR, et al. Evaluation of peak force of a manually operated chiropractic adjusting instrument with an adapter for use in animals. J Manipulative Physiol Ther 2014;37(4):236–41.

19. Paige NM, Miake-Lye IM, Booth MS, et al. Association of spinal manipulative therapy with clinical benefit and harm for acute low back pain: systematic review and meta-analysis. JAMA 2017;317(14):1451–60.

20. Qaseem A, Wilt TJ, McLean RM, et al. Noninvasive treatments for acute, subacute, and chronic low back pain: a clinical practice guideline from the American College of Physicians. Ann Intern Med 2017;166(7):514.

21. LeCouteur R, Grandy J. Diseases of the spinal cord. In: Ettinger S, Feldman E, editors. Textbook of veterinary internal medicine. 6th edition. St Louis (MO): Elsevier Sanders; 2005. p. 871.

22. Makitaipale J, Harcourt-Brown FM, Laitinen-Vapaavuori O. Health survey of 167 pet rabbits (*Oryctolagus cuniculus*) in Finland. Vet Rec 2015;177(16):418.

23. Sharpless SK. Susceptibility of spinal roots to compression block. In: Goldstein M, editor. The Research Status of Spinal Manipulative Therapy. Bethesda (MD): HEW/NINCDS Monograph #15; 1975. p. 976–98.

24. Hobaek Siegnthaler M. Unresolved congenital torticollis and its consequences: a report of 2 cases. J Chiropr Med 2017;16(3):257–61.

25. Hobaek Siegnthaler M. Chiropractic management of infantile torticollis with associated abnormal fixation of one eye: a case report. J Chiropr Med 2015;14(1):51–6.

26. Kaufman R. Co-management and collaborative care of a 20-year-old female with acute viral torticollis. J Manipulative Physiol Ther 2009;32(2):160–5.

27. McWilliams JE, Gloar CD. Chiropractic care of a six-year-old child with congenital torticollis. J Chiropr Med 2006;5(2):65–8.

28. Kukurin GW. Reduction of cervical dystonia after an extended course of chiropractic manipulation: a case report. J Manipulative Physiol Ther 2004;27(6):421–6.

29. Toto BJ. Chiropractic correction of congenital muscular torticollis. J Manipulative Physiol Ther 1993;16(8):556–9.

30. Dadone LI, Haussler KK, Brown G, et al. Successful management of acute-onset torticollis in a giraffe (*Giraffa camelopardalis reticulata*). J Zoo Wildl Med 2013;44(1):181–5.

31. Ness R. Chiropractic care for exotic pets. Exotic DVM 2000;2(1):15–8.

32. Lowell D. Use of chiropractic for therapy and prevention of disease. In: Western Veterinary Conference Proceedings. 2003. Available at: http://www.vin.com/members/cms/project/defaultadv1.aspx?id=3846900&pid=11155. Accessed December 11, 2017.

33. Chiropractic in the NFL. In: Professional Football Chiropractic Society. Available at: http://profootballchiros.com/chiropractic-in-the-nfl/. Accessed December 1, 2017.

34. Hause M. Pain and the nerve root. Spine 1993;18(14):2053.

35. Guidelines on safety of Chiropractic. In: WHO guidelines on basic training and safety in chiropractic. 2005. Available at: http://www.who.int/medicines/areas/traditional/Chiro-Guidelines.pdf. Accessed December 1, 2017.

Printed and bound by CPI Group (UK) Ltd, Croydon, CR0 4YY

03/10/2024

01040391-0009